Female Offenders of Intimate Partner Violence

The perpetration of intimate partner violence by women has long been a controversial topic. More recently, researchers, treatment providers and other professionals have begun to critically examine theoretical research and practice perspectives to gather a better understanding of this controversial issue. The current text will provide the reader with a more thorough discussion on our current understanding of the context and motivation of women's use of violence against intimate partners. This text will discuss the controversies related to the arrest and treatment of women arrested for domestic violence from a variety of theoretical perspectives while also providing updates on the current research focusing on typologies of female offenders. The text also provides a critical review of current treatment strategies for women arrested for domestic violence.

The contributors are the foremost leaders in the field of research and practice on intimate partner violence offending and have written chapters that provide a key review of the work that is currently emerging in the field. As a result, this text is the most comprehensive guide to date that discusses female perpetration of intimate partner violence. Recommendations for specific treatment with this population and implications for practice and policy are provided throughout.

This book was published as a special double issue of the *Journal of Aggression, Maltreatment and Trauma*.

Lisa M. Conradi, PsyD, is a Clinical Psychologist at the Chadwick Center, Rady Children's Hospital, San Diego. She has led multiple projects of national impact designed to improve the service delivery system for children who have experienced trauma. Her interests include domestic violence and working with children affected by trauma.

Robert Geffner, PhD, ABN, ABPP, is the Founder and President of the Family Violence and Sexual Assault Institute in San Diego, CA; President of Alliant International University's (AIU) Institute on Violence, Abuse and Trauma (IVAT); and Clinical Research Professor of Psychology at the California School of Professional Psychology, AIU, San Diego, CA.

Female Offenders of Intimate Partner Violence

Current Controversies, Research and Treatment Approaches

Edited by
Lisa M. Conradi and Robert Geffner

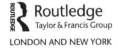

LONDON AND NEW YORK

First published 2012
by Routledge
2 Park Square, Milton Park, Abingdon, Oxfordshire OX14 4RN

Simultaneously published in the USA and Canada
by Routledge
711 Third Avenue, New York, NY 10017

Routledge is an imprint of the Taylor & Francis Group, an informa business

First issued in paperback 2011

This book is a reproduction of the *Journal of Aggression, Maltreatment and Trauma*, vol. 18, issue 6 & 7. The Publisher requests to those authors who may be citing this book to state, also, the bibliographical details of the special issue on which the book was based.

British Library Cataloguing in Publication Data
A catalogue record for this book is available from the British Library

ISBN13: 978-0-415-68127-8 (hbk)
ISBN13: 978-0-415-68168-1 (pbk)

Typeset in Times New Roman
by Taylor & Francis Books

Disclaimer
The publisher would like to make readers aware that the chapters in this book are referred to as articles as they had been in the special issue. The publisher accepts responsibility for any inconsistencies that may have arisen in the course of preparing this volume for print.

Contents

PART II

Introduction to Part I

LISA CONRADI

Chadwick Center for Children and Families, Rady Children's Hospital, San Diego, San Diego, California, USA

ROBERT GEFFNER

Institute on Violence, Abuse and Trauma, Alliant International University, San Diego, California, USA

There are many controversies surrounding women's use of violence in their intimate relationships. This special issue is part one of a two part volume that critically examines the prevalence studies on female offenders of intimate partner violence and addresses the gaps in current research. The six articles contained in this issue provide a description of the controversies surrounding female offenders, and introduces some research examining the role of gender and ethnicity in intimate partner violence.

In its infancy, studies on child abuse, intimate partner violence (IPV), and sexual assault focused on men as perpetrators and women as victims. The historical focus on male perpetrators of IPV has occurred for a variety of reasons. First, it has been found that women are statistically more likely to be victims of IPV than men; according to the National Violence Against Women Survey (Tjaden & Thoennes, 2000), 22.1% of surveyed women, compared with 7.4% of surveyed men, reported they were physically assaulted by a current or former spouse, cohabiting partner, boyfriend or girlfriend, or date in their lifetime. Furthermore, the seriousness of violence against women is increased when the magnitude of injury occurring during an assault is examined. In his meta-analysis of the literature on aggression between heterosexual partners, Archer (2000) found that, overall, when measures were based on specific acts, women were significantly more likely than men to have used physical aggression toward their partners and to have used it more frequently. However, when measures were based on the physical consequences of aggression (including visible injuries or injuries requiring medical treatment), men were more likely than women to have injured their partners.

Only recently has research begun to more carefully study women who perpetrate IPV. There is current controversy among theorists in describing the etiology and motivations for female perpetrators of IPV. While some research indicates that women commit acts of minor and severe violence or aggression as often as men (Straus & Gelles, 1986), other studies describe women as the overwhelming victims in IPV and contend that any harm women inflict on their male partner is likely to be minimal compared to the violence she receives from him (Hamberger, 1997; Saunders, 1986). Based on this research, it has been proposed that female perpetrators of IPV may be categorized into typologies based on the severity, frequency, and motivation for their violence. While these typologies are given different names based on theorists, in general they have been categorized as follows: women who use aggression only in self-defense, women as dominant aggressors committing acts of intimate terrorism (Johnson, 1995), and bi-directional violence or mutually violent control (Johnson, 2001). While these distinctions have been made theoretically and clinically, minimal research exists to support these categories (Swan & Snow, 2002, 2003). Furthermore, there has been minimal research on women's motivation for IPV, particularly within these proposed typologies (Hamberger, 1997).

The issue of female IPV is a contentious one that has many implications for policy and practice (see Straus, this issue). While some research has reported equal use by men and women in intimate relationships, it has been argued that this research ignores the context and motivation of IPV (Hamberger, 1997). Therefore, if policy makers and practitioners acknowledge that women may also use violence in their intimate relationships, there is a fear that there may be a backlash against victim advocacy agencies that provide services to female victims. This may result in decreased funding to provide the necessary services for this population.

ABUSE VERSUS AGGRESSION

A key issue is the definition of abuse as distinct from that of aggression. At times, those debating or researching the issues use these two terms interchangeably. However, abuse and aggression are not the same, although abuse may include physical or sexual aggression and the use of aggression may also be abusive. Geffner and Rosenbaum (2001) discussed abuse as a pattern of behavior in an intimate relationship in which one partner attempts to meet his or her needs at the expense of the other partner utilizing forms of power, coercion, and control. Intimidation is usually the method of operation used by the offender to achieve power and control, and the victim often is traumatized in the process and develops fear. Aggressive behavior may be physical, sexual, or psychological, but does not require elements of power, control, or intimidation, and the victim of aggression may not necessarily experience trauma and fear. Aggression in relationships is not a positive behavior in any case, even if it does not contain the elements of abuse. Mutual or bi-directional abuse would then mean both partners are striving for power and control and both using coercive techniques and behaviors in their relationship. This does not occur often. However, mutual or bi-directional aggression does occur more often in relationships, as shown in the various research articles in this issue.

Thus, using the above (or similar) definitions to argue that females are as abusive in intimate relationships as males ignores much of the research as well as anecdotal reports from agencies dealing with IPV. However, to also suggest that women are never the perpetrators of abuse also denies the data and experiences of those who work in the field. It is also clear, as the articles in this issue describe, that women are often aggressive in many intimate relationships, and some of them are indeed abusive as defined above. It would be helpful if definitions of abuse were described in discussions so that consistency can be achieved in the field. This would eliminate many arguments for those who are trying to understand and deal with IPV. We hope this special issue encourages such a dialogue.

OVERVIEW OF THE ARTICLES IN THIS SPECIAL ISSUE

The current issue is the first part in a two-part series focusing on female offenders of IPV. This issue begins by highlighting the controversial nature of prevalence studies on IPV that have been conducted over the last 30 years. The issue then delves deeper and provides the reader with the most updated research on the role of gender and race/ethnicity in IPV. In the opening article, Murray Straus begins by outlining the controversial aspects of this topic area. He offers explanations for the misperception of these aspects of gender symmetry in partner violence and for the concealment and denial of women's violence by researchers, and discusses how this denial has adversely affected prevention and treatment programs. In the second article, Denise Hines and Emily Douglas discuss the various sources of prevalence rates of IPV by women against men, the dominant theoretical explanation for IPV in general, and its implications for female perpetrators and male victims in the social service and criminal justice systems. They then discuss the current evidence of the consequences of women's use of IPV on the men who sustain it. In the next article, Nicola Graham-Kevan offers an alternative theoretical understanding of women's use of violence. She explores the evidence that finds gender symmetry and the research challenging the conceptualization of women's partner violence as self defensive. Alternative explanations for women's aggression are discussed with a focus on personality traits of psychopathology.

The next group of articles describes recent research on women's use of violence in intimate relationships. Jody Ross and Julia Babcock begin to deconstruct Johnson's (2001) typology of violent couples dimensionally and in the context of the relationship as they relate to injury and observed behavior. Kris Henning, Rochelle Martinsson, and Robert Holdford then examine gender differences in risk factors for IPV recidivism from a criminal justice perspective. In the final article, Tami Sullivan, Courtenay Cavanaugh, Michelle Ufner, Suzanne Swan, and David Snow discuss their research on the relationship between women's use of aggression, their victimization, and substance abuse problems by ethnicity.

Together, this compilation of articles begins to articulate the complexity and controversy surrounding women's use of violence in intimate relationships and describes research on the role of gender and ethnicity in IPV. Too often, researchers, practitioners, policy makers, and advocates have relied upon ideology and assumptions in dealing with this controversial topic. With this issue, it is our hope that readers will critically examine current research and prevalence studies regarding women's use of violence.

REFERENCES

Archer, J. (2000). Sex differences in aggression between heterosexual partners: A meta-analytic review. *Psychological Bulletin*, 126(5), 651–680.

Geffner, R., & Rosenbaum, A. (2001). Domestic violence offenders: Treatment and intervention standards. *Journal of Aggression, Maltreatment & Trauma*, 5(2), 1–9.

Hamberger, L. K. (1997). Female offenders in domestic violence: A look at actions in their context. *Journal of Aggression, Maltreatment and Trauma*, 1(1), 117–129.

Johnson, M. P. (1995). Patriarchal terrorism and common couple violence: Two forms of violence against women. *Journal of Marriage & the Family*, 57(2), 283–294.

Johnson, M. P. (2001). Conflict and control: Symmetry and asymmetry in domestic violence. In A. Booth, A. C. Crouter, & M. Clements (Eds.), *Couples in conflict* (pp. 95–104). Mahwah, NJ: Lawrence Erlbaum Associates.

Saunders, D. G. (1986). When battered women use violence: Husband-abuse or self-defense? *Violence and Victims*, 1(1), 47–60.

Straus, M. A., & Gelles, R. J. (1986). Societal change and change in family violence from 1975 to 1985 as revealed by two national surveys. *Journal of Marriage and the Family*, 48(August), 465–479.

Swan, S. C., & Snow, D. L. (2002). A typology of women's use of violence in intimate relationships. *Violence Against Women*, 8(3), 286–319.

Swan, S. C., & Snow, D. L. (2003). Behavioral and psychological differences among abused women who use violence in intimate relationships. *Violence Against Women*, 9(1), 75–109.

Tjaden, P., & Thoennes, N. (2000). Prevalence and consequences of male-to-female and female-to-male intimate partner violence as measured by the national violence against women survey. *Violence Against Women*, 6(2), 142–161.

CURRENT CONTROVERSIES AND PREVALENCE CONCERNING FEMALE OFFENDERS OF INTIMATE PARTNER VIOLENCE

Why the Overwhelming Evidence on Partner Physical Violence by Women Has Not Been Perceived and Is Often Denied

MURRAY A. STRAUS

University of New Hampshire, Durham, New Hampshire, USA

Over 200 studies have found about the same percentage of women as men physically assault partners, and that the risk factors and motivations are mostly the same as for men. Explanations are suggested for why this fundamental fact has not been perceived by the public and practitioners, including concealment and denial by many academics who know the research. Explanations for concealment and denial are also presented, with discussion of the adverse effect that misperception and denial have had on prevention and treatment programs. The practical implications of recognizing gender symmetry in partner violence are discussed.

The primary purpose of the article is to suggest explanations for the fact that, despite a large body of high-quality evidence, gender symmetry in the perpetration of physical assault against a partner in a marital, cohabiting, or dating relationship has not been perceived by the public or service providers. Moreover, the article also suggests explanations for the fact that research showing symmetry has often been concealed and denied by academics. The term "gender symmetry" will be used to refer to approximately equal rates of perpetration of physical assault by women and men, and similar patterns of motivation and risk factors. To avoid confusion, it is also necessary to identify issues that are *not* among the purposes of the article.

First, the evidence showing gender symmetry has been covered elsewhere (Archer, 2000; Capaldi, Kim, & Shortt, 2007; Capaldi & Owen, 2001; Fiebert, 2004; Moffitt, Caspi, Rutter, & Silva, 2001; Straus, 2005, 2007a), and therefore is not addressed here. Second, this article will not present the evidence and methods used to conceal and deny it (e.g., publishing only the results on perpetration by men, even though results for both genders are available), as that has also been documented previously (Straus, 2007a). Third, the article does not cover sexual assault because there is no controversy concerning the fact that almost all heterosexual rapes are perpetrated by men. When the term "violence" is used, it will refer to nonsexual physical violence. Finally, the article is not intended to change the opinion of those who reject the existence of gender symmetry. Rather, the purpose, as previously stated, is to suggest explanations for the misperception of the high rate of female partner violence (PV) by the public and service providers, and explanations for hiding and denying the evidence on gender symmetry by academics. This will be followed by a discussion of what I believe are some of the consequences of concealment and denial, and my opinion on needed future directions. To put the article in context, it is one of a series of sociology of science essays that have analyzed the development of "family violence" as a field of research (Straus, 1992b, 1999, 2007b).

THE EVIDENCE ON GENDER SYMMETRY

Symmetry in Perpetration

Because concealment and denial of PV by women has been so effective, many readers will not be familiar with the evidence on gender symmetry. Table 1 and Figure 1 provide a small sampling of the basic information. Table 1 presents the gender-specific rates of perpetration from 12 major national epidemiological or longitudinal studies. It shows that the percentage of women who physically assaulted a male partner is as high or higher than the percentage of men who physically assaulted a female partner, and that this applies to severe violence such as kicking, choking, and attacks with objects and

TABLE 1 Twelve Examples of More Than 200 Studies Showing Gender Symmetry in Partner Violence

Study	Severity of assault	Perpetrator	
		Male	Female
1975 National Family Violence Survey (Straus et al., 1980)	Minor	11.6%	12.1%
	Severe	3.8%	4.6%
1985 National Family Violence Survey (Gelles & Straus, 1988)	Minor	11.3%	12.1%
	Severe	3.0%	4.4%
Canadian National Survey (Grandin & Lupri, 1997)	Minor	17.8%	23.3%
	Severe	10.1%	12.9%
Canadian General Social Survey (Fitzgerald, 1999)	Overall rate	7.0%	8.0%
British Crime Survey (Mirrless-Black, 1999)	Overall rate	4.2%	4.2%
National Co-Morbidity Study (Kessler, 2001)	Minor	17.4%	17.7%
	Severe	6.5%	6.2%
National Alcohol and Family Violence Survey (Straus, 1995)	Overall rate	9.1%	9.5%
	Severe	1.9%	4.5%
Dunedin Health and Development Study (Moffitt & Caspi, 1999)	Overall rate	27.0%	34.0%
National Violence Against Women Survey (Tjaden & Thoennes, 2000)	Overall rate	1.3%	0.9%
Youth Risk Behavior Survey (Eaton et al., 2006)	Overall rate	8.8%	8.9%
National Youth Survey (Wofford-Mihalic, Elliott, & Menard, 1994)	Overall rate	20.2%	34.1%
	Severe	5.7%	3.8%
National Longitudinal Study of Adolescent Health (Whitaker et al., 2007)	Overall rate	19.3%	28.4%

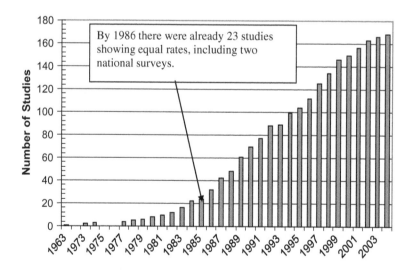

FIGURE 1 Cumulative number of studies showing similar rates of assaulting a partner by women and men.

weapons, as well as to minor violence. Although not shown in Table 1, women *initiate* PV at the same or higher rates as men, and they are the sole perpetrator at the same or higher rates (Capaldi, Shortt, & Crosby, 2003; Kessler, Molnar, Feurer, & Appelbaum, 2001; Straus, 2005; Straus & Ramirez, 2007). Moreover, Figure 1 shows that the evidence demonstrating similar rates of PV perpetration have been available for at least 25 years. One of the earliest studies showing symmetry in both perpetration and risk factors was the 1975 National Family Violence Survey (Straus, Gelles, & Steinmetz, 1980/ 2006). Since then, as shown in Table 1, there have been many other large-scale studies, including a 32-nation study (Straus, 2007a) and about 200 other studies that have found gender symmetry in PV perpetration and a less, but still large, number that have found similar patterns of motivation.

Symmetry in Motives and Risk Factors

While there is beginning to be recognition of gender symmetry in perpetration of PV, those denying symmetry now emphasize the belief that the motives are different for men and women. Although this article will not fully document gender symmetry in risk factors and motivations, it is necessary to provide at least some documentation of symmetry in motives and risk factors because few readers will be familiar with the evidence. An early example is the empirically derived risk factor indices for male violence against female partners and female violence against male partners. The items in these two indices are almost identical (Straus et al., 1980/2006), and have been confirmed by subsequent research. The most commonly reported proximate motivations for violence by both men and women are coercion, anger, and attempts to punish a partner for misbehavior, especially sexual infidelity (Cascardi & Vivian, 1995; Follingstad, Wright, Lloyd, & Sebastian, 1991; Harned, 2001; Hettrich & O'Leary, 2007; Stets & Hammons, 2002). The motive of self-defense, which has often been put forward as an explanation for high rates of female violence, explains only a small proportion of PV perpetrated by women (Carrado, George, Loxam, Jones, & Templar, 1996; Felson & Messner, 1998; Sarantakos, 1999; Sommer, 1996). For example, Follingstad et al.'s (1991) study of college students found that PV perpetrators reported self-defense about 18% of the time (17.7% for men, 18.5% for women). Much other evidence on gender symmetry in motives and risk factors is summarized in Medeiros and Straus (2006).

In contrast to the research evidence showing gender symmetry, public perception of PV and programs to prevent and treat PV are based on the assumption that it is perpetrated almost exclusively by men. This raises the question of why the overwhelming body of evidence on gender symmetry has not been perceived but rather has often been concealed and denied (see Straus, 2007b, for documentation of concealment and denial). This discrepancy is finally starting to be documented and criticized (Dutton, 2006; Felson, 2002;

Hamel & Nicholls, 2006). The following section will suggest explanations for the misperception, followed by a section containing explanations for the fact that, when confronted with the evidence, there has been a 30-year-long effort to hide and deny the evidence (documented in Straus, 2007b).

Asymmetry in Effects

There is one important and consistently reported gender difference in PV: although women engage in both minor and severe violence as often as men, the adverse effects on victims are much greater for women. Attacks by men cause more injury (both physical and psychological), more deaths, and more fear. In addition, women are more often economically trapped in a violent relationship than men because women continue to earn less than men, and because when a marriage ends, women have custodial responsibility for children at least 80% of the time. The greater adverse effect on women is an extremely important difference, and it indicates the need to continue to provide more services for female victims of PV than for male victims. In addition, as will be explained later, the greater adverse effect on women underlies the reluctance to acknowledge the evidence on gender symmetry. However, empathy for women because of the greater injury and the need to help victimized women must not be allowed to obscure the fact that men sustain about a third of the injuries from PV, including a third of the deaths by homicide (Catalano, 2006; Rennison, 2000; Straus, 2005). PV by women is therefore a serious crime, health, and social problem that must be addressed, even though the effects are not as prevalent as assaults perpetrated by male partners. Moreover, the risk of injury and the probability of the violence continuing or escalating is greatest when both partners are violent (Straus, 2007b), as is the case for at least half of violent couples (Feld & Straus, 1989; Ross & Babcock, 2009; Straus & Gozjolko, 2007; Whitaker, Haileyesus, Swahn, & Saltzman, 2007).

EXPLANATIONS OF THE MISPERCEPTION

In contrast to the voluminous empirical evidence on symmetry in perpetration and motivation of PV, the explanations for the misperception described in this section, and the explanation for the concealment described in the following section, are the author's opinions, backed where possible by references to empirical data.

Men Predominate in Almost All Other Crimes

For almost every other type of crime, especially violent crime, men predominate. For some types of crime, such as homicide and sexual assault, the gender ratio is as high as 10 to one (Dawson & Straus, 2007; Ellis & Walsh, 2000). There is naturally a tendency to think that this also applies to PV.

Male Predominance in Police Statistics on Partner Violence

Men also predominate in hospital and police statistics on PV. Most tabulations of police data show that in 80–99% of PV cases reported to police, men are deemed the primary perpetrator of violence. This is not because of more physical attacks by men. It is because of the greater probability of injury from attacks by men and greater fear for safety by women (Straus, 1999), both of which are characteristics that lead to police intervention. In addition, men are even more reluctant than women to report having been assaulted by a partner to the police and hospital staff (Tjaden & Thoennes, 2000). Police are not involved in at least 95% of PV cases (Kaufman Kantor, & Straus, 1990). Despite the unrepresentative nature of police statistics, they are usually taken as representative of all cases of PV. This gives the impression that it is almost exclusively men who physically assault their partner. Similarly, some hospital data show a preponderance of male victims, reflecting the greater probability of injury from an attack by a female, and the fact that the issue is usually investigated only for female patients. But as shown in Table 1, epidemiological surveys of representative samples in western nations have consistently found that the rates of physical PV perpetration by women are about the same as by men.

Women Injured More and Fear More

As noted previously, women are physically injured by PV more frequently than men. Empathy for victims more frequently physically injured thus results in greater concern and sympathy for female victims, and leads the press and the public to focus on assaults perpetrated by male partners. Related to this is the tendency to define physical violence by whether it results in an injury. This combination is probably a large part of the explanation for the greater cultural acceptance of violence by women than by men in developed nations (Straus, 1995; Straus, Kaufman Kantor, & Moore, 1997).

Violence by a male partner produces an appropriate fear of injury among women. However, the much lower but still present probability of injury for men (coupled with greater cultural acceptance of women's PV) leads to trivialization of physical attacks by women and hinders perception of PV perpetrated by women. It also reduces the probability of men (and others) perceiving attacks by women as dangerous or "violent," even though men are victim to a third of the homicides and a third of the nonfatal injuries inflicted by a romantic partner (Catalano, 2006; Rennison, 2000; Straus, 2005). Witnesses are less likely to call police for female-to-male

PV than for male-to-female PV unless the incident is very serious (Felson, 2002). This results in men not fearing injury and neglect of protective steps, such as calling the police or ending the relationship. The fact that about a third of partner homicide victims are men indicates that the neglect of self-protective steps can be fatal.

The Importance of Ending Cultural Norms Tolerating Male Violence

Until nearly the end of the 19th century, husbands were allowed to use "reasonable chastisement" to deal with "errant" wives (Calvert, 1974). Thus, even though female PV has been documented since the Middle Ages (George, 1994), men who "allowed" this were ridiculed. Thus male PV, like corporal punishment of children then and now, has been an accepted part of the culture. It has taken a major effort by feminists and their academic colleagues, including the author (Straus, 1976), to change the continuing implicit cultural norm that accepts a certain amount of male PV. I suggest that the necessary intense focus on this effort interfered with recognizing PV by women, and interfered with recognizing the large body of evidence showing that there are many causes of PV in addition to male dominance (Dutton, 2006; Hamel & Nicholls, 2007; Whitaker & Lutzker, 2009).

Men have the predominant power in society as judged by many indicators (Archer, 2006; Sugarman & Straus, 1988; United Nations Development Programme, 2006; Yodanis, 2004). The cognitive discrepancy between this fact and high rates of PV by females, even in extremely male dominant societies (Douglas & Straus, 2006; Haj-Yahia, 2000; Straus, 2007a; World Health Organization, 2006), blocks recognition of the equal rates of violence. In many societies or segments of societies around the world, high levels of male control over women and of male violence against women is still culturally accepted (Archer, 2006; Sugarman & Straus, 1988; United Nations Development Programme, 2006; Yodanis, 2004). In these countries, there is an urgent need to promote empowerment of women. That need also exists in the United States and other advanced industrial nations, but more as an end in itself than as a means of ending PV.

Gender Stereotypes

Most cultures define women as "the gentle sex," making it difficult to perceive violence by women as being prevalent in any sphere of life. More specifically, there are implicit norms tolerating violence by women, on the assumption that it rarely results in injury (Straus, Kaufman Kantor, & Moore, 1997). This assumption is largely correct, but as previously noted, it is also correct that about a third of homicides of partners are perpetrated by women, as well about a third of nonfatal injuries (Catalano, 2006; Rennison, 2000; Straus, 2005).

Evidence Available to the Public

A major factor in understanding why the public does not perceive the extent of female PV is that the information has not been made available or has been distorted in the media, which are the public's main sources of information. Media coverage of PV reflects and reinforces the gender stereotypes described previously. For example, a study of newspaper coverage of the 785 homicides that occurred in Cincinnati, Ohio over a 17-year period found that 79% of partner homicides perpetrated by men were reported, compared to 50% of the partner homicides perpetrated by women (Lundman, 2000). Moreover, for cases of women killed by a male partner there was a mean of 3.5 articles, compared to a mean of 1.7 articles for men killed by a female partner. Another example (from, literally, thousands) is "And Then He Hit Me" in the *American Association of Retired People Magazine* (France, 2006), which states that the number of woman-on-man incidents of domestic violence among the elderly is "negligible" and cites as the source a study by Pillemer and Finkelhor (1986). But that study found that 43% of the cases of physical violence of the elderly were the wife assaulting the husband, whereas only 17% were husbands assaulting their wife. This probably reflects the fact that many more wives than husbands have the responsibility of providing care for elderly, infirm, and often difficult-to-deal-with partners.

Difficulty of Correcting False Information

Research on persistence of false information has found that it is difficult to correct it. Experiments by Schwarz, Sanna, Skurnik, and Yoon (2007) and others have found that denials and clarifications of false information, although necessary, can paradoxically contribute to the resiliency of popular myths. This may result partly from the fact that denials inherently require repeating the bad information. Consequently, even when the evidence on gender symmetry is presented by an authoritative source such as the Centers for Disease Control and Prevention, there will be only limited success in changing beliefs about female perpetration.

EXPLANATIONS OF THE DENIAL

In addition to failing to perceive the extent of gender symmetry in PV, there have also been strenuous efforts by researchers and other academics to deny the overwhelming evidence, including punishment of researchers who have persisted in publishing results showing gender symmetry, such as denial of tenure. Methods used to deny the evidence and enforce this on others have been described in other articles (Gelles, 2007; Straus, 1990b, 2007b). In this article, the objective is not to repeat the presentation of that evidence, but to suggest why it has occurred. It is important to recognize that the terms "concealment" and "denial" only apply to those who have research evidence that could be concealed or denied. Thus, this section refers to the academic community, not to service providers.

Lack of Attention to Heterogeneity of PV

One of the most important reasons for denial of gender symmetry is failure to adequately recognize heterogeneity in PV. Women's advocates most often focus on the relatively small proportion of overall PV that is visible to justice, shelter, batterer intervention, and other service providers (i.e., cases in which women's injury, fear, and domination are much more common). In contrast, the research showing gender symmetry has been based on general population samples in which the predominant form of PV is minor, bidirectional, not physically injurious, and often not fear provoking for men, even when it should be. The findings of these general population studies are not believed by battered women's advocates because they are inconsistent with the characteristic of the actual cases they work with every day.

Academics are the ones who know or produce the research and are the ones who have concealed, denied, or hidden the evidence. One example is the belief that when women are violent, it is almost always an act of self-defense, whereas the previously cited studies (and others not cited) show that this is rarely the case. Instead of concealing and denying, academic advisors of service providers should help them understand the heterogeneity of severity and motives that characterize PV. This can help provide more effective prevention and treatment programs that take heterogeneity into account.

It is increasingly clear that the characteristics of "clinical" and "nonclinical" levels of PV differ, therefore the interventions also need to differ (Johnson & Ferraro, 2000; Ross & Babcock, 2009; Straus, 1990a; Straus, 2009). This needs to be determined by initial screening, rather than the current practice of proceeding with all offenders as though they were clinical level offenders, motivated by desire to subordinate women as a class. For nonclinical forms of PV, prevention focused on developing healthy relationships, conflict resolution skills, and anger management (usually for both parties, no matter who is the presenting partner) and couple therapy are likely to be most effective. For "clinical-level" cases of PV, where psychopathology is often involved, more intense and evidence-based interventions are required, not just interventions based on the patriarchal theory of PV, but with continued focus on the safety needs of victims (Straus, 2009; Stuart, 2005).

Defense of Feminist Theory

The women's movement brought public attention to the fact that PV may be the most prevalent form of interpersonal violence and to the plight of women victims. The feminist effort created a world-wide determination to cease ignoring PV, and to take steps to combat PV. Feminists have largely been responsible for changing police and court practices from ignoring and minimizing PV (International Association of Chiefs of Police, 1967; Straus, 1976) to compelling the criminal justice system to attend and intervene. That change in police practices is only one of the many ways in which the women's movement has changed social norms tolerating male-to-female PV. In addition, feminists have created two important new social institutions: shelters for battered women and treatment programs for male perpetrators. Because the well- being of women is the primary concern of the feminist effort, their approach appropriately focused on protecting women from male violence.

The problem with this approach is not just the almost exclusive focus on female victims and male perpetrators. The problem is also insistence on a single-cause theory: the belief that PV is a reflection of a patriarchal social and family system (Dobash & Dobash, 1992; Krug, Dahlberg, Mercy, Zwi, & Lozano, 2002; Loseke & Kurz, 2005). Subsequent research has shown that there are many causes of PV and great variability in types of violent relationships. This research has also shown that women perpetrate PV as much as or more than men, and that although some PV is "gendered" in the sense of an effort by men as a category to dominate women as a category, most is traceable to a number of other risk factors. For frequent severe PV, psychopathology such as antisocial personality and borderline personality is frequent (Dutton, 2006); and for "ordinary" (Straus, 1990a) or "situational" (Johnson & Ferraro, 2000) violence, poor anger management, and frustration and anger at misbehavior by the partner are frequent precipitants of PV (see the reviews in Hettrich & O'Leary, 2007, and Straus, 2009). The evidence on these risk factors and motives is difficult to square with the patriarchal theory of PV because the two central tenants of the patriarchal theory are male perpetration, motivated by efforts to maintain a male-dominant family and social system. I suggest that one of reasons for the denial is to maintain adherence to the patriarchal theory of PV.

In addition to being perceived as a threat to the theory that had inspired and sustained the battered women's movement, I suggest that the research showing gender symmetry has been denied because it may have been perceived as a threat to feminism in general. This is because a key step in the effort to achieve an equalitarian society is to bring about recognition of the harm that a patriarchal system causes. The removal of patriarchy as the main cause of PV weakens a dramatic example of the harmful effects of patriarchy. That is unfortunate, but by no means critical because the effort to achieve equality can continue to be made on the basis of many other ways in which women continue to be subordinate to men (e.g., efforts to rectify the differential).

The above discussion only brushes the surface of a complex phenomenon, on which there is a voluminous literature. For example, even though male dominance and male privilege may no longer be the major cause of PV in more egalitarian western societies, dominance by either party, regardless of whether it is the male or female partner, is associated with an increased probability of PV (Straus, 2007a). Moreover, comparative studies have shown that the more male dominant the society or segment of society, the more PV (Archer, 2006; Straus, 1994, 2007a; Yodanis, 2004). Perhaps most important, although ending male dominance and male privilege may not be central to ending PV in western nations, it is central to creating a better society for men as well as women.

Defense of Services and Avoiding Harm to Women Victims

There is a fear that if the public, legislators, and administrators believed the research on gender symmetry, it would weaken support for services to female victims, such as shelters for battered women, and weaken efforts to arrest and prosecute violent men. I know of no cases in which funding for services for female victims has been decreased because "women are also violent." Nevertheless, I have been told on several occasions that I am endangering services for battered women by publishing the results of research showing equal perpetration. One of these was during a panel discussion of PV research at the 1992 meeting of the Society for Study of Social Problems. One panel member said that this type of phalli-centric research was undermining efforts to help battered women. This was followed by vigorous applause.

There is also a fear that efforts to arrest and prosecute male offenders will be undermined by acknowledging female PV, and that women will be unjustly prosecuted for violence perpetrated in self-defense (Feder & Henning, 2005). In fact, a growing number of women are being arrested through the introduction of mandatory or recommended arrest for PV (Martin, 1997; Miller, 2001). For example, in California between 1987 and 1997, the ratio of male and female arrests for PV decreased from 1 female arrest to 18 male arrests to a ratio of 1 to 4.5 (DeLeon-Granados, Wells, & Binsbacher, 2006). It is unlikely that this shift is a result of an increase in female violence. Rates of both fatal and nonfatal PV have been dropping over time (Catalano, 2006; Rennison & Rand, 2003) and such marked shifts in female perpetration are not found for other crimes. I suggest that fear of weakening arrest of men and, more recently, increasing arrest of women is part of the reason for concealing the evidence. However, in my opinion, the main factor contributing to increased arrest of women is the success of the effort by the women's movement to change police practice from one of avoiding interference in "domestic disturbances" to one of mandatory or recommended arrest (DeLeon-Granados et al., 2006).

Another concern that may have motivated the concealment and denial is the fear that recognizing the complexity of PV, including acknowledging female PV, will weaken the ability of the justice system to act on behalf of women victims of PV. The prototypical cases that galvanized efforts to ensure that women received swift police response, followed by arrest and prosecution of their partners, were of nonviolent women who are terrorized by their partners and needed the assistance of the legal system to escape. I suggest that those concerned with protecting female victims fear that if this image of PV is lost—and instead the justice system has to assess the context of the incident, the history of both partners, the motive for the offense, and the level of fear generated—the difficulty and burden of doing that may result in failing to adequately protect women and prosecute male offenders.

CONSEQUENCES OF THE DENIAL

The criticism inherent in this article is directed primarily to the research community. The thousands of dedicated women and their allies who developed and maintain services for battered women are part of a social movement that has benefited the entire society, not just women. The objective of social movements and advocacy groups is to change society. To achieve this, social movements often deny contrary evidence, distort evidence, and exaggerate. This may be necessary to sustain the effort to achieve even modest social changes. But it is the objective of science to explain the way the world works, and for this to be achieved, scientists cannot let their social and moral commitments lead them to deny contrary evidence, to exaggerate, and to penalize those who produce the evidence, as has been the case (Straus, 1990b, 2007b). In a sense, service providers can be considered victims of the denial of the scientific evidence by the academic community concerned with PV.

In denying the evidence, social scientists are also doing a disservice to women. They are hindering efforts to help women avoid engaging in PV. This is important because women, like men, need to be helped to recognize that hitting a partner is morally wrong, criminal, and harmful to the perpetrator as well as to the victim. First, it is associated with lower levels of relationship health. Second, it increases the probability of physical attacks by the woman's partner (Capaldi & Owen, 2001; Straus & Gozjolko, 2007; Whitaker et al., 2007). Third, it exposes children to the well-documented harm from witnessing PV (Jaffe, Wolfe, & Wilson, 1990; Margolin & John, 1997; Wolfe, Wekerle, Scott, Straatman, & Grasley, 2004), and those consequences also apply when the perpetrator is the mother (Straus, 1992a).

Finally, just as denial of painful phenomena by individuals is usually harmful, denial by social groups is likely to be harmful to the group engaged in the denial (Zerubavel, 2006). I am concerned that denial of the evidence on female PV may ultimately interfere with the very goals the denial is intended to achieve because, when the evidence finally prevails, the discrepancy could undermine the credibility of the feminist cause. It may alienate young women from the feminist cause, and it could weaken the public base of feminist support. At the same time, casting PV as almost exclusively a male crime angers men who feel that they are being unjustly accused and provides fuel for the fire of extremist men's groups. These organizations often have a larger antifeminist agenda and publicize feminist denial and distortion of the evidence on PV as part of that larger effort. This is happening in many countries (e.g., see the organization Save India Family Foundation, http://www.saveindianfamily.org). Finally, I am concerned that the denial in the face of overwhelming evidence may reduce the credibility of feminist scholarship among academics.

THE FUTURE

Recent articles and books (e.g., Dutton, 2006; Hamel & Nicholls, 2007; O'Leary & Woodin, 2009; Straus, 2009; Stuart, 2005) indicate a process that is likely to ultimately change the current pattern of denial of gender symmetry in the scholarly literature as well as the current failure to apply what is known about gender symmetry to improving the dismal performance of treatment programs for perpetrators of PV (Babcock, Green, & Robie, 2004; Dutton, 2006). One manifestation of how this denial has interfered with developing effective treatment programs is the deliberate ignoring of evidence from studies that have investigated the issue in the general population and in samples of battered women showing that most PV is bidirectional, and that the bidirectionality is rarely a self-defensive response. This calls for involving both partners in treatment. But legislation or administrative rules in 43% of American states forbid couple therapy in court-mandated treatment of PV.

Almost all batterer intervention programs use the Duluth model for treatment (Rosenbaum & Price, 2007). This model prevents making use of the vast amount of evidence on the etiology of PV accumulated in the past 20 years by excluding from the treatment model any cause except the idea that PV is an effort by men to uphold male privilege in society and the family, and by rejecting any other explanation or treatment modality as excusing male violence. Although replacing patriarchal beliefs and social organization with equalitarian values and equality between men and women is an extremely important goal, it plays a much less important role in explaining individual differences in PV (Sugarman & Frankel, 1996). Instead, the predominant proximal motives for "ordinary" or "common couple" PV by both men and women are frustration and anger at the partner, as well as efforts to coerce the partner into doing or not doing something (Caldwell, Swan, Allen, Sullivan, & Snow, in press; Walley-Jean & Swan, in press). The predominant risk factors for "clinically abusive" PV are antisocial personality traits, excessive drinking, social disadvantage, history of child-hood victimization, and elevated hostility, anger, and other psychological problems (Goldenson, Spidel, Greaves, & Dutton, in press; Straus, 2009). This calls for the development of multiple forms of treatment to address those motives and psychological problems, along with treatments that address the problems of both partners.

At the same time, continued efforts are needed to further the empower-ment of women, especially in less developed nations. Gender equality is a critical part of human rights and a humane society, and it contributes to prevention of PV. Given the fact that patriarchy is not the predominant risk factor for PV, to maximize prevention and treatment of PV it is essential that the effort not be restricted to treatments based on correcting patriarchal beliefs and behavior. For the more common forms of PV, the primary prevention efforts need to focus on reducing acceptance of all forms and levels of violence, starting with corporal punishment by parents (Straus & Yodanis, 1996) and psychological aggression by parents and between part-ners. On the positive side, prevention efforts need to focus on developing the skills needed to manage the inevitable conflicts in relationships, as is exemplified in the *Choose Respect* program of the Centers for Disease Control and Prevention (www.chooserespect.org).

Treatment of existing clinical-level cases of PV requires continuing to include justice system interventions as an expression of social norms con-demning PV, to protect victims, and to mandate treatment. As in the case of the primary prevention, research has shown that psychological problems such as antisocial and borderline personality are major risk factors for clinical-level PV. Consequently, treatment of existing cases needs to expand from efforts to end patriarchal dominance to include diagnosis for these psychological prob-lems and treatment when identified. A tragic irony is that the denial that obstructs this needed fundamental change in prevention and treatment of PV is, in my opinion, largely motivated by a concern with the safety of women. The tragedy associated with this irony is that, rather than enhancing the safety and well-being of women, these denials block key steps that could increase the effectiveness of the effort to reduce violence against women.

REFERENCES

Archer, J. (2000). Sex differences in aggression between heterosexual partners: A meta-analytic review. *Psychological Bulletin, 126*(5), 651–680.

Archer, J. (2006). Cross-cultural differences in physical aggression between partners: A social structural analysis. *Personality and Social Psychology Review, 10*(2), 133–153.

Babcock, J. C., Green, C. E., & Robie, C. (2004). Does batterers' treatment work? A meta-analytic review of domestic violence treatment. *Clinical Psychology Review, 23*(8), 1023–1053.

Caldwell, J. E., Swan, S. C., Allen, C. T., Sullivan, T. P., & Snow, D. L. (in press). Why I hit him: Women's reasons for intimate partner violence. *Journal of Aggression, Maltreatment, & Trauma*.

Calvert, R. (1974). Criminal and civil liability in husband-wife assaults. In S. K. Steinmetz & M. A. Straus (Eds.), *Violence in the family* (pp. 88–97). New York: Harper and Row.

Capaldi, D. M., Kim, H. K., & Shortt, J. W. (2007). Observed initiation and reciprocity of physical aggression in young, at-risk couples. *Journal of Family Violence, 22*(2), 101–111.

Capaldi, D. M., & Owen, L. D. (2001). Physical aggression in a community sample of at-risk young couples: Gender comparisons for high frequency, injury, and fear. *Journal of Family Psychology, 15*(3), 425–440.

Capaldi, D. M., Shortt, J. W., & Crosby, L. (2003). Physical and psychological aggression in at-risk young couples: Stability and change in young adulthood. *Merrill-Palmer Quarterly, 49*(1), 1–27.

Carrado, M., George, M. J., Loxam, E., Jones, L., & Templar, D. (1996). Aggression in British heterosexual relationships: A descriptive analysis. *Aggressive Behavior, 22*, 401–415.

Cascardi, M., & Vivian, D. (1995). Context for specific episodes of marital violence: Gender and severity of violence differences. *Journal of Family Violence, 10*(3), 265–293.

Catalano, S. (2006). *Intimate partner violence in the United States*. Retrieved January 9, 2007, from www.ojp.usdoj.gov/bjs/intimate/ipv.htm.

Dawson, J., & Straus, M. A. (2007, November). *Gender differences and gender convergence in self-reported crime and delinquency: a review of research from 1947 to 2004*. Paper presented at the American Society of Criminology, Atlanta, GA.

Deleon-Granados, W., Wells, W., & Binsbacher, R. (2006). Arresting developments: Trends in female arrests for domestic violence and proposed explanations. *Violence Against Women, 12*(4), 355–371.

Dobash, E. R., & Dobash, R. P. (1992). *Women, violence and social change*. New York: Routledge.

Douglas, E. M., & Straus, M. A. (2006). Assault and injury of dating partners by university students in 19 countries and its relation to corporal punishment experienced as a child. *European Journal of Criminology, 3*, 293–318.

Dutton, D. G. (2006). *Rethinking domestic violence*. Vancouver, BC: University of British Columbia Press.

Eaton, D. K., Kann, L., Kinchen, S., Ross, J., Hawkins, J., Harris, W. A., et al. (2006). Youth risk behavior surveillance–United States, 2005 [MMWR2006: 55]. *Morbidity and Mortality Weekly Report, 55*, No. SS–5.

Ellis, L., & Walsh, A. (2000). *Criminology: A global perspective*. Boston: Allyn & Bacon.

Feder, L., & Henning, K. (2005). A comparison of male and female dually arrested domestic violence offenders. *Violence and Victims, 20*(2), 153–171.

Feld, S. L., & Straus, M. A. (1989). Escalation and desistance of wife assault in marriage. *Criminology, 27*(1), 141–161.

Felson, R. B. (2002). *Violence and gender reexamined*. Washington, DC: American Psychological Press.

Felson, R. B., & Messner, S. F. (1998). Disentangling the effects of gender and intimacy on victim precipitation in homicide. *Criminology, 36*(2), 405–423.

Fiebert, M. S. (2004). References examining assaults by women on their spouses or male partners: an annotated bibliography. *Sexuality and Culture, 8*(3–4), 140–177.

Fitzgerald, R. (1999). *Family violence in Canada: A statistical profile.* Ottawa: Statistics Canada.

Follingstad, D. R., Wright, S., Lloyd, S., & Sebastian, J. A. (1991). Sex differences in motivations and effects in dating violence. *Family Relations, 40*(1), 51–57.

France, D. (2006, January/February). And then he hit me. *American Association of Retired People Magazine.* Retrieved January 26, 2009, from http://www.aarpmagazine.org/family/domestic_violence.html

Gelles, R. J. (2007). The politics of research: The use, abuse, and misuse of social science date—The cases of intimate partner violence. *Family Court Review, 45*(1), 42–51.

Gelles, R., & Straus, M. A. (1988). *Intimate violence: The causes and consequences of abuse in the American family.* New York: Simon & Schuster.

George, M. (1994). Riding the donkey backwards: Men as the unacceptable victims of marital violence. *The Journal of Men's Studies, 3*(2), 137–159.

Goldenson, J., Spidel, A., Greaves, C., & Dutton, D. (in press). Female perpetrators of intimate partner violence: Within-group heterogeneity, related psychopathology, and a review of current treatment with recommendations for the future. *Journal of Aggression, Maltreatment, & Trauma.*

Grandin, E., & Lupri, E. (1997). Intimate violence in Canada and the United States: A cross-national comparison. *Journal of Family Violence, 12*(4), 417–443.

Haj-Yahia, M. M. (2000). The incidence of wife abuse and battering and some sociodemographic correlates as revealed by two national surveys in Palestinian society. *Journal of Family Violence, 15*(4), 347–374.

Hamel, J., & Nicholls, T. (Eds.). (2006). *Family approaches in domestic violence: A practitioner's guide to gender-inclusive research and treatment.* New York: Springer.

Hamel, J., & Nicholls, T. (Eds.). (2007). *Family interventions in domestic violence: A handbook of gender-inclusive theory and treatment.* New York: Springer.

Harned, M. S. (2001). Abused women or abused men? An examination of the context and outcomes of dating violence. *Violence and Victims, 16*(3), 269–285.

Hettrich, E. L., & O'Leary, K. D. (2007). Females' reasons for their physical aggression in dating relationships. *Journal of Interpersonal Violence, 22*(9), 1131–1143.

International Association of Chiefs of Police. (1967). *Training Kely 16: Handling domestic disturbance calls.* Gaithersburg, MD: Author.

Jaffe, P. G., Wolfe, D. A., & Wilson, S. K. (1990). *Children of battered women.* Newbury Park, CA: Sage.

Johnson, M. P., & Ferraro, K. J. (2000). Research on domestic violence in the 1990's: Making distinctions. *Journal of Marriage and the Family, 62*(4), 948–963.

Kaufman Kantor, G., & Straus, M. A. (1990). Response of victims and the police to assaults on wives. In M. A. Straus & R. J. Gelles (Eds.), *Physical violence in American families: Risk factors and adaptations to violence in 8,145 families* (pp. 473–487). New Brunswick, NJ: Transaction Publishers.

Kessler, R. C., Molnar, B. E., Feurer, I. D., & Appelbaum, M. (2001). Patterns and mental health predictors of domestic violence in the United States: Results from the National Comorbidity Survey. *International Journal of Law and Psychiatry, 24*(4–5), 487–508.

Krug, E. G., Dahlberg, L. L., Mercy, J. A., Zwi, A. B., & Lozano, R. (2002). *World report on violence and health*. Geneva: World Health Organization.

Loseke, D. R., & Kurz, D. (2005). Men's violence toward women is the serious problem. In D. R. Loseke, R. J. Gelles, & M. M. Cavanaugh (Eds.), *Current controversies on family violence* (pp. 79–95). Thousand Oaks, CA: Sage Publications.

Lundman, R. J. (2000, March 3). *Selection bias in newspaper coverage of homicide: Intersections of newsworthiness, market factors, and typifications with race and gender stereotypes*. Paper presented at the Eastern Sociological Society Meeting, Baltimore, MD.

Margolin, G., & John, R. S. (1997). Children's exposure to marital aggression: Direct and mediated effects. In G. K. Kantor, & J.L. Jasinski (Eds.), *Out of the darkness: Contemporary perspectives on family violence* (pp. 90–104). Thousand Oaks, CA: Sage Publications.

Martin, M. E. (1997). Double your trouble: Dual arrest in family violence. *Journal of Family Violence, 12*(2), 139–157.

Medeiros, R. A., & Straus, M. A. (2006). Risk factors for physical violence between dating partners: Implications for gender-inclusive prevention and treatment of family violence. In J. C. Hamel & T. Nicholls (Eds.), *Family approaches to domestic violence: A practitioners guide to gender-inclusive research and treatment* (pp. 59–87). New York: Springer (also available at http://pubpages. unh.edu/~mas2).

Miller, S. L. (2001). Paradox of women arrested for domestic violence: Criminal justice professionals and service providers respond. *Violence Against Women, 7*(12), 1339–1376.

Mirrless-Black, C. (1999). *Domestic violence: Findings from a new British Crime Survey Self-Completion Questionnaire*. London: Great Britian Home Office.

Moffitt, T. E., & Caspi, A. (1999). Findings about intimate partner violence from the Dunedin Multidisciplinary Health and Development Study (No. NCJ 170018). Washington DC: National Institute of Justice.

Moffitt, T. E., Caspi, A., Rutter, M., & Silva, P. A. (2001). *Sex differences in antisocial behavior*. Cambridge, UK: Cambridge University Press.

O'Leary, K. D., & Woodin, E. M. (2009). *Psychological and physical aggression in couples*. Washington, DC: American Psychological Association.

Pillemer, K., & Finkelhor, D. (1986). The prevalence of elder abuse: A random sample survey. *The Gerontologist, 28*(1), 51–57.

Rennison, C. M. (2000). *Intimate partner violence* (Special Report No. NCJ, 178247). Washington, DC: Bureau of Justice Statistics.

Rennison, C. M., & Rand, M. R. (2003). *Crime victimization, 2002*. Washington, DC: U.S. Department of Justice.

Rosenbaum, A., & Price, B. (2007, July). *National Survey of Perpetrator Intervention Programs*. Paper presented at the International Family Violence Research Conference, Portsmouth, NH.

Ross, J. M., & Babcock, J. C. (2009). Gender differences in partner violence in context: Deconstructing Johnson's (2001) control-based typology of violent couples. *Journal of Aggression, Maltreatment, & Trauma, 18*(6), 604–622.

Sarantakos, S. (1999). Husband abuse: Fact or fiction? *Australian Journal of Social Issues, 34*(3), 231–252.

Schwarz, N., Sanna, L. J., Skurnik, I., & Yoon, C. (2007). Metacognitive experiences and the intricacies of setting people straight: Implications for debiasing and public information campaigns. In M. Zanna (Ed.), *Advances in experimental social psychology* (Vol. 39, pp. 127–161). San Diego: Elsevier Academic Press, Inc.

Sommer, R. (1996). *Male and female perpetrated partner abuse: Testing a diathesis-stress model.* Unpublished doctoral dissertation, University of Manitoba, Winnepeg, Manitoba.

Stets, J. E., & Hammons, S. A. (2002). Gender, control, and marital commitment. *Journal of Family Issues, 23*(1), 3–25.

Straus, M. A. (1976). Sexual inequality, cultural norms, and wife-beating. In E. C. Viano (Ed.), *Victims and society* (pp. 543–559). Washington, DC: Visage Press.

Straus, M. A. (1990a). Injury, frequency, and the representative sample fallacy in measuring wife beating and child abuse. In M. A. Straus & R. J. Gelles (Eds.), *Physical violence in American families: Risk factors and adaptations to violence in 8,145 families* (pp. 75–89). New Brunswick, NJ: Transaction Publications.

Straus, M. A. (1990b). The National Family Violence Surveys. In M. A. Straus & R. J. Gelles (Eds.), *Physical violence in American families: Risk factors and adaptations to violence in 8,145 families* (pp. 3–16). New Brunswick, NJ: Transaction Publishers.

Straus, M. A. (1992a). Children as witnesses to marital violence: A risk factor for life long problems among a nationally representative sample of American men and women. In D. F. Schwartz (Ed.), *Children and violence: Report of the Twenty Third Ross Roundtable on Critical Approaches to Common Pediatric Problems* (pp. 98–109). Columbus, OH: Ross Laboratories.

Straus, M. A. (1992b). Sociological research and social policy: The case of family violence. *Sociological Forum, 7*(2), 211–237.

Straus, M. A. (1994). State-to-state differences in social inequality and social bonds in relation to assaults on wives in the United States. *Journal of Comparative Family Studies, 25*(1), 7–24.

Straus, M. A. (1995). Trends in cultural norms and rates of partner violence: An update to 1992. In J. A. Mancini (Series Ed.) & S. Stith & M. A. Straus (Vol. Eds.), *Families in Focus, Vol. 2. Understanding partner violence: Prevalence, causes, consequences, and solutions* (pp. 30–33). Minneapolis, MN: National Council on Family Relations.

Straus, M. A. (1999). The controversy over domestic violence by women: A methodological, theoretical, and sociology of science analysis. In X. Arriaga & S. Oskamp (Eds.), *Violence in intimate relationships* (pp. 17–44). Thousand Oaks, CA: Sage.

Straus, M. A. (2005). Women's violence toward men is a serious social problem. In D. R. Loseke, R. J. Gelles & M. M. Cavanaugh (Eds.), *Current controversies on family violence* (2nd ed., pp. 55–77). Newbury Park, CA: Sage Publications.

Straus, M. A. (2007a). Dominance and symmetry in partner violence by male and female university students in 32 nations. *Children and Youth Services Review, 30*, 252–275.

Straus, M. A. (2007b). Processes explaining the concealment and distortion of evidence on gender symmetry in partner violence. *European Journal of Criminal Policy and Research, 13*, 227–232.

Straus, M. A. (2009). Gender symmetry in partner violence: The evidence and the implications for primary prevention and treatment. In J. R. Lutzker & D. J. Whitaker (Eds.), *Prevention of partner violence*. Washington DC: American Psychological Association.

Straus, M. A., Gelles, R. J., & Steinmetz, S. K. (1980/2006). *Behind closed doors: Violence in the American family*. New York: Doubleday/Anchor Books. (Reissued by Transaction Publications, 2006, with a new foreword by R. J. Gelles & M. A. Straus.)

Straus, M. A., & Gozjolko, K. L. (2007, June). *Intimate terrorism and injury of dating partners by male and female university students*. Paper presented at the Stockholm Criminology Prize Symposium, Stockholm, Sweden.

Straus, M. A., Kaufman Kantor, G., & Moore, D. W. (1997). Change in cultural norms approving marital violence from 1968 to 1994. In G. Kaufman Kantor & J. L. Jasinski (Eds.), *Out of the darkness: Contemporary perspectives on family violence* (pp. 3–16). Thousand Oaks, CA: Sage Publications.

Straus, M. A., & Ramirez, I. L. (2007). Gender symmetry in prevalence, severity, and chronicity of physical aggression against dating partners by University students in Mexico and USA. *Aggressive Behavior, 33*, 281–290.

Straus, M. A., & Yodanis, C. L. (1996). Corporal punishment in adolescence and physical assaults on spouses later in life: What accounts for the link? *Journal of Marriage and the Family, 58*(4), 825–841.

Stuart, R. B. (2005). Treatment for partner abuse: Time for a paradigm shift. *Professional Psychology-Research and Practice, 36*(3), 254–263.

Sugarman, D. B., & Frankel, S. L. (1996). Patriarchal ideology and wife-assault: A meta-analytic review. *Journal of Family Violence, 11*(1), 13–40.

Sugarman, D. B., & Straus, M. A. (1988). Indicators of gender equality for American states and regions. *Social Indicators Research, 20*, 229–270.

Tjaden, P., & Thoennes, N. (2000). *Full report of the prevalence, incidence, and consequences of violence against women: Findings from the National Violence Against Women Survey* (No. NCJ 183781). Washington, DC: U.S. Department of Justice, Office of Justice Programs.

United Nations Development Programme. (2006). *Human development report*. Retrieved September 20, 2007, from http://hdr.undp.org/hdr2006/statistics/indicators/230.html.

Walley-Jean, J. C., & Swan, S. (in press). Motivations and justifications for partner aggression in a sample of African American college women. *Journal of Aggression, Maltreatment, & Trauma*.

Whitaker, D. J., Haileyesus, T., Swahn, M., & Saltzman, L. S. (2007). Differences in frequency of violence and reported injury between relationships with reciprocal and nonreciprocal intimate partner violence. *American Journal of Public Health, 97*(5), 941–947.

Whitaker, D. J., & Lutzker, J. R. (Eds.). (2009). *Prevention of partner violence.* Washington, DC: American Psychological Association.

Wolfe, D. A., Wekerle, C., Scott, K., Straatman, A.-L., & Grasley, C. (2004). Predicting abuse in adolescent dating relationships over 1 year: The role of child maltreatment and trauma. *Journal of Abnormal Psychology, 113*(3), 406–415.

World Health Organization. (2006). *Global School-based Health Survey.* Geneva: World Health Organization. Retrieved from http://www.who.int/school_youth_health/gshs.

Yodanis, C. (2004). Gender inequality, violence against women, and fear: A cross-national test of the feminist theory of violence against women. *Journal of Interpersonal Violence, 19*(6), 655–675.

Zerubavel, E. (2006). *The elephant in the room: Silence and denial in everyday life.* New York: Oxford University Press.

Women's Use of Intimate Partner Violence against Men: Prevalence, Implications, and Consequences

DENISE A. HINES

Clark University, Worcester, Massachusetts, USA

EMILY M. DOUGLAS

Bridgewater State College, Bridgewater, Massachusetts, USA

Evidence showing that women use intimate partner violence (IPV) against their male partners has existed since the 1970s when IPV was first systematically examined. This article discusses the various sources of prevalence rates of IPV by women against men, the dominant theoretical explanation for IPV in general, and its implications for female perpetrators and male victims in the social service and criminal justice systems, as well as the current evidence of the consequences of women's use of IPV to the men who sustain it. Finally, we discuss directions for future research, including our own study focusing on men who sustain IPV.

Intimate partner violence (IPV) used by women against men is a phenomenon that has received little attention, both within the scholarly literature and the popular media. Despite this lack of attention, for nearly three decades research on IPV has shown that men are frequently the targets of IPV by their female partners. Estimates from national family violence surveys show that within a given year, at least 12% of men are the targets of some sort of physical aggression from their female partners, and 4% (or over 2.5 million men in the United States) sustain severe violence (Straus, 1995). Despite declines in other forms of family violence (e.g., against women or children), rates of nonlethal IPV by women against men have remained steady for the past 30 years (Straus, 1995; U. S. Department of Health and Human Services, 2004).[1] In addition, the National Violence Against Women Survey (NVAWS; Tjaden & Thoennes, 2000) showed that female-perpetrated violence accounts for 40% of all injuries due to IPV during a 1-year time period, 27% of all injuries requiring medical attention, and 31% of all victims fearing bodily harm (calculated from NVAWS).

Preliminary research also shows that IPV by women against men is associated with various mental health problems in men, such as depression, stress, psychosomatic symptoms, and general psychological distress (Cascardi, Langhinrichsen, & Vivian, 1992; Simonelli & Ingram, 1998; Stets & Straus, 1990). Thus, IPV by women against men, like other forms of family violence, can be considered a significant health and mental health problem in this country. Scholars, community providers, and mental health practitioners, however, still have much to learn about this social problem. The purpose of the present article is to summarize various estimates of the extent to which women use IPV against male partners. We then discuss how the conceptualization of IPV from a strict feminist viewpoint has hampered the ability of women who use IPV and men who sustain it to seek and get help from the social service and criminal justice systems. It has also hampered our ability to develop programs that can address this issue. We then end with a discussion of our current knowledge of the mental health consequences for men who sustain IPV from women and directions for future research.

EXTENT OF IPV BY WOMEN AGAINST MEN

Incidence reports of women physically aggressing toward their male partners have appeared since studies of IPV began in the early to mid-1970s. For example, in his groundbreaking study of domestic violence, Gelles (1974) found that "the eruption of conjugal violence occurs with equal frequency among both husbands and wives" (p. 77). Since then, information regarding rates of IPV by women toward men has come from multiple sources. First, crime statistics from the U.S. Department of Justice's National Crime Victimization Survey (NCVS) have shown that in 2004, over 1.3 per 1,000 men were assaulted by an intimate partner, most of whom were women (Catalano, 2007). Moreover, in contrast to the dramatic declining rates of reported IPV toward women between 1993 and 2004 (from 9.8 to 3.8 women per 1,000), the rates for men did not decline quite so precipitously

---

[1]   Rates of IPV-related deaths, however, have been declining for both genders. In 1976, 1,357 men and 1,600 women were killed by intimate partners, whereas in 2001, 440 men and 1,247 women were killed by an intimate partner (Rennison, 2003).

(from 1.6 to 1.3 men per 1,000). Crime surveys, however, are likely to underestimate the number of people who sustain IPV because many people, both men and women, often do not conceptualize the physical violence they sustain from their intimate partner as a "crime." This reluctance may be even more pronounced in men because men are commonly expected to be physically dominant; consequently, admitting to sustaining IPV from a woman and labeling it a "crime" may be viewed as emasculating (Steinmetz, 1977). Indeed, studies show that men are not only reluctant to report assaults by women, they are also unlikely to report assaults by other men, even when severe injuries result (Henman, 1996). Furthermore, when marital violence is conceptualized as a crime in surveys, women are significantly less likely than men to report their use of IPV, and some research shows that women fail to report as much as 75% of their use of IPV (Mihalic & Elliott, 1997).

A second source of data on violence by female partners has come from the NVAWS, which showed that 0.8% of men reported being physically assaulted by a current or former intimate partner in the previous year, most of whom were women (Tjaden & Thoennes, 2000). Straus (1999) argued that the NVAWS may have underestimated the amount of IPV that all participants experienced (1.8% of women reported sustaining IPV) for several reasons, including the fact that the respondents were asked first if they were assaulted by anyone and subsequently asked who the assaulter was; however, when thinking about assaults, many people may fail to think of aggressive acts on the part of family members or intimate partners as assaults or violence. Also, in the introductory and subsequent sections of the NVAWS, participants were told that the survey was on personal safety, then were asked if they perceived that violence by men was more or less of a problem "these days." These two components of the survey may lead to underestimates of IPV by women toward men because (a) violence by women is less likely than violence by men to lead to an injury, thus, when considering assaults, men are unlikely to think of the physical aggression their intimate partners may have used; and (b) by framing the study as one concerned with violence by men, all respondents were primed to think of assaults that were committed only by men. The fact that the NVAWS is likely underestimating the extent of IPV experienced by both men and women is further highlighted by the fact that these estimates are one fifteenth of those obtained in hundreds of family conflict studies on IPV (Straus, 1999).

A final source of data on violence by women toward men comes from family conflict studies, many of which use the Conflict Tactics Scales (CTS; Straus, Hamby, Boney-McCoy, & Sugarman, 1996). In contrast to the NVAWS, the instructions for the CTS prompt participants to think about their relationships first and conflicts that may be occurring within those relationships, then report the number of times specific behaviors—such as slapping, punching, and beating—were used. The words "assault," "violence," or "crime" are never used, but the behaviors are commensurate with the criminal classifications of simple and aggravated assaults. National studies (National Family Violence Surveys [NFVS] of 1975 and 1985; 1992 National Alcohol and Family Violence Survey) conducted by researchers at the University of New Hampshire in the 1970s to 1990s showed that in contrast to declining rates of violence by men toward women, violence by women toward men has remained stable over the 17-year period that spans the time between the first (1975) and last (1992) surveys (Straus, 1995). These trends mirror those found in the NCVS, only the rates of IPV in the family violence surveys are much higher. Specifically, after controlling for age and socioeconomic status, minor assaults (e.g., slapping, pushing) by wives toward husbands were reported to have occurred at a rate of approximately 75 per 1,000 in 1975 and 1985; reports then increased to approximately 95 per 1,000 in 1992. Rates of severe assaults (e.g., punching, beating up) by wives toward husbands reportedly remained constant at approximately 45 per 1,000 in all study years. These rates of severe assaults projected into approximately 2.6 million men per year who sustained IPV that had a high likelihood of causing an injury (Straus & Gelles, 1986).

Rates of sexual and psychological IPV by women toward male partners are harder to obtain because they have rarely been systematically investigated, even though studies show women use both of these types of IPV toward male partners. Studies of college women show that as many as 33% report using aggression (either verbal or physical) to coerce men into engaging in sexual behavior or intercourse (Anderson, 1998; Hines & Saudino, 2003; Struckman-Johnson, 1988), and 20% of men report sustaining such sexual aggression from a woman (Hines & Saudino, 2003; Struckman-Johnson, 1988). Percentages differ based on the exact operational definition of "sexual aggression," and although most of the aggressive tactics used by the women in these encounters to coerce men into sex were verbal, a few women and men indicated that women sometimes use physical force to achieve their sexual goals (Anderson, 1998; Struckman-Johnson & Struckman-Johnson, 1998). Reports of the prevalence of psychological aggression by women toward men estimate that at least half, and as much as 90%, of men are the recipients of some type of psychologically aggressive act (e.g., being threatened, called names, or being insulted or sworn at) in their relationships (Hines & Malley-Morrison, 2001; Hines & Saudino, 2003; Simonelli & Ingram, 1998; Straus & Sweet, 1992).

SOCIAL SERVICE AND CRIMINAL JUSTICE IMPLICATIONS

Taken together, our best population-based surveys show that between 25% and 50% of victims of IPV are men, yet the policy and practice responses to

IPV from the social service and criminal justice professions have been based on a response to patriarchy theory (Dutton & Corvo, 2006). In these arenas, patriarchal theorists assert that the sole cause of IPV is the gendered structure of society. Men have economic, political, social, and occupational power over women, a power structure that is reflected in heterosexual romantic and sexual relationships. To maintain their power in heterosexual relationships, men strategically use IPV and have been socialized to believe that IPV is justified to maintain their dominance (e.g., Dobash & Dobash, 1979; Hammer, 2003). This perspective dominates because feminist advocates were the leaders in enlightening the public, lawmakers, and scholars during the feminist movement of the 1970s to the problem of IPV against women, changing IPV laws and policies, and developing programs to help female victims of IPV and reform male batterers (see Straus, 2009).

The patriarchal theoretical framework is exemplified in the Duluth Model (Pence & Paymar, 1983), the long-standing and dominant model for treating IPV perpetrators, which stresses that battering is a calculated choice by men to exert their power and control over women. According to the Duluth Model, women do not and would not use IPV against men because IPV is an issue of power and control of which only men in a system of patriarchy are capable. Thus, women who use IPV face considerable barriers when seeking help within the current domestic-violence service system because it does not allow for their existence. The following quote exemplifies the experiences of some of these women: "[Now] he tries to understand my side of the argument. He talks to me rather than hits me. I still hit him, however. I would like to enroll in a class in anger management, but the [local] shelter for battered women does not help women with this problem" (Stacey, Hazlewood, & Shupe, 1994, p. 63).

The predominant criminal justice policy that has affected female perpetrators of IPV has been mandatory arrest policies, which mandate (or in some states, strongly encourage) police officers to make an arrest in any call involving IPV. These policies have led to an increase in women being arrested for IPV, particularly in "dual-arrest" situations—those that are seemingly mutually volatile and in which the police cannot determine whether one party is the perpetrator of assault, and therefore arrest both parties (Buzawa & Buzawa, 2003). Dual-arrest situations have allowed many researchers to investigate possible gender differences between male and female perpetrators of IPV, which could have implications for differential treatment programs. Arrest data from one midwestern city in 1997 (Melton & Belknap, 2003) showed the types of violence used by male versus female perpetrators. Male perpetrators seemed to engage in more severe violence than female perpetrators. For example, men were more likely to have used lethal and nonlethal threats; attempted to prevent their female partners from calling the police; and shoved, grabbed, dragged, pulled the hair of, physically restrained, or strangled their partners. Female perpetrators were more likely than male perpetrators to have hit their male partners with an object, thrown an object at him, struck him with a vehicle, bit him, and used a weapon against him. There were no gender differences in whether the perpetrator slapped, punched, hit, knifed, or stabbed the victim, or in injury rates for cuts, abrasions, broken bones, or broken teeth.

A study of IPV offenders in Shelby County, Tennessee, from December 1997 and March 2001 found similar results for levels of violence, but also extended our knowledge by analyzing other perpetrator and victim data (Henning & Feder, 2004). Male perpetrators engaged in more serious violence—such as choking, forcing sexual activity, and threatening homicide—and engaged in such violence more frequently than female perpetrators, but female perpetrators were more likely to have used a weapon. Male perpetrators had a longer criminal history and more substance abuse problems. The authors found no gender differences in victim injury rates, frequency or severity of psychological abuse, suicidal threats, stalking behaviors, or juvenile arrest rates.

A final study investigated gender differences among 45 male and 45 female IPV primary perpetrators in North Carolina who were mandated to attend treatment as part of their probation (Busch & Rosenberg, 2004). This study showed that although men had a longer history of domestic violence offenses and other nonviolent criminal offenses than women, the majority of women did have criminal histories. There were no gender differences in the number of previous domestic violence arrests among perpetrators with a prior offense or in a history of violent crime outside the home. In addition, men used more violent acts in the arrest incident, but men and women were equally likely to use a severely violent act. There were no gender differences in the injury rates of the victims, but there were gender differences in the method used to inflict injury: women tended to use a weapon or object, whereas men tended to use their bodies alone, to injure their victims. Finally, there were no gender differences in substance abuse problems, the use of substances at the time of arrest, or the types of substances that the perpetrators abused.

Overall, these studies show that there may be some gender differences in the way men and women use IPV and in the events that precipitate their use of IPV. At the same time, these studies present information concerning documented instances of criminal-level IPV perpetration by women. This research demonstrates the importance of studying women who use IPV because the service needs for women may differ from those of men.

These studies also allude to the potential problems that men who sustain IPV from their female partners may face when encountering the social service and criminal justice systems as an IPV victim. Men who sustain IPV from their female partners face several potential internal and external barriers to seeking help from social services and the criminal justice system. For example, men, in general, are not likely to seek help for issues that society deems nonnormative or for which society deems they should be able to handle themselves (Addis & Mihalik, 2003). Men who sustain IPV may not seek help because of fears that they will be ridiculed and experience shame and embarrassment (McNeely, Cook, & Torres, 2001).

If they do overcome these internal barriers, they may experience external barriers when contacting social services or the police. They may have trouble locating the few resources that are available specifically for male victims of IPV and may encounter resistance by those providing IPV services. For example, when calling domestic violence hotlines, men who sustained IPV have reported that hotline workers indicate that they only help women or infer that the men must be the actual abuser. Male help-seekers report that hotlines will sometimes refer them to batterers' programs. Some men have reported that when they call the police during an incident in which their female partners are violent, the police sometimes fail to respond or take a report. Other men report being ridiculed by the police or being incorrectly arrested and convicted as the violent perpetrator, even when there is no evidence of injury to the female partner (Cook, 1997; Hines, Brown, & Dunning, 2007; McNeely et al., 2001). There are also policies in some regions that discourage the arrest of women as the primary perpetrators of IPV. For example, in Massachusetts, instances involving male victims were five times less likely to end in an arrest than similar instances involving female victims. Furthermore, in some instances involving male victims, officers either made no arrest or arrested the male victims— presuming that they were the primary aggressors (Buzawa & Hotaling, 2000).

Anecdotal studies, in which self-identified male victims described their experiences with the criminal justice system, provide some indication that within the judicial system, some men who sustained IPV may be treated unfairly because of their gender. Even with apparent corroborating evidence that their female partners were violent and that the help-seekers were not violent toward their partners or children, male help-seekers reported that they have lost custody of their children and have been falsely accused by their female partners of violence and of sexually abusing their children. Male help-seekers have reported that their complaints concerning their female partners' violence have not always been taken seriously, yet their partner's false accusations have reportedly been given serious weight during the judicial process (Cook, 1997). Other men have reported similar experiences in which their female partners misused the legal or social service systems to inappropriately block access between them and their children or to file false allegations with child welfare services (Hines et al., 2007). According to some experts, the burden of proof for IPV victimization is high for men because it falls outside of our common understanding of gender roles (Cook, 1997); this can make leaving a violent female partner that much more difficult. For example, many men who sustained IPV report that they stayed with their violent female partners in order to protect the children from their partner's violence. The men worried that if they left their violent wives, the legal system could still grant custody of the children to their wives and that perhaps even their custody rights would be blocked by their wives as a continuation of the controlling behaviors that their wives used during the marriage (McNeely et al., 2001).

CONSEQUENCES TO MEN WHO SUSTAIN IPV

Most research concerning the outcomes and consequences for men who sustain IPV typically have been conducted on men in community- or population-based samples, thus, these results cannot necessarily be generalized to all men seeking help for IPV victimization. Furthermore, many of these studies compare the relative consequences of female versus male victims, and because the female victims tend to have worse outcomes, the problematic outcomes that men experience are typically glossed over. Nonetheless, these studies are useful for elucidating possible outcomes on men who sustain IPV. Overall, results have shown that many men are physically injured and sometimes even killed as a result of IPV (Mann, 1996; Stets & Straus, 1990). Emergency room doctors have reported treating many types of injuries to men who sustained IPV, including ax injuries, burns, injuries with fireplace pokers and bricks, and gunshot wounds (Duminy & Hudson, 1993; Krob, Johnson, & Jordan, 1986; McNeely et al., 2001). Reports of men being physically injured by their female partners are also evident in the literature on community samples of couples. For example, Cascardi and colleagues (1992) found that 2% of men who reported experiencing minor or severe IPV also reported suffering broken bones, broken teeth, and/or an injury to a sensory organ. Similarly, data from the 1985 NFVS showed that 1% of the men who reported being severely assaulted needed medical attention (Stets & Straus, 1990). Morse (1995) and Makepeace (1986) found higher rates of injury among men: between 10% and 20% of the men who sustained IPV reported some type of injury. These higher injury rates could be a function of the different measures of injuries among the studies and/or the different types of samples (e.g., Morse sampled younger adults, whereas Stets and Straus studied a U.S. population–based sample).

Research on the possible psychological outcomes on men who sustain physical IPV shows that many report experiencing anger, emotional hurt, shame, and fear as a result of IPV (Follingstad, Wright, Lloyd, & Sebastian, 1991; Morse, 1995). Studies also show that in comparison to men who have not experienced IPV, men who sustained IPV experienced greater levels of depression, stress, psychological distress, and psychosomatic symptoms (Cascardi et al., 1992; Simonelli & Ingram, 1998; Stets & Straus, 1990). Men who experienced psychological maltreatment from a partner have been shown to display depressive symptoms and psychological distress (Simonelli & Ingram, 1998; Vivian & Langhinrichsen-Rohling, 1994). Little work has been done on the mental health status of men who sustained sexual aggression from a female intimate partner, although preliminary research does indicate that the majority of these men are upset by these experiences (Struckman-Johnson & Struckman-Johnson, 1998).

The studies reviewed here are valuable in addressing possible outcomes of IPV toward men, but they are limited. For example, these studies focused primarily on internalizing symptoms, which women experience at two times the rate of men in the population as a whole. The studies did not examine more externalizing symptoms, such as alcoholism, which are more characteristic of how men respond to stressful events (Comer, 1992), and they did not assess symptoms of post-traumatic stress disorder (PTSD), which have been found in women who sustain IPV (Walker, 1993), as well as men who have been exposed to other types of traumatic events (Kulka et al., 1990). Also, none of the studies on mental health status were of men who sustained IPV and sought help; help-seeking men may experience more physical and psychological injuries than men in a community- or population-based sample, in the same way that samples of women who use shelters experience more injuries than women who sustain IPV in community- or population-based studies.

The experience of IPV is generally considered to be a traumatic event, and many men who sustain IPV and seek help view their IPV experiences as traumatic (Cook, 1997). People who experience traumatic events are at increased risk for a range of psychological disorders, such as those discussed above. However, more common types of traumatic responses include symptoms of PTSD and alcohol/substance abuse (American Psychiatric Association, 1994). PTSD is a psychiatric condition that can follow the experience of a traumatic incident, and its symptoms tend to cluster on three dimensions: persistent re-experiencing of the trauma, persistent avoidance of stimuli associated with the trauma, and persistent increased arousal (American Psychiatric Association, 1994). Severe and persistent symptoms are needed for one to be diagnosed with PTSD (Wakefield & Spitzer, 2002); however, many people who experience a traumatic event respond with at least some of the symptoms of PTSD. PTSD has consistently been found among women who experience IPV. For example, among battered women, about 30–60% evidence PTSD (Astin, Lawrence, & Foy, 1993; Cascardi, O'Leary, Lawrence, & Schlee, 1995; Gleason, 1993; Saunders, 1994). Moreover, increased symptoms are positively correlated with greater severity of IPV exposure, although even psychological or mild IPV can elicit PTSD symptoms (Astin et al., 1993; Housekamp & Foy, 1991; Kemp, Rawlings, & Green, 1991; Woods & Isenberg, 2001). Little work has been conducted on whether men could have similar mental health reactions. Preliminary work suggests that greater severity of IPV experiences among men is associated with increased PTSD symptoms (Hines, 2007; Hines & Malley-Morrison, 2001); however, these studies used only university students in their subject pools. It is unknown whether this association would generalize to the larger population and/or to a population of men who sustain IPV and seek help. Moreover, research has not examined whether PTSD symptoms would be more severe among male help-seekers than among men sustaining IPV in the general population.

In addition, alcohol and substance abuse are common means of coping with the experience of a traumatic event. Stress-coping models of alcohol and substance use suggest that increases in the use of these substances may be associated with the psychological sequelae of a traumatic experience (Jacobsen, Southwick, & Kosten, 2001; Simons, Gaher, Jacobs, Meyer, & Johnson-Jimenez, 2005; Stewart, 1996). Indeed, research consistently shows that victims of abuse in both childhood and adulthood have higher rates of alcohol and substance abuse than nonvictims, and that the severity of abuse is related to the severity of trauma exposure (Stewart, 1996). Thus, the use of alcohol or other substances is a maladaptive mechanism for coping with the negative emotions associated with a traumatic event (Jacobsen et al., 2001). However, no studies to our knowledge have investigated the association between sustaining IPV and alcohol/substance abuse among men.

Not only are both PTSD and alcohol/substance abuse independent sequelae of traumatic exposure, but in both clinical and nonclinical samples, they are highly comorbid disorders that are functionally related (Chilcoat & Breslau, 1998; Jacobsen et al., 2001; Stewart, 1996; Stewart, Pihl, Conrod, & Dongier, 1998). Studies consistently have shown that alcohol and substance abuse are most often associated with the re-experiencing and hyperarousal symptoms of PTSD (Shipherd, Stafford, & Tanner, 2005; Stewart, 1996; Stewart et al., 1998). Although the functional relationship between PTSD and alcohol/substance abuse could follow one of many causal pathways, the dominant model in the field that receives the overwhelming majority of research support is the self-medication model (Chilcoat & Breslau, 1998; Jacobsen et al., 2001; Stewart, 1996; Stewart et al., 1998). In this model, alcohol and other substances seem to provide acute-symptom relief of PTSD. In particular, they seem to lessen the hyperarousal components and facilitate the forgetting of traumatic memories through their effects on the central nervous system (Chilcoat & Breslau, 1998; Jacobsen et al., 2001; Stewart, 1996; Stewart, Conrod, Pihl, & Dongier, 1999; Stewart et al., 1998). In other words, alcohol and other substances seem to be used in an effort to provide relief from the distressing symptoms of PTSD (Chilcoat & Breslau, 1998). Thus, PTSD seems to serve as a partial mediator for the association between the experience of a traumatic event and alcohol/substance abuse. Although studies indicate that many trauma victims will abuse alcohol and substances as a result of the trauma independent of PTSD symptoms, the more severe the trauma, the more likely both PTSD and alcohol/substance abuse will develop (Kilpatrick & Resnick, 1993). However, no studies have investigated whether men who sustain IPV are at risk for PTSD and alcohol/substance abuse comorbidity, and if greater IPV severity is associated with PTSD–alcohol/substance abuse comorbidity.

CONCLUSION

Overall, there is evidence that women use IPV against their male partners. The evidence also suggests that criminal justice and social service agencies are unsure of how to respond to or provide services to female perpetrators or male victims. Given the potentially serious physical and mental health consequences this can have, particularly for victims, there are compelling reasons why research in this area needs to move beyond the argument over who perpetrates more IPV and who suffers more as a consequence of IPV. As shown above, the majority of research thus far on men who sustain IPV makes these comparisons, and because the prevalence of male victimization may be lower and the injuries and mental health consequences to male victims may be less widespread or severe on average, the very severe consequences suffered by many men who sustain IPV have been largely overlooked. It is time that these men get the attention and services they need regardless of the prevalence of their experiences in comparison to others.

We are currently conducting a study on men who sustain IPV and seek help that is funded by the National Institute of Mental Health. Our goal is to move research in this field beyond arguments over who perpetrates the most IPV and who suffers most. We are concentrating on men who seek help for IPV issues so that we can better understand the dynamics of their relationships (e.g., the extent of physical, psychological, and sexual abuse by both the female and male partners; the details of their last physical argument; the extent to which alcohol and drug abuse are involved in arguments; and the extent to which children witness IPV); the physical injuries men sustain and the possible mental health issues men experience in these relationships, particularly PTSD symptoms and alcohol/substance abuse; and the help-seeking experiences of men who sustain IPV (e.g., the extent to which they find domestic violence helplines, domestic violence programs, and the police to be helpful or barriers in their quest to end the IPV in their relationships) and the potential mental health problems that may be related to or correlated with barriers to seeking help. Data collection was completed in early January 2009; we will begin to make preliminary results available on our study Web site and at national professional conferences (see http://www.clarku.edu/faculty/dhines). We are hopeful that this study will provide solid groundwork for future studies on women's IPV against male partners.

REFERENCES

Addis, M. E., & Mihalik, J. R. (2003). Men, masculinity, and the contexts of help seeking. *American Psychologist, 58*, 5–14.

American Psychiatric Association. (1994). *Diagnostic and statistical manual of mental disorders* (4th ed.). Washington, DC: Author.

Anderson, P. B. (1998). Women's motives for sexual initiation and aggression. In P. B. Anderson & C. Struckman-Johnson (Eds.), *Sexually aggressive women: Current perspectives and controversies* (pp. 79–93). New York: Guilford.

Astin, B., Lawrence, K. J., & Foy, D. W. (1993). Posttraumatic stress disorder among battered women: Risk and resiliency factors. *Violence and Victims, 8,* 17–28.

Busch, A., & Rosenberg, M. (2004). Comparing women and men arrested for domestic violence: A preliminary report. *Journal of Family Violence, 19,* 49–58.

Buzawa, E. S., & Buzawa, C. G. (2003). *Domestic violence: The criminal justice response.* Thousand Oaks, CA: Sage.

Buzawa, E. S., & Hotaling, G. (2000). *The police response to domestic violence calls for assistance in three Massachusetts towns: Final report.* Washington, DC: National Institute of Justice.

Cascardi, M., Langhinrichsen, J., & Vivian, D. (1992). Marital aggression: Impact, injury, and health correlates for husbands and wives. *Archives of Internal Medicine, 152,* 1178–1184.

Cascardi, M., O'Leary, K. D., Lawrence, E. E., & Schlee, K. A. (1995). Characteristics of women physically abused by their spouses and who seek treatment regarding marital conflict. *Journal of Consulting and Clinical Psychology, 63,* 616–623.

Catalano, S. (2007). *Intimate partner violence in the United States* [Electronic Version]. Washington, DC: U.S. Department of Justice, Office of Justice Programs, Bureau of Justice Statistics. Retrieved October 1, 2007 from http://www.ojp.usdoj.gov/bjs/intimate/ipv.htm.

Chilcoat, H. D., & Breslau, N. (1998). Investigations of causal pathways between PTSD and drug use disorders. *Addictive Behaviors, 23*(6), 827–840.

Comer, R. J. (1992). *Abnormal psychology.* New York: Freeman.

Cook, P. W. (1997). *Abused men: The hidden side of domestic violence.* Westport, CT: Praeger.

Dobash, R. E., & Dobash, R. P. (1979). *Violence against wives: A case against the patriarchy.* New York: Free Press.

Duminy, F. J., & Hudson, D. A. (1993). Assault inflicted by hot water. *Burns, 19,* 426–428.

Dutton, D. G., & Corvo, K. (2006). Transforming a flawed policy: A call to revive psychology and science in domestic violence research and practice. *Aggression and Violent Behavior, 11,* 457–483.

Follingstad, D. R., Wright, S., Lloyd, S., & Sebastian, J. A. (1991). Sex differences in motivations and effects in dating violence. *Family Relations, 40,* 51–57.

Gelles, R. J. (1974). *The violent home: A study of physical aggression between husbands and wives.* Beverly Hills, CA: Sage.

Gleason, W. J. (1993). Mental disorders in battered women: An empirical study. *Violence and Victims, 8,* 53–68.

Hammer, R. (2003). Militarism and family terrorism: A critical feminist perspective. *The Review of Education, Pedagogy, and Cultural Studies, 25*, 231–256.

Henman, M. (1996). Domestic violence: Do men under report? *Forensic Update, 47*, 3–8.

Henning, K., & Feder, L. (2004). A comparison of men and women arrested for domestic violence: Who presents the greater threat? *Journal of Family Violence, 19*(2), 69–80.

Hines, D. A. (2007). Post-traumatic stress symptoms among men who sustain partner violence: A multi-national study of university students. *Psychology of Men and Masculinity, 8*, 225–239.

Hines, D. A., Brown, J., & Dunning, E. (2007). Characteristics of callers to the Domestic Abuse Helpline for Men. *Journal of Family Violence, 22*, 63–72.

Hines, D. A., & Malley-Morrison, K. (2001, August). *Effects of emotional abuse against men in intimate relationships.* Paper presented at the American Psychological Association's Annual Convention, San Francisco, CA.

Hines, D. A., & Saudino, K. J. (2003). Gender differences in psychological, physical, and sexual aggression among college students using the Revised Conflict Tactics Scales. *Violence and Victims, 18*, 197–218.

Housekamp, B. M., & Foy, D. W. (1991). The assessment of posttraumatic stress disorder in battered women. *Journal of Interpersonal Violence, 6*, 367–375.

Jacobsen, L. K., Southwick, S. M., & Kosten, T. R. (2001). Substance use disorders in patients with posttraumatic stress disorder: A review of the literature. *American Journal of Psychiatry, 158*(8), 1184–1190.

Kemp, A., Rawlings, E. I., & Green, B. L. (1991). Post-traumatic stress disorder (PTSD) in battered women: A shelter sample. *Journal of Traumatic Stress, 4*, 137–148.

Kilpatrick, D. G., & Resnick, H. S. (1993). Posttraumatic stress disorder associated with exposure to criminal victimization in clinical and community populations. In J. R. T. Davidson & E. B. Foa (Eds.), *Posttraumatic stress disorder: DSM-IV and beyond* (pp. 113–143). Washington, DC: American Psychiatric Press.

Krob, M. J., Johnson, A., & Jordan, M. H. (1986). Burned and battered adults. *Journal of Burn Care and Rehabilitation, 7*, 529–531.

Kulka, R. A., Schlenger, W. E., Fairbank, J. A., Hough, R. L., Jordan, B. K., Marmar, C. R., et al. (1990). *Trauma and the Vietnam War generation: Report of the findings from the National Vietnam Veterans Readjustment Study.* New York: Brunner/Mazel.

Makepeace, J. M. (1986). Gender differences in courtship violence victimization. *Family Relations, 35*, 383–388.

Mann, C. R. (1996). *When women kill.* New York: State University of New York Press.

McNeely, R. L., Cook, P. W., & Torres, J. B. (2001). Is domestic violence a gender issue, or a human issue? *Journal of Human Behavior in the Social Environment, 4*, 227–251.

Melton, H. C., & Belknap, J. (2003). He hits, she hits: Assessing gender differences and similarities in officially reported intimate partner violence. *Criminal Justice and Behavior, 30*(3), 328–348.

Mihalic, S. W., & Elliott, D. (1997). If violence is domestic, does it really count? *Journal of Family Violence, 12*, 293–311.

Morse, B. J. (1995). Beyond the Conflict Tactics Scales: Assessing gender differences in partner violence. *Violence and Victims, 10*, 251–272.

Pence, E., & Paymar, M. (1983). *Education groups for men who batter: The Duluth Model.* New York: Springer.

Rennison, C. M. (2003). *Intimate partner violence, 1993–2001* (Special Report, NCJ 197838). Washington, DC: U.S. Department of Justice, Office of Justice Programs, Bureau of Justice Statistics.

Saunders, D. G. (1994). Post-traumatic stress symptom profiles of battered women: A comparison of survivors in two settings. *Violence and Victims, 9*, 31–44.

Shipherd, J. C., Stafford, J., & Tanner, L. R. (2005). Predicting alcohol and drug abuse in Persian Gulf War veterans: What role do PTSD symptoms play? *Addictive Behaviors, 30*, 595–599.

Simonelli, C. J., & Ingram, K. M. (1998). Psychological distress among men experiencing physical and emotional abuse in heterosexual dating relationships. *Journal of Interpersonal Violence, 13*, 667–681.

Simons, J. S., Gaher, R. M., Jacobs, G. A., Meyer, D., & Johnson-Jimenez, E. (2005). Associations between alcohol use and PTSD symptoms among American Red Cross disaster relief workers responding to the 9/11/2001 attacks. *American Journal of Drug and Alcohol Abuse, 31*, 385–304.

Stacey, W. A., Hazlewood, L. R., & Shupe, A. (1994). *The violent couple.* Westport, CT: Praeger.

Steinmetz, S. K. (1977). Wifebeating, husbandbeating: A comparison of the use of physical violence between spouses to resolve marital fights. In M. Roy (Ed.), *Battered women: A psychosociological study of domestic violence* (pp. 63–72). New York: Van Nostrand Reinhold Co., Inc.

Stets, J. E., & Straus, M. A. (1990). Gender differences in reporting marital violence and its medical and psychological consequences. In M. A. Straus & R. J. Gelles (Eds.), *Physical violence in American families: Risk factors and adaptation to violence in 8,145 families* (pp. 151–166). New Brunswick, NJ: Transaction.

Stewart, S. H. (1996). Alcohol abuse in individuals exposed to trauma: A critical review. *Psychological Bulletin, 120*(1), 83–112.

Stewart, S. H., Conrod, P. J., Pihl, R. O., & Dongier, M. (1999). Relations between posttraumatic stress syndrome dimensions and substance dependence in a community-recruited sample of substance-abusing women. *Psychology of Addictive Behaviors, 13*, 78–88.

Stewart, S. H., Pihl, R. O., Conrod, P. J., & Dongier, M. (1998). Functional associations among trauma, PTSD, and substance-related disorders. *Addictive Behaviors, 23*(6), 797–812.

Straus, M. A. (1995). Trends in cultural norms and rates of partner violence: An update to 1992. In National Council on Family Relations (Series Ed.) & S. Stith & M. A. Straus (Vol. Eds.), *Families in Focus, Vol. 2. Understanding partner violence: Prevalence, causes, consequences, and solutions* (pp. 30–33). Minneapolis, MN: National Council on Family Relations.

Straus, M. A. (1999). The controversy over domestic violence by women: A methodological, theoretical, and sociology of science analysis. In X. B. Arriaga & S. Oskamp (Eds.), *Violence in intimate relationships* (pp. 17–44). Thousand Oaks, CA: Sage.

Straus, M. A. (2009). Why the overwhelming evidence on partner physical violence by women has not been perceived and is often denied. *Journal of Aggression, Maltreatment, & Trauma, 18*(6), 552–571.

Straus, M. A., & Gelles, R. J. (1986). Societal change and change in family violence from 1975 to 1985 as revealed by two national surveys. *Journal of Marriage and the Family, 48*, 465–479.

Straus, M. A., Hamby, S. L., Boney-McCoy, S., & Sugarman, D. B. (1996). The Revised Conflict Tactics Scales (CTS2): Development and preliminary psychometric properties. *Journal of Family Issues, 17*, 283–316.

Straus, M. A., & Sweet, S. (1992). Verbal/symbolic aggression in couples: Incidence rates and relationships to personal characteristics. *Journal of Marriage and the Family, 54*, 346–357.

Struckman-Johnson, C. (1988). Forced sex on dates: It happens to men, too. *Journal of Sex Research, 24*, 234–241.

Struckman-Johnson, C., & Struckman-Johnson, D. (1998). The dynamics and impact of sexual coercion of men by women. In P. B. Anderson & C. Struckman-Johnson (Eds.), *Sexually aggressive women: Current perspectives and controversies* (pp. 121–143). New York: Guilford.

Tjaden, P., & Thoennes, N. (2000). *Extent, nature, and consequences of intimate partner violence: Findings from the National Violence Against Women Survey.* Washington, DC: U.S. Department of Justice. Retrieved September 9, 2003, from http://www.ojp.usdoj.gov/nih/victdocs.htm#2000.

U. S. Department of Health and Human Services. (2004). *Child maltreatment, 2002.* Washington, DC: Administration on Children, Youth, and Families. Retrieved September 11, 2004, from http://www.acf.hhs.gov/programs/cb/publications/cmreports.htm.

Vivian, D., & Langhinrichsen-Rohling, J. (1994). Are bi-directionally violent couples mutually victimized? A gender sensitive comparison. *Violence and Victims, 9*, 107–124.

Wakefield, J. C., & Spitzer, R. L. (2002). Lowered estimates—but of what? *Archives of General Psychiatry, 59*, 129–130.

Walker, L. E. (1993). The battered woman syndrome is a psychological consequence of abuse. In R. J. Gelles & D. R. Loseke (Eds.), *Current controversies on family violence* (pp. 133–153). Newbury Park, CA: Sage.

Woods, S., & Isenberg, M. A. (2001). Adaptation as a mediator of intimate abuse and traumatic stress in battered women. *Nursing Science Quarterly, 14*, 215–221.

The Psychology of Women's Partner Violence: Characteristics and Cautions

NICOLA GRAHAM-KEVAN

University of Central Lancashire, Preston, Lancashire, United Kingdom

This article provides an overview of research on women's partner violence as well as the literature that investigates the developmental pathway to women's aggressive behavior. While women are known to commit partner violence toward their male partners, the prevalence and motivations for such behavior is still debated. Evidence that finds gender symmetry is reviewed and alternative literature discussed. Research challenging the conceptualization of women's partner violence as self-defensive is explored. The literature on the veracity of women partner violence offenders' explanations for their aggression is contrasted with the tendency within the literature to treat women's accounts as unproblematic. Alternative explanations for women's aggression are discussed with a focus on personality traits of psychopathology. Implications for interventions are also discussed.

Any scholar who researches the psychology of women quickly realizes that it is a highly politicized arena. One the most contentious topics within this arena is women's use of violence within intimate relationships with men (Straus, 2005; Straus, 2009),with women's mental health coming a close second (Padgett, 1997). In this article, women's use of partner violence (PV) and its relationship to personality and psychopathology will be discussed. While the aim of this article is not controversy, there is an urgent need to advance our understanding of women's PV. This article presents a review of the different types of research that can be utilized to enhance our understanding of women's aggression toward their male partners and to illustrate how related research, such as developmental origins of aggression, can be applied to specific types of aggression, such as women's partner violence, to stimulate novel and potentially rewarding avenues for future research. The article adds to the growing call for PV research and policy to be informed by sound and empirically supported research. To this aim, the research on sex similarities in PV prevalence, self-defense and other attributions, developmental research on female aggression, and the relationship between psychopathology and women's PV will be reviewed.

SEX SIMILARITIES IN THE USE OF PARTNER VIOLENCE

Studies using unbiased sampling procedures, including several longitudinal ones (Capaldi, Kim, & Shortt, 2004; Ehrensaft, Moffitt, & Caspi, 2004; Moffitt, Caspi, Rutter, & Silva, 2001; Serbin et al., 2004), found that men and women use similar amounts of physical aggression toward their partners (Archer, 2000; Chermack, Walton, Fuller, & Blow, 2001; Graham, Wells, & Jelley, 2002; Hird, 2000; Katz, Kuffel, & Coblentz, 2002; Ross & Babcock, 2009). The data are dominated by U.S. samples, but similar patterns are also found in Europe (Archer, 2006). Samples from the Western world that find men to be the primary aggressors typically derive from court samples of men convicted of PV and their female victims, self reports from men in treatment for PV, and victim reports from women in refuges (see Archer, 2000). That men are more aggressive in such samples is hardly surprising. What is surprising are the conclusions that authors have drawn from such data, such as "[T]he findings suggest that intimate partner violence is primarily an asymmetrical problem of men's violence to women, and that women's violence does not equate to men's in terms of frequency, severity, and consequences . . . " (Dobash & Dobash, 2004, p. 324). Although such study designs may be appropriate when exploring the dynamics of relationships in which the man is identified as the primary aggressor, research utilizing such a sampling procedure should be rejected by scholars studying sex differences in PV, as they effectively sample on the dependent variable (Felson, 2005), which negates subsequent analysis. With the exception of such studies, gender symmetry in PV is the norm (see Fiebert, 2006, for an annotated bibliography), which has led to an interest in women who perpetrate PV.

SELF-DEFENSE AND ALTERNATIVE EVIDENCE

Feminist theories have typically explained women's PV as defensive and men's aggression as coercive (e.g., Dobash, Dobash, Cavanagh, & Lewis,

1998). Henning, Jones, and Holdford (2003) embraced this approach when they stated, " . . . many, if not most women arrested for intimate partner violence are victims of abuse who may have been acting in self-defense" (p. 841). This has led to calls for partner-violent women to be treated as victims (Hamberger & Potente, 1994). In studies in which men and women involved with the criminal justice system for their use of PV have actually been compared using police reports and validated measures, few differences are found (e.g., Busch & Rosenberg, 2004; Dunning, 2004; McFarlane, Wilson, Malecha, & Lemmey, 2000; McLeod, 1984; Simmons, Lehmann, Cobb, & Fowler, 2005). Evidence for women's "victim" status usually comes from the female perpetrators' own reports. Such attributions by male perpetrators would be challenged and probably labeled "minimization" or "victim blaming"; indeed, many authors insist that collateral information from partners is essential in assessing male perpetrators' reports of their violent behavior (Austin & Dankwort, 1999; Hamberger, 1997). Such caution is rarely exercised when discussing women's accounts. However, research has found that women's reports are likely to suffer from similar biases to men's (Sugarman & Hotaling, 1997). Henning, Jones, and Holdford (2005) found in their sample of women and men convicted of a partner assault that there were no sex differences in self blame for the index offense, but that women blamed their victim significantly more than did men. They also found that both partner-violent women and men showed evidence of socially desirable responding, an effect subsequently replicated by Simmons et al. (2005). Consistent with this finding, Dunning (2002) asked his sample of women in treatment for PV how many had acted violently due to fear. He found that initially 92% of his sample indicated that they had acted in self-defense. Upon elaboration, however, it became apparent that they were responding in a way consistent with the perceived demand characteristics of the situation and were aware that calling their aggression self-defensive was not accurate. This suggests that women's self reports should be treated with the same caution as men's.

Convergent evidence against such blanket explanations can be found in research that investigates the nature of PV. For example, some study designs investigate one-sided assaults, the rationale being that where there is only one combatant, self-defense is not a viable explanation. Such studies frequently find that when one sex is the sole perpetrator, it is more likely to be a woman than a man (Anderson, 2002; DeMaris, 1987; Gray & Foshee, 1997; Morse, 1995; O'Leary, Barling, Arias, & Rosenbaum, 1989; Riggs, 1993; Roscoe & Callahan, 1985). Studies of women who have been arrested for PV find that women are equally likely to be the sole aggressor as are male arrestees (Simmons et al., 2005), which does not support Henning et al.'s (2003) assertion quoted above.

Instead of relying on inferences, other approaches have asked women and men why they used PV. Such studies typically find that self-defense is cited by only a minority of women (Foo & Margolin, 1995; Sommer, 1994), and that the prevalence of self-defense attributions women make are similar to men's (Carrado, George, Loxam, Jones, & Templar, 1996; Harned, 2001). In clinical populations, such as perpetrator programs for men and women's refuge samples, women do describe their aggression as sometimes being self-defensive but they also use descriptions that are more consistent with retaliation, retribution, and vigilantism (Dasgupta, 1999; Dobash & Dobash, 1984, 2004; Dunning, 2002; Felson, 2002). These studies suggest that women's PV cannot be explained as purely defensive, even in samples of highly victimized women. The reasons women and men give for their own PV are many and include control, anger, jealousy, and a lack of commitment from their partner (Carrado et al., 1996; Dasgupta, 1999; Fiebert & Gonzalez, 1997; Harned, 2001; Henning et al., 2005).

Interestingly, women in nonselected samples appear to be similar to men in their attributions and beliefs about their own PV. Research suggests that physical aggression toward a male victim is associated with instrumental beliefs in women (Archer & Graham-Kevan, 2003; Archer & Haigh, 1997a, 1997b; Campbell, Muncer, & Odber, 1997), and that men and women do not differ in their instrumentality when the type of violence is PV (Archer & Haigh, 1999). Behavioral measures of instrumentality such as controlling behavior also show that men and women are similar, and the relationship between using PV and controlling behaviors holds for men *and* women (e.g., Caldwell, Swan, Allen, Sullivan, & Snow, in press; Graham-Kevan & Archer, 2005a, 2008; Molidor, 1995; Rouse, 1990; Stets, 1988; Stets & Pirog-Good, 1990; Walley-Jean & Swan, in press). There are generally no sex differences in controlling behavior when sampling is unbiased (e.g., Hamby & Sugarman, 1999; Statistics Canada, 2000; Stets, 1991), and they are an important predictor of physical aggression for both sexes (e.g., Follingstad, Bradley, Helff, & Laughlin, 2002; Graham-Kevan & Archer, 2008; White, Merrill, & Koss, 2001). This is in contrast to the work of Michael Johnson, who proposed that highly controlling aggressors (termed "intimate terrorists") were almost universally men, whereas those who use lower levels of control in conjunction with PV were equally likely to be men or women (Johnson, 1995). Although his proposition has enjoyed some empirical support (e.g., Graham-Kevan & Archer, 2003a, 2003b; Johnson, 1999; Johnson & Leone, 2005), this support has been contingent on sampling methods that greatly increase the likelihood of sampling victimized women and highly aggressive men. When men and women are sampled in the same way, the difference between the proportion of men and women classified as intimate terrorists is greatly reduced (e.g., LaRoche, 2008) or disappears entirely (e.g., Bates & Graham-Kevan, in press; Graham-Kevan & Archer, 2005b). If women's PV cannot be explained as simply arising from purely defensive motivations, then there is a need to explore what factors may help to explain women's use of aggression toward their male intimates.

WOMEN'S VIOLENCE: THE EMPIRICAL EVIDENCE

The risk factors that have been identified in the literature for later aggressive behavior are generally shared by both girls and boys. More important for the study of women's PV, these risk factors appear to predict both general and partner aggression (Moffitt, Krueger, Caspi, & Fagan, 2000; Tremblay et al., 2004). Risk factors that have been identified include low intelligence, impulsivity, fearlessness, a general lack of empathy, and negative emotionality. Those who use aggression as adults are extremely likely to have a long history of oppositional and aggressive behavior beginning very early in life (Conradi, Geffner, Hamberger, & Lawson, in press; Hay, 2005).

Early Risk Factors for Aggression

Although many studies investigating the development of aggressive behavior and predictors of adult personality disorders do not include female participants, there are sufficient exceptions for consistent trends to be identified. Tremblay and colleagues (2004) investigated ante- and postnatal risk factors for the development of aggressive behavior using developmental trajectories. They found that risk factors for being on the high aggression trajectory in middle childhood are present before birth (e.g., mother's antisocial behavior, young motherhood, low income, and smoking during pregnancy) or within the first two years of life (mothers' coercive parenting behavior and family dysfunction). Children whose mothers had high levels of antisocial behavior and began childbearing early in life were 11 times more likely to be on this trajectory than children without these two risk factors (controlling for all other predictors such as SES and gender). Similar results were found by Moffitt et al. (2001). What these studies tell us is that adolescent girls' (and boys') antisocial behavior usually can be predicted by factors present either before birth or within the first two years of life and that such traits are stable across childhood (Broidy et al., 2003).

Conduct disorder is a constellation of problematic behaviors manifested in childhood that are reliable predictors of adult women's aggression problems and personality disorder (Burnett & Newman, 2005). Twin studies have found that there are both genetic and environmental contributions to conduct-disordered behavior (Slutske et al., 1997; Slutske, Heath, Madden, Bucholz, Statham, & Martin, 2002). In particular, negative emotionality and behavioral undercontrol have been found to be important predictors, with the latter showing a substantial genetic influence (Slutske et al., 2002). Côté, Tremblay, Nagin, Zoccolillo, and Vitaro (2002) found that the combination of a girl's high hyperactivity and low helpfulness at age six increased the odds of subsequent conduct disorder in adolescence 4.6 times (in contrast to boys, whose conduct disorder was primarily predicted by hyperactivity alone). Côté et al. (2002) suggested that girls' (and boys') childhood behavioral problems " . . . are likely to be the continuation of a preschool development associated with difficult temperament, neurodevelopmental deficits, poor emotional regulation, poor executive functioning, and poor socialization practices" (p. 1092). Findings from longitudinal studies that measured adolescent (14 years) to adult (27 years) aggression have found that women's (and men's) use of aggression is relatively stable (Pulkkinen & Pitkänen, 1993). Kukko and Pulkkinen (2005) extended this investigation and found that aggression was stable for women from ages 8 to 42. Interestingly, all types of aggression measured by Pulkkinen and Pitkänen (verbal, physical, indirect, self-defensive, and proactive) were found to be correlated with externalizing problems, hyperactivity-impulsivity, and inattentiveness, which suggests that different types of aggressive behavior are not developmentally distinct and are likely to co-occur. This is relevant to adult women's use of PV because these same risk factors have been found to predict this as well. Moffitt et al. (2001) found that conduct problems were a strong predictor of women's use of PV at age 21. However, adolescent conduct problems also predicted PV victimization at 21 years. These data may therefore be interpreted as showing that girls with conduct problems pair up with abusive men and then use PV in self-defense. What is both unusual and refreshing with Moffitt et al.'s analysis, however, is rather than accept this assumption, they instead tested it. What they found was that adolescent conduct problems not only predicted pairing up with a similarly antisocial partner but also independently predicted the woman's PV As Moffitt et al. stated, " . . . pre-existing characteristics such as approval of the use of violence, excessive jealousy and suspiciousness, a tendency to experience intense and rapid negative emotions, poor behavioral control, predicted which...women were to engage in violent behavior towards their partners" (p. 65). These partner-violent women were also 4.4 times more likely than nonpartner-violent women to assault nonfamily members. A follow-up analysis at 24–26 years old found consistent results (Ehrensaft, Cohen, & Johnson, 2006). Similar results have been found in other longitudinal studies (e.g., Giordano, Millhonin, Cernokovich, Pugh, & Rudolph, 1999). Findings from longitudinal studies represent the most rigorous design for investigating causal relationships. Scholars and practitioners should be cautious of claims that women's PV can be explained purely in terms of self defense or that the psychopathology of women involved in PV is in some way "different" to that reliably documented to be present in men who assault their partners.

Personality Disorders (PD) and Partner Violence Perpetration

Evidence from cross-sectional and longitudinal studies suggests that like their male counterparts, women who use PV show evidence of personality disorders (PDs). Although some authors have posited that PD may be a consequence of PV victimization, this is inconsistent with both diagnostic criteria for some disorders (e.g., antisocial PD) and with findings from longitudinal studies (some of which were reviewed above) that found that risk factors such as conduct problems predate the onset of dating relationships and thus cannot be solely a consequence of victimization from boyfriends and husbands (Babcock, Miller, & Siard, 2003; Capaldi et al., 2004; Ehrensaft, Cohen, et al., 2006; Ehrensaft et al., 2004; Giordano et al., 1999; Moffitt et al., 2001; Serbin et al., 2004). Retrospective accounts of mental illness also suggest that this is likely to predate PV victimization (e.g., Cascardi, O'Leary, Lawrence, & Schlee, 1995; Gleason, 1993; Rounsaville, 1978). Such research suggests that preexisting PD traits (in particular Cluster B) leave the recipient vulnerable to experiencing high levels of chronic interpersonal stress (Daley, Hammen, Davila, & Burge, 1998), relationship conflict and abuse (Daley, Burge, & Hammen, 2000; Goldenson, Spidel, Greaves, & Dutton, in press), and marital dissatisfaction (Whisman, 1999). PD in women is not confined to only those who offend against their partner but is also the norm in samples of violent female offenders (e.g., Weizmann-Henelius, Viemerö, & Eronen, 2004). PD, particularly the presence of Axis II disorders such as antisocial PD and borderline PD, may also partially or wholly account for the relationship between depression and PV involvement (Coolidge & Anderson, 2002; Daley et al., 2000).

Ehrensaft, Cohen, et al. (2006) used a longitudinal design to explore the causal relationship between PD and PV. They found that Clusters A and B were both associated with women's (and men's) increased risk of PV being used 10 years later, whereas Cluster C traits appeared to be protective. Interestingly, antisocial PD mediated these relationships. As the authors commented, this suggests that "...individuals who go on to perpetrate partner violence are more stably impulsive, angry, self-centered and experience greater affective instability" (p. 480). Studies that assess PD in PV offenders find that its presence is the norm rather than the exception in female and male perpetrators (e.g., Simmons et al., 2005).

Criminality of Women Perpetrators of Partner Violence

Consistent with the longitudinal and retrospective data suggesting that women involved in PV have a history of antisocial behavior are studies that have investigated the criminality of women arrested for PV. These studies have found that such women (or at least a substantial subgroup of them) frequently have prior criminal convictions not related to partner assaults (Babcock et al., 2003; Busch & Rosenberg, 2004; Henning & Feder, 2004; Moffitt et al., 2001). These women are less likely to have a prior conviction for PV than men; however, it is likely that lower rates of prior PV convictions are at least partly an artifact of criminal justice policy that has traditionally ignored women's aggression to men. Support for this explanation comes from the statistics that have found that mandatory arrest policies in many states in the United States have resulted in a disproportionate increase in women coming into contact with the criminal justice system (Martin, 1997; State of California, 1999). This suggests that police were previously using their discretion to not arrest women. As population studies suggest that the proportion of PV perpetrators who are women is close to 50% (e.g., Archer, 2006) but that women still typically only constitute approximately 20% of those arrested, it is likely that police will continue to do so (Simmons et al., 2005).

Women "Victims" of Partner Violence

Authors such as Abel (2001), Back, Post, and D'Arcy (1982), and Walker (1991) reported that PV victimization of women can result in the development of psychopathology. However, studies that have investigated the effects of PV victimization have frequently ignored the wealth of studies that have found that most PV is mutual (e.g., Anderson, 2002; Davies, Ralph, & Hawton, 1995; Graham, Plant, & Plant, 2004; Graham-Kevan & Archer, 2003a, 2003b, 2005b; Johnson, 1995). This failure means that conclusions drawn from victimization studies are flawed unless the victim's own use of PV is controlled for. This may explain why many authors suggest that PV victimization is a risk factor for developing personality disorders, whereas the available evidence suggests that many victims are likely to be both perpetrators of PV and have a history of aggressive behavior that predates the current relationship (see above). Support for the need to assess a women's involvement in PV both as the victim and the perpetrator comes from studies that compare women "victims" with women "perpetrators." These studies frequently find a large overlap between the experiences of these two supposedly separate groups and use these findings to suggest that women perpetrators are really as much victim as aggressor (e.g., Abel, 2001). However, the converse is equally likely to be true. Studies have found that some women who identify themselves or are labeled as victims are also aggressors, which is consistent with the research that has actually asked about female victims' use of aggression (e.g., Dobash & Dobash, 2004; Giles-Sims, 1983; Graham-Kevan & Archer, 2003a, 2005b; Johnson, 1999; Johnson & Leone, 2005). This is also consistent with research that has assessed female victims for PD (e.g., Back et al., 1982; Faulkner, Cogan, Nolder, & Shooter, 1991), although this relationship may be more representative of women who report more than one physically abusive relationship (Coolidge & Anderson, 2002).

Women are also referred to as victims if they have a history of victimization in their childhood; however, this label is rarely applied to violent men, even though men in treatment for PV also frequently have childhood abuse histories and exposure to violence (e.g., Dixon & Browne, 2003;

Holtzworth-Munroe & Stuart, 1994). Indeed, there is evidence that prior victimization is a stronger risk factor for men than women (e.g., Bergen, Martin, Richardson, Allison, & Roeger, 2004). Experiencing childhood victimization is so consistently found in violent offenders, including murderers (Lewis, Yeager, Swica, Pincus, & Lewis, 1997), that it forms part of violence risk assessments (e.g., HCR-20; Webster, Douglas, Eaves, & Hart, 1997). However, articles that detail women's past victimization experiences rarely refer to this extensive research area. Typical is the following conclusions: "[T]hese findings suggest that women who are involved in domestic violence situations, whether labeled 'victims' or 'batterers,' have experienced heightened victim-related exposure to violence . . . Although victimization issues are addressed in programs for battered women, they are not covered in the traditional curricula offered to batterers [i.e., men]. This study suggests that curricula for helping women to cope with past victimization might be developed and offered to women in batterer intervention groups" (Abel, 2001, p. 414). An uninformed reader may infer from this that women, unlike men, have additional needs, whereas the literature is clear that men also have these needs, which are recognized in the nonintimate aggression literature (e.g., Bergen et al., 2004), though rarely addressed within PV treatment programs for men.

PD and Women

The role of PD in women's PV represents an extremely important emerging research area. However, researchers and clinicians should be careful when reviewing the empirical evidence, as there are two potential problems. The first concerns sex bias in diagnosis (Ford & Widiger, 1989), with women being significantly less likely than men to be given a diagnosis of antisocial PD and more likely to be diagnosed as histrionic PD, in spite of the presentation being the same. The second concerns feminist therapists who reject the use of PDs such as borderline PD on the ideological grounds that it is a form of characterological blame. These therapists instead suggest the use of post-traumatic stress disorder (PTSD) as a "non-blaming" alternative (Becker, 2000). Both these trends potentially obscure the contribution that PDs such as antisocial and borderline can make to understanding the function aggression serves for the perpetrator, thus successfully treating women's PV. This ultimately does a great disservice to women (and their therapists) who need to understand this behavior in order to be able to benefit from appropriate treatment.

CONCLUSIONS

The research reviewed in this article suggests that women who use physical aggression toward a male partner cannot be routinely excused as victims fighting back. That such claims are still made in spite of the evidence to the contrary is a cause for concern. It also highlights a tendency within the PV literature toward "special pleading" in regard to women's aggression. This distorts the literature and misinforms practice. Longitudinal studies are probably best placed to inform on predictors and consequences of partner violence involvement, and evidence from them suggests that women and men who are involved as perpetrators and victims may have multiple problems, including suffering from psychopathology. Denying such problems and instead offering a simplistic, ideologically based assessment such as PTSD is not helpful to these women or their victims.

The implications for the diagnosis and treatment of women who perpetrate PV is that there is clear evidence to suggest that partner aggression cannot be understood by self-defensive explanations alone. PV interventions need to be informed by empirical research, including the general violence literature. This research suggests that interventions must address psychological risk factors such as negative emotionality and impulsivity to adequately understand and successfully treat PV. Existing violence programs developed for nonpartner-violence offenders should be investigated with a view to adapting those practices found to be effective for use with PV perpetrators. For policy makers and clinicians, current and future interventions should be judged on whether they offer well-designed programs developed through a thorough review of the empirical research. It is only such programs that can accurately assess the risk and needs of women and men who offend against their intimate partners. Programs that meet these standards of treatment are likely to be effective, whereas those treatments based on political theory unfortunately are not (Babcock, Green, & Robie, 2004; Gilchrist et al., 2003; Jackson et al., 2003).

REFERENCES

Abel, E. M. (2001). Comparing the Social Service utilization, exposure to violence, and trauma symptomology of domestic violence female "victims" and female "batterers." *Journal of Family Violence, 16,* 401–420.

Anderson, K. (2002). Perpetrator or victim? Relationships between intimate partner violence and well-being. *Journal of Marriage and Family, 64,* 851–863.

Archer, J. (2000). Sex differences in aggression between heterosexual partners: A meta-analytic review. *Psychological Bulletin, 126,* 651–580.

Archer, J. (2006). Cross-cultural differences in physical aggression between partners: A social-role analysis. *Personality and Social Psychology Review, 10,* 133–153.

Archer, J., & Graham-Kevan, N. (2003). The association between beliefs about aggression and partner physical aggression. *Aggressive Behavior, 29,* 41–54.

Archer, J., & Haigh, A. (1999). Sex differences in beliefs about aggression: Opponent's sex and the form of aggression. *British Journal of Social Psychology, 38,* 71–84.

Archer, J., & Haigh, A.M. (1997a). Do beliefs about aggressive feelings and actions predict reported levels of aggression? *British Journal of Social Psychology, 36,* 83–105.

Archer, J., & Haigh, A. (1997b). Beliefs about aggression among male and female prisoners. *Aggressive Behavior, 23,* 405–415.

Austin, J., & Dankwort, J. (1999). Standards for batterer programs: A review and analysis. *Journal of Interpersonal Violence, 14,* 152–168.

Babcock, J. C., Green, C. E., & Robie, C. (2004). Does batterers' treatment work? A meta-analytic review of domestic violence treatment. *Clinical Psychology Review, 23,* 1023–1053.

Babcock, J. C., Miller, S., & Siard, C. (2003). Toward a typology of abusive women: Differences between partner-only and generally violent women in the use of violence. *Psychology of Women Quarterly, 13,* 46–59.

Back, S. M., Post, R. D., & D'Arcy, G. (1982). A study of battered women in a psychiatric setting. *Women in Therapy, 1,* 13–26.

Bates, E., & Graham-Kevan, N. (in press). Testing Johnson's hypothesis on a large community sample. *Partner Abuse.*

Becker, D. (2000). When she was bad: Borderline Personality Disorder in a posttraumatic age. *American Journal of Orthopsychiatry, 70,* 422–432.

Bergen, H. A., Martin, G., Richardson, A. S., Allison, S., & Roeger, L. (2004). Sexual abuse, antisocial behavior and substance use: gender differences in young community adolescents. *Australian and New Zealand Journal of Psychiatry, 38,* 34–41.

Broidy, L., Nagin, D., Tremblay, R., Bates, J., Brame, B., Dodge, K., et al. (2003). Developmental trajectories of childhood disruptive behaviors and adolescent delinquency: A six-site, cross-national study. *Developmental Psychology, 39,* 222–245.

Burnett, M. L., & Newman, D. L. (2005). The natural history of Conduct Disorder symptoms in female inmates: On the predictive utility of the syndrome in severely antisocial women. *American Journal of Orthopsychiatry, 75,* 421–430.

Busch, A. L., & Rosenberg, M. S. (2004). Comparing women and men arrested for domestic violence: A preliminary report. *Journal of Family Violence, 19,* 49–57.

Caldwell, J. E., Swan, S. C., Allen, C. T., Sullivan, T. P., & Snow, D. L. (in press). Why I hit him: Women's reasons for intimate partner violence. *Journal of Aggression, Maltreatment, & Trauma.*

Campbell, A., Muncer, S., & Odber, J. (1997). Aggression and testosterone: Testing a bio-social model. *Aggressive Behavior, 23,* 229–238.

Capaldi, D. M., Kim, H. K., & Shortt, J. W. (2004). Women's involvement in aggression in young adult romantic relationships. In M. A. B. Putallaz, K.L. (Ed.), *Aggression, antisocial behavior, and violence among girls* (pp. 223–242). New York: Guilford. Carrado, Follinstad, Wright, & Sebastian, 1991

Carrado, M., George, M. J., Loxam, E., Jones, L., & Templar, D. (1996). Aggression in British heterosexual relationships: A descriptive analysis. *Aggressive Behavior, 22,* 401–415.

Cascardi, M., O'Leary, D., Lawrence, E. E., & Schlee, K. A. (1995). Characteristics of women physically abused by their spouses and who seek treatment regarding marital conflict. *Journal of Consulting and Clinical Psychology, 63,* 616–623.

Chermack, S. T, Walton, M. A., Fuller, B. E., & Blow, F. C. (2001). Correlates of expressed and received violence across relationship type among men and women substance abusers. *Psychology of Addictive Behaviors, 15,* 140–151.

Coolidge, F. L., & Anderson, L. W. (2002). Personality profiles of women in multiple abusive relationships. *Journal of Family Violence, 17,* 117–131.

Conradi, L. M., Geffner, R., Hamberger, L. K., & Lawson, G. (in press). An exploratory study of women as dominant aggressors of physical violence in their intimate relationships. *Journal of Aggression, Maltreatment, & Trauma.*

Côté, S., Tremblay, R. E., Nagin, D. S., Zoccolillo, M., & Vitaro, F. (2002). Childhood behavioral profiles leading to adolescent conduct disorder: Risk trajectories for boys and girls. *Journal of American Academic Child Adolescent Psychiatry, 41,* 1086–1094.

Daley, S. E., Burge, D., & Hammen, C. (2000). Borderline Personality Disorder symptoms as predictors of 4-year romantic relationship dysfunction in young women: Addressing issues of specificity. *Journal of Abnormal Psychology, 109,* 451–460.

Daley, S. E., Hammen, C., Davila, J., & Burge, D. (1998). Axis II symptomatology, depression, and life stress during the Transition. *Journal of Consulting and Clinical Psychology, 66,* 595–603.

Dasgupta, S. D. (1999). Just like men? A critical view of violence by women. In M. E. Shephard & E. L. Pence (Eds.), *Coordinating community responses to domestic violence* (pp. 195–222). Thousand Oaks, CA: Sage Publications.

Davies, B., Ralph, S., & Hawton, M. (1995). A study of client satisfaction with family court counseling in cases involving domestic violence. *Family & Conciliation Courts Review, 33,* 324–341.

DeMaris, A. (1987). The efficacy of a spouse abuse model in accounting for courtship violence. *Journal of Family Issues. 8,* 291–305.

Dixon, L., & Browne, K. (2003). The heterogeneity of spouse abuse: a review. *Aggression and Violent Behavior, 8,* 107–130.

Dobash, R. E., & Dobash, R. P (1984). The nature and antecedents of violent events. *British Journal of Criminology, 24,* 269–287.

Dobash, R. P., & Dobash, R. E. (2004). Women's violence to men in intimate relationships: Working on a puzzle. *British Journal of Criminology, 44,* 324–349.

Dobash, R. P., Dobash, R. E., Cavanagh, K., & Lewis, R. (1998). Separate and intersecting realities: A comparison of men and women's accounts of violence against women. *Violence Against Women, 4,* 382–414.

Dunning, E. (2002). *Contemporary perspectives on batterers' intervention: An exploratory study.* Unpublished manuscript.

Ehrensaft, M. K., Cohen, P., & Johnson, J. G. (2006). Development of personality disorder symptoms and the risk for partner violence. *Journal of Abnormal Behavior, 115,* 474–483.

Ehrensaft, M. K., Moffitt, T. E., & Caspi, A. (2004). Clinically abusive relationships in an unselected birth cohort: Men's and women's participation and developmental antecedents. *Journal of Abnormal Psychology, 113,* 258–270.

Ehrensaft, M. K., Moffitt, T. E., & Caspi, A. (2006). Is domestic violence followed by an increased risk of psychiatric disorders among women but not men? A longitudinal cohort study. *The American Journal of Psychiatry, 163,* 885–893.

Faulkner, K. K., Cogan, R., Nolder, M., & Shooter, G. (1991). Characteristics of men and women completing cognitive/behavioral spouse abuse treatment. *Journal of Family Violence, 6,* 243–254.

Felson, R. B. (2002). *Violence and gender reexamined.* Washington, DC: American Psychological Association.

Felson, R. B. (2005, July). *How is couple violence different from other forms of violence?* Paper presented at the 9th International Family Violence Research Conference, Durham, NH.

Fiebert, M. S. (2006). *References examining assaults by women on their spouses or male partners: An annotated bibliography.* Retrieved July 12, 2006, from www.csulb.edu/~mfiebert

Fiebert, M. S., & Gonzalez, D. M. (1997). College women who initiate assaults on their male partners and the reasons offered for such behavior. *Psychological Reports, 80,* 583–590.

Follingstad, D. R., Bradley, R. G., Helff, C. M., & Laughlin, J. E. (2002). A model for predicting dating violence: Anxious attachment, angry temperament, and the need for relational control. *Violence and Victims, 17,* 35–47.

Foo, L., & Margolin, G. (1995). A multivariate investigation of dating aggression. *Journal of Family Violence, 10,* 351–377.

Ford, M. R., & Widiger, T. A. (1989). Sex bias in the diagnosis of histrionic and antisocial personality disorders. *Journal of Consulting and Clinical Psychology, 57,* 301–305.

Gilchrist, E., Johnson, R., Takriti, R., Weston, S., Beech, T., & Kebbell, M. (2003). Domestic violence offender: Characteristics and offending related needs. *Home Office Research Findings No 217,* London: Home Office.

Giles-Sims, J. (1983). *Wife battering: A systems theory approach.* New York: The Guilford Press.

Giordano, P. C., Millhonin, T. J., Cernokovich, S. A., Pugh, M. D., & Rudolph, J. L. (1999). Delinquency, identity and women's involvement in relationship violence. *Criminology, 37,* 17–40.

Goldenson, J., Spidel, A., Greaves, C., & Dutton, D. (in press). Female perpetrators of intimate partner violence: Within-group heterogeneity, related psychopathology, and a review of current treatment with recommendations for the future. *Journal of Aggression, Maltreatment, & Trauma.*

Gleason, W. J. (1993). Mental disorders in battered women: An empirical study. *Violence and Victims, 8,* 53–68.

Graham, K., Plant, M., & Plant, M. (2004). Alcohol, gender and partner aggression: A general population study of British adults. *Addiction Research and Theory, 12,* 385–401.

Graham, K., Wells, S., & Jelley, J. (2002). The social context of physical aggression among adults. *Journal of Interpersonal Violence, 17,* 64–83.

Graham-Kevan, N., & Archer, J. (2003a). Patriarchal terrorism and common couple violence: A test of Johnson's predictions in four British samples. *Journal of Interpersonal Violence, 18,* 1247–1270.

Graham-Kevan, N., & Archer, J. (2003b). Physical aggression and control in heterosexual relationships: The effect of sampling procedure. *Violence and Victims, 18,* 181–198.

Graham-Kevan, N., & Archer, J. (2005a). Investigating three explanations of women's relationship aggression. *Psychology of Women Quarterly, 29,* 270–277.

Graham-Kevan, N., & Archer, J. (2005b, July). *Using Johnson's domestic violence typology to classify men and women in a non-selected sample.* Paper presented at the 9th International Family Violence Research Conference, Durham, NH.

Graham-Kevan, N., & Archer, J. (2008). Does controlling behavior predict partner aggression? *Journal of Family Violence, 23,* 539–548.

Gray, H. M., & Foshee, V. (1997). Adolescent dating violence: Differences between one-sided and mutually violent profiles. *Journal of Interpersonal Violence, 12,* 126–141.

Hamberger, K. (1997). Cognitive behavioral treatment of men who batter their partners. *Cognitive Behavior Practice, 4,* 147–169.

Hamberger, L., & Potente, T. (1994). Counseling heterosexual women arrested for domestic violence: Implications for theory and practice. *Violence and Victims, 9,* 125–137.

Hamby, S. L., & Sugarman, D. B. (1999). Acts of psychological aggression against a partner and their relation to physical assault and gender. *Journal of Marriage and the Family, 61,* 959–970.

Harned, M. S. (2001). Abused women or abused men? An examination of the context and outcomes of dating violence. *Violence and Victims, 16,* 269–285.

Hay, D. F. (2005). The beginnings of aggression in infancy. In R. E. Tremblay, W. W. Hartup, & J. Archer (Eds.), *Developmental origins of aggression* (pp. 107–132). New York: The Guildford Press.

Henning, K., & Feder, L. (2004). A comparison of men and women arrested for domestic violence: Who presents the greater threat? *Journal of Family Violence, 19,* 69–80.

Henning, K., Jones, A., & Holdford, R. (2003). Treatment needs of women arrested for domestic violence: A comparison with male offenders. *Journal of Interpersonal Violence, 18,* 839–856.

Henning, K., Jones, A., & Holdford, R. (2005). 'I didn't do it, but if I did I had a good reason': Minimization, denial, and attributions of blame among male and female domestic violence offenders. *Journal of Family Violence, 20,* 131–139.

Hird, M. J. (2000). An empirical study of adolescent dating aggression in the U.K. *Journal of Adolescence, 23,* 69–78.

Holtzworth-Munroe, A., & Stuart, G. L. (1994). Typologies of male batterers: Three subtypes and the differences among them. *Psychological Bulletin, 116,* 476–497.

Jackson, S., Feder, L., Forde, D. R., Davis, R. C., Maxwell, C. D., & Taylor, B. G. (2003). *Batterer intervention programmes: Where do we go from here?* Washington, DC: Office of Justice Programs, National Institute of Justice. Retrieved May 5, 2009, from http://www.ojp.usdoj.gov/nij.

Johnson, M. P. (1995). Patriarchal terrorism and common couple violence: Two forms of violence against women. *Journal of Marriage and the Family, 57,* 283–294.

Johnson, M. P. (1999, November). *Two types of violence against women in the American family: Identifying intimate terrorism and common couple violence.* Paper presented at the Annual Meetings of the National Council on Family Relations, Irvine, CA.

Johnson, M. P., & Leone, J. M. (2005). The differential effects of intimate terrorism and common couple violence: Findings from the National Violence Against Women Survey. *Journal of Family Issues, 26,* 322–349.

Katz, J., Kuffel, S. W., & Coblentz, A. (2002). Are there gender differences in sustaining dating violence? An examination of frequency, severity and relationship satisfaction. *Journal of Family Violence, 17,* 247–271.

Kukko, K., & Pulkkinen, L. (2005). Stability of aggressive behavior from childhood to middle age in women and men. *Aggressive Behavior, 31,* 485–497.

LaRoche, D. (2008). *Context and consequences of domestic violence against men and women in Canada in 2004.* Québec, Canada: Institut de la statistique du Québec.

Lewis, D. O., Yeager, C. A., Swica, Y., Pincus, J. H., & Lewis, M. (1997). Objective documentation of child abuse and dissociation in 12 murderers with dissociative identity disorder. *American Journal of Psychiatry, 154,* 1703–1710.

Martin, M. (1997). Double your trouble: Dual arrest in family violence. *Journal of Family Violence, 12,* 139–157.

McFarlane, J., Wilson, P., Malecha, A., & Lemmey, D. (2000). Intimate partner violence. A gender comparison. *Journal of Interpersonal Violence, 15,* 158–169.

McLeod, M. (1984). Women against men: An estimation of domestic violence based on an analysis of official data and national victimization data. *Justice Quarterly, 1,* 171–193.

Moffitt, T. E., Caspi, A., Rutter, M., & Silva, P. A. (2001). *Sex differences in antisocial behavior.* Cambridge: Cambridge University Press.

Moffitt, T. E., Krueger, R. F., Caspi, A., & Fagan, J. (2000). Partner abuse and general crime: How are they the same? How are they different? *Criminology, 38,* 199–232.

Molidor, C. E. (1995). Gender differences of psychological abuse in high school dating relationships. *Child and Adolescent Social Work Journal, 12,* 119–134.

Morse, B. J. (1995). Beyond the conflict tactics scale: Assessing gender differences in partner violence. *Violence and Victims, 10,* 251–272.

O'Leary, K. D, Barling, J., Arias, I., & Rosenbaum, A. (1989). Prevalence and stability of physical aggression between spouses: A longitudinal analysis. *Journal of Consulting and Clinical Psychology, 57,* 263–268.

Padgett, D. K. (1997). Women's mental health: Some directions for research. *American Journal of Orthopsychiatry, 6,* 521–534.

Pulkkinen, L., & Pitkänen, T. (1993). Constitution in aggressive behavior from childhood to adulthood. *Aggressive Behavior, 19,* 249–263.

Riggs, D. S. (1993). Relationship problems and dating aggression: A potential treatment target. *Journal of Interpersonal Violence, 8,* 18–35.

Roscoe, B., & Callahan, J. E. (1985). Adolescent's self-reports of violence in families and dating relationships. *Adolescence, 79,* 545–553.

Ross, J. M., & Babcock, J. C. (2009). Gender differences in partner violence in context: Deconstructing Johnson's (2001) control-based typology of violent couples. *Journal of Aggression, Maltreatment, & Trauma, 18*(6), 604–622.

Rouse, L. P. (1990). The dominance motive in abusive partners: Identifying couples at risk. *Journal of College Student Development, 31,* 330–335.

Rounsaville, B. (1978). Theories in marital violence: Evidence from a study of battered women. *Victimology: An International Journal, 3*, 11–31.

Serbin, L., Stack, D., De Genna, N., Grunzeweig, N., Temcheff, C. E., Schwartzmann, A. E., et al. (2004). When aggressive girls become mothers. In M. Putallaz & K. L. Bierman (Eds.), *Aggression, antisocial behavior and violence among girls* (pp. 262–289). New York: The Guilford Press.

Simmons, C., Lehmann, P., Cobb, N., & Fowler, C. (2005). Personality profiles of women and men arrested for domestic violence: An analysis of similarities and differences. *Journal of Offender Rehabilitation, 41*, 63–81.

Slutske, W., Heath, A., Dinwiddie, S., Madden, P., Bucholz, K. K., Dunne, M. P., et al. (1997). Modeling genetic and environmental influences in the etiology of conduct disorder: A study of 2,682 adult twin pairs. *Journal of Abnormal Psychology, 106*, 266–279.

Slutske, W., Heath, A., Madden, P., Bucholz, K., Statham, D., & Martin, N. (2002). Personality and the genetic risk for alcohol dependence. *Journal of Abnormal Psychology, 111*, 124–133.

Sommer, R. (1994). Male and female perpetrated partner abuse. *Dissertation Abstracts International, 56*(9–B), 5185.

State of California. (1999). *Report on arrest for domestic violence in California, 1998* (Office of the Attorney General). Criminal Justice Statistics Center, at.Cent.3, 1–20.

Statistics Canada. (2000). Family violence in Canada: A statistical profile. *Canadian Centre for Justice Statistics*, No. 85.

Stets, J. E. (1988). *Domestic violence and control*. New York: Springer-Verlag.

Stets, J. E. (1991). Psychological aggression in dating relationship: The role of interpersonal control. *Journal of Family Violence, 6*, 97–114.

Stets, J. E., & Pirog-Good, M. A. (1990). Interpersonal control and courtship aggression. *Journal of Social and Personal Relationships, 7*, 371–394.

Straus, M. A. (2005). Women's violence toward men is a serious social problem. In R. J. Gelles & D. R. Loseke (Eds.), *Current controversies on family violence* (2nd ed., pp. 55–77). Newbury Park, CA: Sage Publications.

Straus, M. A. (2009). Why the overwhelming evidence on partner physical violence by women has not been perceived and is often denied. *Journal of Aggression, Maltreatment, & Trauma, 18*(6), 552–571.

Sugarman, C. B., & Hotaling, G. T., (1997). Intimate violence and social desirability: A meta-analytic review. *Journal of Interpersonal Violence, 12*, 275–290.

Tremblay, T. E., Nagin, D. S., Séguin, J. R., Zoccolillo, M., Zelazo, P. D., Boivin, M., et al. (2004). Physical aggression during early childhood: Trajectories and predictors. *Pediatrics, 114*, 43–50

Walker, L. E. A. (1991). Post-traumatic stress disorder in women: Diagnosis and treatment of battered women syndrome. *Psychotherapy, 28*, 21–29.

Walley-Jean, J. C., & Swan, S. (in press). Motivations and justifications for partner aggression in a sample of African American college women. *Journal of Aggression, Maltreatment, & Trauma*.

Webster, C. D., Douglas, K. S., Eaves, D., & Hart, S. D. (1997). *The HCR-20: Assessing the Risk for Violence (Version 2)*. Vancouver, Canada: Mental Health, Law and Policy Institute, Simon Fraser University.

Weizmann-Henelius, G., Viemerö, V., & Eronen, M. (2004). Psychological risk markers in violent female behavior. *International Journal of Forensic Health*, *3*, 185–196.

Whisman, M. A. (1999). Marital dissatisfaction and psychiatric disorders: Results from the National Comorbidity Survey. *Journal of Abnormal Psychology*, *108*, 701–706.

White, J. W., Merrill, L. L., & Koss, M. P. (2001). Predictors of courtship violence in a Navy recruit sample. *Journal of Interpersonal Violence*, *16*, 910–927.

RESEARCH EXAMINING THE ROLE OF GENDER AND RACE/ETHNICITY IN INTIMATE PARTNER VIOLENCE

Gender Differences in Partner Violence in Context: Deconstructing Johnson's (2001) Control-Based Typology of Violent Couples

JODY M. ROSS

Indiana University–Purdue University, Fort Wayne, Indiana, USA

JULIA C. BABCOCK

University of Houston, Houston, Texas, USA

We examined the variables comprising Johnson's (2001) typology of violent couples dimensionally and in the context of the relationship as they relate to injury and observed behavior. A community sample of couples (N = 281) reported on self- and partner-perpetrated violence, control, and injury, and engaged in a conflict discussion. Women reported engaging in more violent acts and as much control as their partners and were more hostile than men during the conflict discussion. Twelve percent of women reported being the sole aggressor. For women, controlling but not violent behavior predicted observed, hostile behavior. For men, violence and control predicted hostility during the discussion. Clinically, both genders may benefit from treatments aimed at reducing violence and control.

Intimate partner violence (IPV) in the United States has typically been associated with wife abuse and commonly is perceived as exclusively or predominantly a crime against women. Feminist scholars of IPV (e.g., Dobash & Dobash, 1977–1978) assume that women are the sole victims of partner violence and that aggression perpetrated by them is enacted either in self-defense or in retaliation for past abuse (Dobash & Dobash, 1977–1978; Hamberger & Potente, 1994). The patriarchal traditions of our society and the resulting inequalities between men and women are viewed as the root cause of IPV (Johnson, 1995). IPV perpetrated by men is considered a power and control tactic used to dominate a female partner (Yllö, 1993) or to punish her unwanted behavior (Hamberger, Lohr, Bonge, & Tonlin, 1997). For feminist researchers, domestic violence remains a deeply gendered phenomenon, as "spousal violence is to all extents and purposes wife beating" (Dobash & Dobash, 1977–1978, p. 439).

More recently, a different view of IPV has emerged that regards partner abuse as a human and not simply a gender or women's issue (McNeely, Cook, & Torres, 2001). From "the family violence perspective," IPV is one of many forms of abuse that occurs within families that can be perpetrated by both men and women. Although it is women who primarily seek shelter from family violence, survey research has found that women engage in IPV at equal or higher rates compared to men (Straus & Gelles, 1986). Women are also arrested for IPV (Muftic, Bouffard, & Bouffard, 2007) and their violence is not solely in self-defense; some women use violence in order to control their mates (Babcock, Miller, & Siard, 2003; Leisring, in press). Researchers from the family violence perspective commonly employ large-scale community surveys and often assess IPV via the Conflict Tactics Scales (CTS; Straus, 1979; Straus, Hamby, Boney-McCoy, & Sugarman, 1996; Straus, Hamby, & Warren, 2003). Many also criticize the methodology of feminist scholars for neglecting to systematically assess for female perpetration of IPV and examining only samples representing the extreme end of the partner violence continuum (i.e., women in battered women's shelters; Graham-Kevan, this issue; Hines & Douglas, this issue; Straus, 2009).

In turn, feminist researchers have criticized the methodology and findings of family violence researchers. They assert that the CTS is flawed in that it does not assess motivation, meaning, or context of violent incidents (Dobash, Dobash, Wilson, & Daly, 1992) and that partners' reports are often discrepant (Dobash, Dobash, Cavanagh, & Lewis, 1998). They also point out that, despite the findings of similarity in frequency counts of male and female aggression, women are still at an increased risk of injury, more fearful of their partners, and generally more physically and psychologically harmed by IPV (Melton & Belknap, 2003). Family violence researchers agree that women suffer greater financial and emotional strain and are "more often the victims of severe partner assault and injury not because men strike more often, but because men strike harder" (Morse, 1995, p. 251).

JOHNSON'S TYPOLOGIES

In order to reconcile some of the findings of feminist and family violence researchers, Johnson (1995) developed a theoretical typology of violent couples based on violence and control. These two camps, according to Johnson, are actually investigating distinct forms of IPV. Feminist researchers, collecting data mainly from samples of female victims of abuse who are seeking assistance from shelter facilities, are studying severe abuse that Johnson termed "patriarchal" or "intimate terrorism" (IT). Conversely, the large, national, random samples utilized by family violence researchers represent couples engaged in what Johnson called "common couple violence" (CCV). Johnson (2001) later added two additional groups to his typology, which he named "mutual violent control" (MVC) and "violent resistance" (VR).

According to Johnson's original typology, CCV is characterized by similar levels of IPV perpetrated by both partners (Johnson, 1995). The violence in CCV is infrequent and typically the result of an argument getting out of hand. CCV is not characterized by high levels of severe violence or control and typically does not escalate over time (Johnson, 2001). In contrast to CCV, patriarchal terrorists (Johnson, 1995), or more recently renamed intimate terrorists (Johnson, 2001), utilize physical aggression as well as nonviolent methods of control in order to dominate their partners (Johnson, 1995). In these relationships, violence is asymmetrical and can be severe in nature. Intimate terrorists are often emotionally as well as physically abusive (Johnson & Ferraro, 2000) and the abuse in many of these relationships escalates over time (Johnson, 2001). The major distinction between CCV and IT is the motive of control by the primary aggressor. Despite the name being changed from "patriarchal terrorism," IT is still thought to be "essentially perpetrated by men" (Johnson & Ferraro, 2000, p. 950). In MVC, both partners are highly violent and controlling. Finally, with VR the individual's violence is thought to be enacted in self-defense.

CATEGORIES VERSUS DIMENSIONS

While Johnson's typology of violent couples has intuitive appeal, categorical approaches within the field of psychology have been increasingly criticized as poor representations of reality (Jablensky, 2005). Dimensional approaches to the study of human behavior are thought to be methodologically superior (Widiger, 2005). The theory behind Johnson's typology of violent couples can be conceptualized dimensionally. Essentially, Johnson's typology is about severity and symmetry of violence and control. CCV couples show low levels of both physical abuse and controlling behaviors (low severity) and both partners engage in similar levels of violence and controlling (high symmetry). MVC is typified by high severity as well as high symmetry. Both partners tend to be highly violent and both are controlling. CCV and MVC describe both partners' behavior. In contrast, IT and VR are defined as low symmetry but then focus on the behavior of just one partner. Along with low symmetry, IT is defined as high severity of violence and control by only one partner. Like IT, VR couples show low symmetry, high severity of violence, and control by one perpetrator, with the addition of the other partner using violence (but not control) in self-defense.

The aims of the current study are two-fold. First, we attempt to test within a community sample whether women as well as men engage in IT by examining both men's and women's perpetration of IPV and of control. Second, rather than typing violent couples into broad, mutually exclusive groups, we examine severity and symmetry of physical abuse and controlling behavior, the major variables composing Johnson's typology, adopting a dimensional approach to the study of male and female perpetrated IPV. We investigate how severity and symmetry of violence and control, examined with the couple serving as the unit of analysis, relate to partner injury and observed hostile behavior toward one's partner. Specifically we ask: Are both men and women equally domineering, belligerent, and contemptuous in their interactions with their partners? Do perpetration of IPV and control have different correlates (e.g., hostility and injury) depending on whether the perpetrator is a man or woman? Can women be intimate terrorists?

Severe violence, regardless of gender of the perpetrator, was expected to be related to greater physical injury. While women have often been shown to suffer more severe injuries than men at the hand of intimate partners, researchers have proposed that the use of weapons by some women may serve to equalize the size differential between the sexes (McNeely et al., 2001). Furthermore, the more asymmetrical the IPV in a relationship, the higher the number of injuries expected of the less violent partner.

During observed laboratory interactions with their partners, abusive husbands exhibit more aversive behaviors such as criticisms and put downs (Cordova, Jacobson, Gottman, Rushe, & Cox, 1993; Margolin, John, & Gleberman, 1988) and tend to be more domineering, belligerent, and contemptuous than nonviolent husbands (Jacobson et al., 1994). To our knowledge, no research has examined the aversive behaviors of female perpetrators during a conflict discussion with their partners. We expected that both men's and women's IPV perpetration and control tactics would be related to observed hostile behaviors in the lab. We also expected that the more physically aggressive and controlling participants (relative to their partners) would display the most domineering, belligerence, and contempt.

METHOD

Participants

Participants were recruited via ads in free newspapers and flyers soliciting "couples experiencing conflict." Couples were required to be at least 18 years of age and married or living together as if married for at least six months. Women were phoned by trained undergraduate interviewers who administered the violence subscale of the CTS (Straus, 1979) and one item from the Dyadic Adjustment Scale (DAS; Spanier, 1976) to recruit a sample of violent couples and distressed but nonviolent couples. Data were collected as part of a larger study on psychophysiological reactivity as it relates to IPV (Babcock, Green, & Webb, 2008; Babcock, Green, Webb, & Yerington, 2005; Babcock, Roseman, Green, & Ross, 2008). Couples were eligible to participate in the larger study if (a) the female partner reported any male-to-female IPV in the past year or (b) the woman reported no violence but being "a little unhappy" or worse on the following DAS global item: "On a scale from 1 to 7 where 1 is 'very unhappy,' 4 is 'happy,' and 7 is 'perfectly happy,' where would you rate your present relationship?" This item has been shown to correlate highly with the total DAS score (Goodwin, 1992). The goal was to recruit a nonviolent sample matched to the IPV sample on levels of relationship distress (i.e., a distressed/nonviolent comparison group). Final categorization was based on men's and women's reports of their own and their partner's IPV on the longer CTS2 (Straus et al., 1996, 2003) in the lab. Nonviolent couples ($n = 67$) were excluded from all analyses.

Overview of Procedures

Data were collected during a 3-hour assessment period. Couples were separated to complete a series of questionnaires and then reunited to engage in a conflict discussion. Graduate student researchers helped couples identify topics of conflict in their current relationships. In no case did either partner become physically aggressive. Participants were each paid $10 per hour.

Questionnaire Measures

INTIMATE PARTNER VIOLENCE

All participants completed the CTS2 (Straus et al., 1996), a widely used 78-item questionnaire that assesses frequency of male-to-female and female-to-male physically, sexually, and psychologically abusive acts in the past year. For the present study, the CTS2 physical assault and injury subscales were used. There appears to be agreement about which items on the CTS tap more or less severe forms of intimate partner aggression. For example, both Marshall (1992) and Archer (2002) discussed the various types of aggressive acts from least to the most severe as pushing, shoving, grabbing, and handling forcefully, slapping, kicking, hitting with an object, choking and beating up, and using a knife or gun on one's partner. Still, the CTS has been criticized for only measuring counts of violent incidents without adequate consideration of differences in severity of items. In this way, individuals who admit to pushing their partner 10 times obtain the same score as those who admit to using a knife or gun on their partner 10 times. For the present study, the CTS2 physical assault items were weighted in accordance with the physical harm impact weights derived for the Severity of Violence Against Women Scales (Marshall, 1992) so that the total score for this subscale reflected not only counts but also the severity of the violent acts. For example, pushing/shoving one's partner was weighted .586, whereas using a knife or gun on one's partner was weighted .970. A man reporting that he pushed his wife 10 times would earn a score of 5.86, while a man who used a knife on his partner 10 times would earn a score of 9.7. In this way, higher CTS2 physical assault scores in the current study do not simply represent a greater number of violent acts but more severe levels of IPV perpetration.

CONTROLLING BEHAVIOR

A subset (n = 175) of female participants reported their own and their partner's controlling behaviors as part of a larger questionnaire assessing emotional abuse (Emotional Abuse Scale, EAS; Murphy & Hoover, 1999). Four subscales compose this measure, including Dominance/Intimidation (D/I), Restrictive Engulfment (RE), Denigration (D), and Hostile Withdrawal (HW). The subscales of the EAS have good psychometric properties (alphas ranging from .85 to .91). In the current study, the first three EAS subscales were used as an index of control, based on the content overlap between the items on these scales and the eight true/false items used to measure control in Leone, Johnson, and Cohan's (2004) study. These three EAS subscales are intended to measure (a) fear-inducing or submission-inducing behaviors (D/I); (b) isolating, restrictive, or possessive behaviors (RE); and (c) humiliating and degrading behaviors (D; Murphy & Hoover, 1999). The eight items used by Leone and colleagues to measure intimate partner control included "insult you, swear at you, or call you out of your name," "accuse you of being with another man," "do or say something just to spite you," "try to control your every move," "withhold money, make you ask for money, or take yours," "threaten you with a knife or gun," "threaten to kill you," and "threaten to hurt your family or friends" (Leone et al., 2004, p. 478). Because men did not complete the EAS, intimate partner control as a predictor was based on women's reports exclusively.

Observational Measures

SPECIFIC AFFECT

Displayed affect was coded by 11 trained observers (8 female, 3 male) using the Specific Affect Coding System (SPAFF 16-code version; Gottman, McCoy, Coan, & Collier, 1996) during a conflict discussion. Graduate student researchers administered the Play-by-Play Interview (Hooven, Rushe, & Gottman, 1996) to each couple in order to clarify two topics of conflict within the relationship. Videotaped conversations were later coded by trained research assistants using the Video Coding System (VCS; Long, 1998). SPAFF 16-code version is composed of 10 negative codes (disgust, anger, defensiveness, domineering, contempt, stonewalling, belligerence, whining, fear/tension, and sadness); five positive codes (validation, interest, humor, affection/caring, and joy/surprise); and a neutral code. Three of the negative codes (belligerence, domineering, and contempt) were combined and summed to produce frequency counts for men's and women's observed behavior. Interrater reliability for the combined code was kappa = .71.

Data Analysis

Men's and women's reports of IPV were analyzed in separate multiple regression analyses to determine if findings differed due to a gender-based reporting bias. Men's and women's reports on the CTS2 and women's reports on the EAS were used to construct the predictor variables. Sum and difference scores were computed from CTS2 and EAS data as indicators of the total amount of violence and control within the relationship (severity scores) and the difference between men's and women's perpetrated violence and men's and women's use of control (symmetry scores). Specifically, female report–based violence severity scores were computed by adding a woman's report of her own violence to her report of her partner's violence to get an indicator of the sum total amount of violence in the relationship. Weighting of CTS2 physical abuse items as described above resulted in a "severity" subscale, as opposed to simple summed frequency counts of IPV. Control severity scores were computed by adding a woman's report of her own controlling behavior to her report of her partner's controlling behavior. Female report–based symmetry scores were obtained by subtracting a woman's report of her own violence (or control) from her report of her partner's violence (or control). A positive difference score indicated a couple with more male- than female-perpetrated physical aggression (or control). A negative difference score indicated that the woman was more violent (or controlling) than her partner. The closer the difference score to zero, the more similar the partners were in their use of violence or control. The steps for computing sum and difference scores were repeated using men's reports on the CTS2. These sum and difference scores served as predictor variables in several multiple regressions. The outcomes of interest include partner injury and observed belligerence and domineering toward one's partner during a conflict discussion.

RESULTS

The final sample consisted of 281 couples in which at least one partner reported some IPV in the current relationship in the past year. Just over 50% of the participants were African American, 27% were Caucasian, 16% were Hispanic, and 7% were from other racial or ethnic origins. The average age was 32 (SD = 10.04) for men and 29 (SD = 9.12) for women, and the average family income was $32,224 ($SD$ = $21,535.36) per year. Participants' responses on the CTS2 revealed that the most common physically aggressive behaviors were the same for men and women (Table 1).

While this sample was recruited for relationship dissatisfaction or male-to-female IPV, several couples indicated that only the woman was violent. According to women, 12% of the couples were classified as female-only violent, while the man was the sole aggressor in nearly 16.5% of the couples. Based on men's reports, the woman was the only violent partner in 11% and the man in nearly 9% of couples. Additionally, both men and women reported that, on average, women engaged in more acts of physical aggression as compared to men (see Table 2). However, while men reported women to be significantly more violent (t[278] = 2.27, p = .02), women reported small differences between their own and their partner's IPV (t[280] = 0.30, p = .77). Additionally, after weighting of the CTS2 items to reflect severity of IPV, women's reports indicated similar severity of violence for men and women, while men's reports painted a picture of women as both more frequently *and* more severely violent. While men and women agreed on rates of IPV perpetrated by each partner, they were in less agreement about symmetry of IPV (see Table 2).

On average, both partners tended to agree that the woman was the more frequently violent partner; however, men and women disagreed about who experienced the most injuries. On average, men reported more injuries

TABLE 1 Means and Standard Deviations of the Most Common Aggressive Behaviors by Reporter

| | Men's report of: | | Women's report of: | |
| | Self Mean (SD) | Partner Mean (SD) | Self Mean (SD) | Partner Mean (SD) |
Behavior				
Threw something at	1.13 (3.48)	2.40 (4.95)	2.52 (5.61)	1.38 (3.46)
Pushed/shoved	2.73 (5.12)	3.42 (5.56)	2.94 (5.25)	2.96 (5.02)
Grabbed	3.39 (5.52)	2.90 (5.74)	2.53 (4.68)	2.95 (4.71)

TABLE 2 Means, Standard Deviations, and Correlations for IPV Predictors and Outcomes by Reporter

Variable	Men's (report)		Women's (report)		r^1
	Mean	SD	Mean	SD	
CTS2 Counts of men's violence	12.05	(22.14)	12.62	(19.63)	0.41***
CTS2 Counts of women's violence	17.87	(33.48)	13.17	(21.57)	0.35***
Severity of men's violence[2]	8.11	(14.64)	9.26	(15.34)	0.42***
Severity of women's violence	12.12	(24 .02)	9.24	(15.73)	0.36***
Total relationship IPV severity	20.27	(34.37)	18.53	(27.66)	0.46***
Symmetry of violence[3]	−4.06	(20.17)	0.01	(14.25)	0.07
Men's injuries	2.48	(7.54)	1.91	(4.71)	0.20**
Women's injuries	2.14	(4.90)	2.97	(6.61)	0.18**
Observed hostility[4]	120.19	(88.52)	148.22	(93.29)	0.19**

[1]Correlations between men's and women's reports.
[2]Severity variables were calculated by summing CTS2 items weighted in accordance with the impact weights derived for the Severity of Violence Against Women Scales (Marshall, 1992).
[3]Symmetry variables were calculated by subtracting counts of women's behavior from counts of men's behavior. Positive symmetry scores indicate male predominance for this behavior; negative symmetry scores indicate female predominance for this behavior.
[4]Values here represent the mean number of seconds men and women displayed hostility during a conflict discussion with their partner.
*$p < .05$, **$p < .01$, ***$p < .001$.

for themselves than for their partners, whereas women, who reported more frequent perpetration of IPV for themselves but similar severity of IPV for both partners, reported experiencing more injuries than men (see Table 2). Despite agreement about who is the most frequently violent, both men and women claimed themselves to be the most injured. Objective laboratory observation showed that women were more domineering, belligerent, and contemptuous toward their partner in the lab as compared to men (see Table 2).

With regard to intimate partner control, women reported similar levels of overall control for themselves and their partners (see Table 3). Women endorsed significantly higher rates of perpetrating restrictive engulfment for themselves, significantly higher rates of domination-intimidation for their partners, and similar rates of denigration for both partners (see Table 3). In order to see what proportion of the sample might be considered intimate terrorists, we examined the number of partner-violent men and partner-violent women who scored more than one standard deviation (SD) above the mean (>150.44) on control, in accordance with the recommendations of Leone et al. (2004), that control (and not severity of violence) be used to differentiate "types" of batterers. Note that the more stringent cutoff based on the mean plus SD for men's scores (150.44, versus mean plus SD of women's scores, 144.49) was used for both men and women so that both were held to the same standard. Using these criteria, 23 (13%) women and

TABLE 3 Means and Standard Deviations of MEA Subscales & Overall Control Score

	Men		Women		
	Mean	SD	Mean	SD	t(1,174)
Restrictive engulfment	26.95	(35.20)	33.46	(37.34)	2.27*
Denigration	19.57	(29.49)	19.92	(29.13)	0.15
Domination/intimidation	24.03	(35.70)	16.43	(28.85)	2.91**
Overall control[1]	68.97	(81.47)	69.31	(75.18)	0.06

*$p < .05$, **$p < .01$.
[1]Overall control combines restrictive engulfment, denigration, and domination/intimidation.

21 (12%) men could potentially be considered intimate terrorists. Eight of these were from the same couple, possibly representing MVC. When these eight couples were removed, men in the male IT group were significantly more violent than their partners (t[12] = 4.21, $p < .01$) and women in the female IT group were significantly more violent than their partners (t[14] = 3.56, $p < .01$), confirming that one can identify groups of both men and women who engage in both IPV and control (i.e., IT) within a community sample.

Women's Injuries

WOMEN'S REPORTS

As expected, physical aggression was a significant predictor of women's injuries (see Table 4). Approximately 45% of the variance in women's injuries was accounted for by the physical violence predictors (F[2,241] = 98.51, $p < .001$). Both symmetry and severity of IPV significantly predicted women's injuries. As severity of violence in the relationship increased, women's injuries increased ($\beta = 0.60$, $p < .001$). Also, as asymmetry increased so that the man was increasingly more violent than the woman (i.e., a positive difference score), women's injuries increased ($\beta = 0.33$, $p < .001$).

TABLE 4 Summary of Regression Analyses for Variables Predicting Women's Injuries

Variable	B	SE B	β
Women's reports			
Symmetry of violence	0.15	0.02	0.33***
Severity of violence	0.14	0.01	0.60***
Men's reports			
Symmetry of violence	0.03	0.02	0.14*
Severity of violence	0.08	0.01	0.53***

*$p < .05$, **$p < .01$, ***$p < .001$.

Men also reported that IPV significantly predicted women's injuries (F[2,239] = 34.18, $p < .001$). As severity of the violence within a relationship increased, women's injuries increased ($\beta = 0.53$, $p < .001$). Based on men's reports, symmetry of IPV was also significantly related to women's injuries. As asymmetry increased so that the man was increasingly more violent than the woman, women's injuries increased ($\beta = 0.14$, $p < .05$), although the relation here was notably weaker (see Table 4).

Men's Injuries

WOMEN'S REPORTS

IPV was also a significant predictor of men's injuries (see Table 5). Combined symmetry and severity of IPV accounted for approximately 31% of the variance in men's injuries (F[2,232] = 52.37, $p < .001$). Severity, but not symmetry, of violence significantly predicted men's injuries. As severity of IPV increased, men experienced more injuries ($\beta = 0.55$, $p < .001$).

Men's reports. Men and women appeared to be in agreement that IPV was a significant predictor of men's injuries. Also, both men's and women's reports indicated that only severity and not symmetry of IPV was a significant predictor here. Together, the violence predictors accounted for 35% of the variance in men's injuries (F[2,240] = 64.83, $p < .001$). As severity of IPV in the relationship increased, men's injuries increased ($\beta = 0.62$, $p < .001$).

Observed Women's Behavior

Women's reports of their own and their partner's controlling behaviors were better predictors of behavior observed during the conflict discussion (belligerence, domineering, and contempt) than were physical violence scores (see Table 6). Women's reports of IPV severity and their reports of control severity and symmetry significantly predicted women's hostile behavior

TABLE 5 Summary of Regression Analyses for Variables Predicting Men's Injuries

Variable	B	$SE\ B$	β
Women's reports			
Symmetry of violence	−0.02	0.02	−0.07
Severity of violence	0.09	0.01	0.55***
Men's reports			
Symmetry of violence	0.02	0.02	0.04
Severity of violence	0.13	0.01	0.62***

*$p < .05$, **$p < .01$, ***$p < .001$.

TABLE 6 Summary of Regression Analyses for Variables Predicting Observed Women's Behavior

Variable	B	$SE\ B$	β
Women's reports			
Symmetry of violence	−0.26	0.40	−0.04
Severity of violence	0.60	0.21	0.18*
Symmetry of control	−0.28	0.13	−0.19*
Severity of control	0.15	0.06	0.23**
Men's reports			
Symmetry of violence	0.16	0.35	0.04
Severity of violence	0.40	0.21	0.15

*$p < .05$, **$p < .01$, ***$p < .001$.

observed during a conflict discussion with their partners. As severity of relationship violence increased, so did women's observed domineering, belligerence, and contempt toward their partner in the lab (see Table 6). Symmetry and severity of control together accounted for approximately 5% of the variance in observed women's behavior ($F[2,131] = 4.76$, $p = .01$). As the total amount of control in the relationship increased, women were observed to be more belligerent, domineering, and contemptuous toward their partners during the conflict discussion ($\beta = 0.23$, $p < .01$). Also, as symmetry decreased such that the woman was relatively more controlling than her partner, the woman was observed to be more interpersonally hostile toward her partner ($\beta = -0.19$, $p < .05$). Men, reporting only on physical aggression, indicated that neither IPV severity nor asymmetry was significantly related to women's observed belligerence, domineering, or contempt toward her partner in the lab (see Table 6).

Observed Men's Behavior

A different pattern of results emerged when the models predicting observed women's behavior were compared to the models predicting observed men's behavior (see Tables 6 and 7). Whereas women's observed behavior was more related to severity of IPV and control, men's observed behavior was related to asymmetry of these behaviors. Together, severity and symmetry of IPV accounted for nearly 4% of the variance in observed men's behavior ($F[2,240] = 5.91$, $p < .01$. The relation between symmetry of violence and observed men's control was in the predicted direction: the higher the ratio of the man's violence (relative to his partner), the more belligerent, domineering, and contemptuous he was toward his partner in the lab ($\beta = 0.19$, $p < .01$). Similarly, men reported by their wives or girlfriends to be the more controlling partner in the relationship were observed to be the most belligerent, domineering, and contemptuous during the conflict discussion ($\beta = 0.24$, $p < .01$). Severity of either IPV or control was not a significant predictor of

TABLE 7 Summary of Regression Analyses for Variables Predicting Observed Men's Behavior

Variable	B	SE B	β
Women's reports			
Symmetry of violence	1.18	0.38	0.19**
Severity of violence	0.33	0.20	0.11
Symmetry of control	0.35	0.12	0.24**
Severity of control	0.11	0.06	0.17
Men's reports			
Symmetry of violence	0.32	0.34	0.07
Severity of violence	0.27	0.20	0.11

*$p < .05$, **$p < .01$, ***$p < .001$.

men's observed behavior in the lab. Based on men's reports, IPV was not significantly related to men's hostile behavior (see Table 7).

DISCUSSION

Although it was predicted that women would experience more injuries in relationships predominated by male-perpetrated violence and that men would sustain more injuries in relationships predominated by female-perpetrated violence, these hypotheses were only partially supported. As expected, participants agreed that IPV predicts both men's and women's injuries. However, while we predicted that asymmetry of violence would put the less violent partner at risk for more injuries, this held true only for women's injuries. Women's injuries did increase as asymmetry was skewed toward the man being the more violent partner, although the relation here was weaker when analyses were based exclusively on men's reports. In contrast, men's injuries were related to the cumulative severity of violence within a relationship and not to the gendered asymmetry of IPV. Men and women agreed that, regardless of which partner was more violent, men were increasingly injured as total violence within the relationship increased.

These findings support the importance of looking at symmetry and severity of violence as separate variables, as they appear to predict injury outcomes by gender differentially—that is, while women do seem to suffer more injuries in relationships predominated by male IPV (violence in accordance with male IT), men seem to suffer more injuries when both partners are highly violent (violence expected in MVC relationships). An additional difference here relates to the notably weaker relation between women's injuries and male-perpetrated asymmetrical violence based on men's versus women's reports. One possible explanation for differences here is that men may have been attempting to minimize their violence or shift the blame for their partners' injuries to the partner by implicating her own violence in her injuries. Men may have been attempting to justify their physically abusive behavior by pointing out that they were not the only violent partner in the relationship. Finally, both men and women seemed to agree that men were more likely to be injured when both partners were highly violent. Thus, the hypothesis that men would experience the most injuries in relationships predominated by female violence was not supported by the data.

In the present study, while women's and men's reports of IPV were similar, the correlates of IPV differed depending on the respondent. Overall, female reports of IPV were a better predictor of outcomes than were men's reports of IPV. The failure of men's reports of their own IPV to predict other variables suggests that men may have been underreporting their own violence. Certainly, most men understand that hitting their female partners is socially unacceptable and may be reluctant to admit to their own IPV. The different pattern of results that emerged when asking identical questions of men and women suggests that gaining an accurate picture of IPV may require the input of both partners (Moffitt et al., 1997). On the other hand, because women's reports showed more construct validity, these findings may justify the exclusive use of women's reports of IPV.

While thought to stem from patriarchal, sexist beliefs, intimate partner control does not appear to be gender based. According to women's reports, women and men engaged in similar levels of intimate partner control. Additionally, a similar number of the partner-violent men and women in this sample could potentially be considered intimate terrorists. These intimate-terrorist individuals were highly controlling and significantly more violent than their partners. Thus, even though this community sample was originally recruited with a focus on male-perpetrated IPV, there did appear to be sizable number of violent and controlling women (female intimate terrorists).

Control, as measured by three EAS subscales, was the best predictor of women's hostile behavior during a conflict discussion with an intimate partner. Considering levels of control in the relationship, women in relationships with high cumulative rates of control were observed to be highly belligerent, domineering, and contemptuous toward their partners in the lab. Women in highly violent relationships were also observed to be hostile toward their partners in the lab. Other studies have found similarly high rates of controlling, belligerent, and psychologically abusive behavior among battered women during interactions with a violent partner (e.g., Jacobson et al., 1994). As the majority of men in the current sample had been violent toward their partner, women's observed domineering, belligerence, and contempt toward the man may reflect women's anger at their partner's past IPV. In fact, women may have responded to the advertisement for "couples experiencing conflict" because they were angry with their partners. Still, those women observed to be the most hostile toward their partner during the conflict discussion also self-reported that they were more controlling, in general, than their partners.

For both men and women, observed hostility was predicted by their asymmetrical use of intimate partner control. Like women, the most hostile men were those described as being relatively more controlling than their partners. However, the most hostile men were also relatively more violent than their partners. The finding that only women's controlling behavior predicted their observed hostility, whereas both men's physical aggression and control predicted their hostility, is an interesting gender difference. Women's perpetration of violence was unrelated to women's belligerence, contempt, and domineering behaviors during conflict. Observed hostility can be thought of as an index of relationship distress. Perhaps women express their frustration or dissatisfaction with their relationship by becoming controlling and psychologically abusive toward their partner, while men act out their frustration and dissatisfaction physically in addition to becoming more controlling. Findings that women's violence did not predict their observed hostility and asymmetrical violence did not predict men's injury suggests different context and meaning of women's perpetration of IPV.

These data support Johnson's theory that violence and control are both important variables of interest in the study of IPV. Deconstructing the typology to examine men's and women's violence and control as continuous measures is an important step, as not all couples will fit neatly into the theorized categories (Johnson & Ferraro, 2000; Leone et al., 2004). As typologies and categorical representations of behavior decline in popularity within the behavioral sciences, some researchers have modified their own typologies to be less restrictive. Johnson's typology has undergone such a change, as the original typology, containing just two categories (IT and CCV), was broadened to include two additional categories (VR and MVC). Examining dimensionally the variables that compose typologies may prove to be a more parsimonious approach than adding additional categories. Moving away from the categorical nature of Johnson's theory also allows researchers to examine violence and control as independent predictors of behavior, as these variables are differentially related to several outcomes associated with IPV for men and women. Similarly, symmetry and severity of violence and control are unique predictors, suggesting that there is merit in considering the context of abuse within the relationship rather than examining violent men or women individually. These data also reveal that women as well as men perpetrate acts of violence and control, although the meaning and impact may be different by gender.

Limitations

A number of considerations limit the present study. First, the sample was prescreened using women's reports only of relationship dissatisfaction and men's violence. This may have limited the number of couples with an exclusively or severely violent woman. Screening procedures that assess both partners' IPV may be better suited to capture possible female intimate terrorists. While this sample included subjects engaging in a range of IPV and control, it is not a representative community sample nor is it generalizable to batterers arrested for IPV or victims recruited from shelters or social service agencies. Another limitation is that control was assessed using a measure designed to study male forms of emotionally abusive control tactics. Women's control tactics may differ. Future research is needed to investigate gender differences in control tactics. Additionally, as only women in the present sample completed the EAS (Murphy & Hoover, 1999), it was not possible to assess reporting biases by comparing men's and women's reports of control. As with all research on sensitive topics, such as IPV and control, there is the potential for subjects to present themselves in a favorable light while impugning their partners. Future studies may consider collecting collateral reports and assessment of impression management to further help to control for reporting biases.

Clinical Implications and Future Directions

The current findings support other studies of community samples of violent couples, suggesting that rates of IPV between men and women actually are quite similar (Malone, Tyree, & O'Leary, 1989; Straus & Gelles, 1986). Despite the fact that female-to-male IPV was not originally screened for, women were shown, on average, to be at least as violent as men. The presence of couples in which the woman was the sole perpetrator of physical abuse may refute claims that women's violence is simply enacted in self-defense. At the same time, the data support feminists' claims that intimate partner control should be a major target of intervention in the treatment of male batterers (e.g., Adams & Cayouette, 2002; Pence, 2002).

Control is thought to be more important than violence in differentiating CCV from IT (M. Johnson, personal communication, March 7, 2008), and women acknowledged engaging in at least as much controlling behavior as men. Furthermore, when held to the same standard, similar numbers of men and women in the current sample were highly controlling of their partners. Like men, the most highly controlling women were significantly more violent than their partners, according to the women's own reports. The use of control tactics also significantly predicted women's use of caustic relationship communication behaviors. While control is commonly a target in treating partner assaultive men, these data suggest that it should also be a treatment target for partner-violent women, and that IPV interventions should be available to both genders (see Tutty, Babins-Wagner, & Rothery, in press, for research on an available intervention for women). Finally, while men's IPV predicted his hostility in the lab, women's violence did not predict her observed behavior. This suggests gender differences in the meaning and context of violence and highlights the need for more research that goes beyond frequency counts of IPV to dig deeper into the meaning, context, and consequences of IPV perpetrated by women.

REFERENCES

Adams, D., & Cayouette, S. (2002). Emerge—A group education model for abusers. In E. Aldarondo & F. Mederos (Eds.), *Programs for men who batter: Intervention and prevention strategies in a diverse society* (pp. 4-1–4-32). Kingston, NJ: Civic Research Institute.

Archer, J. (2002). Sex differences in physically aggressive acts between heterosexual partners: A meta-analytic review. *Aggression & Violent Behavior, 7*(4), 313–351.

Babcock, J. C., Green, C. E., & Webb, S.A. (2008). Decoding deficits of different types of batterers during presentation of facial affect slides. *Journal of Family Violence, 23*(5), 295–302.

Babcock, J. C., Green, C. E., Webb, S. A., & Yerington, T. P. (2005). Psychophysiological profiles of batterers: Autonomic emotional reactivity as it predicts antisocial spectrum behavior among intimate partner abusers. *Journal of Abnormal Psychology, 11*, 445–455.

Babcock, J. C., Miller, S. A., & Siard, C. (2003). Toward a typology of abusive women: Differences between partner-only and generally violent women in the use of violence. *Psychology of Women Quarterly, 27*(2), 153–161.

Babcock, J. C., Roseman, A. C., Green, C. E., & Ross, J. M. (2008). Intimate partner abuse and PTSD symptomology: Examining mediators and moderators of the abuse-trauma link. *Journal of Family Psychology, 22*(6), 809–818.

Cordova, J. V., Jacobson, N. S., Gottman, J. M., Rushe, R., & Cox, G. (1993). Negative reciprocity and communication in couples with a violent husband. *Journal of Abnormal Psychology, 102*(4), 559–564.

Dobash, R. E., & Dobash, R. P. (1977–78). Wives: The 'appropriate' victims of marital violence. *Victimology, 2*(3–4), 426–442.

Dobash, R. P., Dobash, R. E., Cavanagh, K., & Lewis, R. (1998). Separate and intersecting realities: A comparison of men's and women's accounts of violence against women. *Violence Against Women, 4*(4), 382–415.

Dobash, R. P., Dobash, R. E., Wilson, M., & Daly, M. (1992). The myth of sexual symmetry in marital violence. *Social Problems, 39*(1), 71–91.

Goodwin, R. (1992). Overall, just how happy are you? The magical question 31 of the Spanier Dyadic Adjustment Scale. *Family Therapy, 19*, 273–275.

Gottman, J. M., McCoy, K., Coan, J., & Collier, H. (1996). The Specific Affect Coding System (SPAFF). In J. M. Gottman (Ed.), *What predicts divorce? The measures* (pp. 1–169). Mahwah, NJ: Lawrence Erlbaum.

Graham-Kevan, N. (2009). The psychology of women's partner violence: Characteristics and cautions. *Journal of Aggression, Maltreatment, & Trauma, 18*(6), 587–603.

Hamberger, L. K., & Potente, T. (1994). Counseling heterosexual women arrested for domestic violence: Implications for theory and practice. *Violence & Victims, 9*(2), 125–137.

Hamberger, L. K., Lohr, J. M., Bonge, D., & Tonlin, D. F. (1997). An empirical classification of motivations for domestic violence. *Violence Against Women, 3*(4), 401–423.

Hines, D. A., & Douglas, E. M. (2009). Women's use of intimate partner violence against men: Prevalence, implications, and consequences. *Journal of Aggression, Maltreatment & Trauma, 18*(6), 572–586.

Hooven, C., Rushe, R., & Gottman, J. M. (1996). The Play-by-Play Interview. In J. M. Gottman (Ed.), *What predicts divorce? The measures* (pp. PPIM-1–26). Mahwah, NJ: Lawrence Erlbaum.

Jablensky, A. (2005). Boundaries of mental disorders. *Current Opinion in Psychiatry, 18*, 653–658.

Jacobson, N. S., Gottman, J. M., Waltz, J., Rushe, R., Babcock, J.C., & Holtzworth-Munroe, A. (1994). Affect, verbal content, and psychophysiology in the arguments of couples with a violent husband. *Journal of Consulting and Clinical Psychology, 62*, 982–988.

Johnson, M. P. (1995). Patriarchal terrorism and common couple violence: Two forms of violence against women. *Journal of Marriage & the Family, 57*(2), 283–294.

Johnson, M. P. (2001). Conflict and control: Symmetry and asymmetry in domestic violence. In A. Booth, A. C. Crouter, & M. Clements (Eds.), *Couples in conflict* (pp. 95–104). Mahwah, NJ: Lawrence Erlbaum Associates.

Johnson, M. P., & Ferraro, K. J. (2000). Research on domestic violence in the 1990s: Making distinctions. *Journal of Marriage & the Family, 62*(4), 948–963.

Leisring, P. A. (in press). What will happen if I punch him? Expected consequences of female violence against male dating partners. *Journal of Aggression, Maltreatment, & Trauma.*

Leone, J. M., Johnson, M. P., & Cohan, C. L. (2004). Consequences of male partner violence for low-income minority women. *Journal of Marriage & Family, 66*(2), 472–490.

Long, J. (1998). *Video Coding System: Reference guide.* Caroga Lake, NY: James Long Co.

Malone, J., Tyree, A., & O'Leary, K. D. (1989). Generalization and containment: Different effects of past aggression for wives and husbands. *Journal of Marriage & the Family, 51*(3), 687–697.

Margolin, G., John, R. S., & Gleberman, L. (1988). Affective responses to conflictual discussions in violent and nonviolent couples. *Journal of Consulting & Clinical Psychology, 56*(1), 24–33.

Marshall, L. L. (1992). Development of the severity of violence against women scales. *Journal of Family Violence, 7*(2), 103–121.

McNeely, R. L., Cook, P. W., & Torres, J. B. (2001). Is domestic violence a gender issue or a human issue? *Journal of Human Behavior in the Social Environment, 4*(4), 227–251.

Melton, H. C., & Belknap, J. (2003). He hits, she hits: Assessing gender differences and similarities in officially reported intimate partner violence. *Criminal Justice & Behavior, 30*(3), 328–348.

Moffitt, T. E., Caspi, A., Krueger, R. F., Magdol, L, Margolin, G., Silva, P. A., et al. (1997). Do partners agree about abuse in their relationship? A psychometric evaluation of interpartner agreement. *Psychological Assessment, 9*, 47–56.

Morse, B. J. (1995). Beyond the Conflict Tactics Scale: Assessing gender differences in partner violence. *Violence & Victims, 10*(4), 251–272.

Muftic', L. R., Bouffard, J. A., & Bouffard, L. A. (2007). An exploratory study of women arrested for intimate partner violence: Violent Women or Violent Resistance. *Journal of Interpersonal Violence, 22*(6), 753–774.

Murphy, C., & Hoover, S. (1999). Measuring emotional abuse in dating relationships as a mulitfactorial construct. *Violence and Victims, 14*(1), 39–53.

Pence, E. (2002). The Duluth Domestic Abuse Intervention Project. In E. Aldarondo & F. Mederos (Eds.), *Programs for men who batter: Intervention and prevention strategies in a diverse society* (pp. 6-1–6-46). Kingston, NJ: Civic Research Institute.

Spanier, G. B. (1976). Measuring dyadic adjustment: New scales for assessing the quality of marriage and similar dyads. *Journal of Marriage and the Family, 38*, 15–28.

Straus, M. A. (1979). Measuring intrafamily conflict and violence: The Conflict Tactics (CT) Scales. *Journal of Marriage and the Family, 41*, 75–88.

Straus, M. A. (2009). Why the overwhelming evidence on partner physical violence by women has not been perceived and is often denied. *Journal of Aggression, Maltreatment, & Trauma, 18*(6), 552–571.

Straus, M. A., & Gelles, R. J. (1986). Societal change and change in family violence from 1975 to 1985 as revealed by two national surveys. *Journal of Marriage & Family, 48*, 465–479.

Straus, M. A., Hamby, S. L., Boney-McCoy, S., & Sugarman, D. B. (1996). The revised Conflict Tactics Scales (CTS2): Development and preliminary psychometric data. *Journal of Family Issues, 17*(3), 283–316.

Straus, M. A., Hamby, S. L., & Warren, W.L. (2003). *The Conflict Tactics Scales handbook*. Los Angeles, CA: Western Psychological Services.

Tutty, L. M., Babins-Wagner, R., & Rothery, M. A. (in press). Responsible choices for women: A treatment comparison of mandated and non-mandated aggressive women. *Journal of Aggression, Maltreatment, & Trauma*.

Widiger, T. A. (2005). A dimensional model of psychopathology. *Psychopathology, 38*, 211–214.

Yllö, K. A. (1993). Through a feminist lens: Gender, power, and violence. In R. J. Gelles & D. R. Loseke (Eds.), *Current controversies on family violence* (pp. 47–62). Newbury Park: Sage.

Gender Differences in Risk Factors for Intimate Partner Violence Recidivism

KRIS HENNING and ROCHELLE MARTINSSON

Portland State University, Portland, Oregon, USA

ROBERT HOLDFORD

Exchange Club Family Center, Memphis, Tennessee, USA

Risk assessment measures are increasingly used to evaluate offenders charged with intimate partner violence (IPV). Scales currently available for this purpose suffer from two important limitations: First, several well-established risk factors from research with general offenders are excluded from most IPV scales, including age, deviant peer associations, and antisocial attitudes. Further research is needed to determine whether these factors should be included in the next generation of IPV risk measures. Second, all of the existing scales have been validated solely for use with males despite increased arrests among women. This study sought to investigate both of these issues using a large sample of male and female IPV offenders. The results highlight gender differences in risk factors for recidivism.

In the 1970s, family violence researchers and victim advocates began exposing long-standing biases in the U.S. criminal justice system that minimized the seriousness of intimate partner violence (IPV) and its impact on victims (Fagan, 1996). Many of those involved in this movement successfully lobbied to expand the criminalization of this behavior, hoping that such actions would contribute to broader social change and reduce the likelihood of recidivism on the part of individual offenders. One outcome of the resulting policy changes has been a dramatic increase in the number of cases entering the criminal justice system (Hirschel & Buzawa, 2002). Increases like these present a serious challenge to most jurisdictions, because resources allocated to the management of these offenders have rarely expanded to the same degree. In response to rising caseloads, some jurisdictions have begun to use formal risk assessment scales to classify IPV offenders based on their risk for recidivism or dangerousness, a practice that is common in managing other offender populations. However, there are a couple of important limitations with existing IPV risk scales that merit further discussion and are addressed in the present study.

Consideration of an offender's dangerousness and likelihood for recidivism has always played an important role in the decision-making of criminal justice professionals. Police officers are more likely to arrest suspects who they believe are dangerous, prosecutors pursue charges against defendants who they feel will recidivate, and judges consider risk when determining sentences (Steffensmeier & Demuth, 2000; Vigorita, 2003). Until fairly recently, most of these assessments were unstructured and based largely on professional opinion. This is concerning, as major flaws have been identified with this type of subjective risk assessment (Quinsey, Harris, Rice, & Cormier, 1998). One problem is that decision-makers are often acutely concerned with false negatives, or underestimating someone's risk for recidivism and failing to take appropriate action to prevent further offenses (Cunningham & Reidy, 1999). As a result, assessments based solely on professional opinion often overestimate risk for offenders, leading to unnecessarily severe sanctions and increased caseloads and expenditures. A second concern involves the poor reliability of these informal decisions: different raters often come to very different conclusions regarding an individual's risk for recidivism. Finally, the most significant challenge for professional judgments is that they offer limited improvement in predicting recidivism beyond what could be expected by chance alone (Grove & Meehl, 1996).

Not surprisingly given its limitations, the past few decades have seen a movement away from sole reliance on professional judgment, particularly in correctional practice with general, mentally ill, and sexual offenders. Taking its place are structured decision-making guides and actuarial risk instruments like the Level of Service Inventory-Revised (LSI-R; Andrews & Bonta, 1995), Historical, Clinical, and Risk Management-20 (HCR-20; Webster, Douglas, Eaves, & Hart, 1997), and the Violence Risk Appraisal Guide (VRAG; Quinsey et al., 1998), scales that are based on empirical research. Most of the items comprising these scales have been repeatedly validated as predictors of reoffending (e.g., Bonta, Law, & Hanson, 1998; Hanson & Bussiere, 1998). Static risk factors for violent recidivism, or characteristics that cannot be changed through intervention, include an offender's current age, severity of juvenile and adult criminal behavior, and family history (e.g., parental criminality, child abuse, broken home). Dynamic risk factors, or characteristics that can be impacted through intervention, include delinquent peer associations, cognitive functioning, antisocial attitudes, alcohol and drug abuse, personality functioning, and social achievement (e.g., marital status, education, employment). Studies suggest that structured clinical scales and actuarial measures using factors such as these are considerably more reliable and accurate in predicting recidivism than professional opinion (Andrews, Bonta, & Wormith, 2006; Grove & Meehl, 1996; Hanson & Bussiere, 1998). Using these scales allows practitioners to classify offenders more efficiently and assign individuals to appropriate supervision levels. Attention to varying risk levels is also consistent with current best practices in offender rehabilitation. Andrews and colleagues (Andrews, Bonta, & Hoge, 1990; Andrews & Dowden, 2006) have demonstrated that correctional interventions are most effective when they are provided to high-risk offenders and when the treatment attempts to modify dynamic risk factors.

Despite decades of advancement in risk assessment with general, mentally ill, and sexual offenders, comparatively little research has been done to develop and validate risk scales for those who engage in IPV (Kropp, 2004). Delays in the development of IPV risk scales may be due in part to the unique history of this offense within our criminal justice system. Prior to the 1980s, law enforcement officers, prosecutors, and judges were granted a significant degree of autonomy in deciding how to handle domestic conflicts. Because many criminal justice professionals considered IPV to be a less serious crime, very few perpetrators were ever arrested or prosecuted (Sherman, 1992). As such, there was little need for risk assessment scales to use in managing this population.

A combination of increased victim advocacy, pending lawsuits, and research highlighting the harms of IPV led states and local municipalities to enact new policies throughout the 1980s and 1990s that served to criminalize IPV (Fagan, 1996). Many of these policies either removed or limited the discretionary powers of criminal justice agents when it came to handling physical assaults between intimates. Police were now required to arrest a suspect if an assault occurred, prosecutors were trained to proceed with litigation aggressively regardless of whether the victim cooperated, and offenders were ordered to attend batterer intervention programs, the content and length of which were increasingly regulated by state law (Holtzworth-Munroe, 2002). Within this new system, minimal regard was paid to varying levels of risk; instead, most IPV offenders were treated alike once prosecuted.

The predominant theory used to explain IPV during this time may also have contributed to the one-size-fits-all approach that has developed in many jurisdictions (Corvo & Johnson, 2003; Dutton & Corvo, 2006). Feminist scholars have argued that IPV is the result of broader socialization condoning men's use of abusive tactics to maintain power in their intimate relationships (Pence & Paymar, 1993). Given that all men were traditionally believed to be subject to the same socialization forces, it stood to reason that everyone arrested for IPV needed the same intervention. Further, because IPV was seen as distinct from general offending, minimal efforts were made during this earlier period to draw upon the broader rehabilitation literature, work that was increasingly emphasizing the need to differentiate offenders based on their risk for recidivism (e.g., Andrews et al., 1990).

Only in the past decade has there been a noticeable increase in efforts to validate and implement risk assessment tools for use with IPV offenders. There are several good reasons to support continued work in this area. First, as mentioned previously, IPV caseloads at all stages of the criminal justice system expanded dramatically following the implementation of mandatory arrest laws (Hirschel & Buzawa, 2002). In the context of stable or, in some cases, diminishing resources for handling these cases, it has become necessary in some communities to prioritize cases in some meaningful way (Roehl & Guertin, 2000). Based on the broader risk assessment literature, it is unlikely that informal professional judgments will be a productive means for achieving this end (Quinsey et al., 1998). Second, IPV recidivism rates are high, ranging from one quarter to one half of offenders when measured using official reports (Gondolf, 1997; Grann & Wedin, 2002; Renauer & Henning, 2005). While a 50% recidivism rate is certainly not desirable, it does provide a unique statistical advantage that has the potential to make risk assessment more useful in this area (Dutton & Kropp, 2000). In contrast to most other violent crimes, the likely victim of an IPV offender's next offense is also already known. This provides a unique opportunity for the criminal justice system to enact measures to prevent the reoccurrence of violence.

The intimate nature of the relationship between victim and offender in IPV cases presents a third justification for continued efforts to develop risk scales. Unlike victims of extrafamilial assaults, IPV victims have extensive knowledge of their attacker, some of which could be particularly useful in predicting recidivism (Dutton & Kropp, 2000). Indeed, studies have already shown that IPV victims have some skill in determining whether their spouse/partner will recidivate (Cattaneo, Bell, Goodman, & Dutton, 2007; Heckert & Gondolf, 2004; Weisz, Tolman, & Saunders, 2000). A final and perhaps the most important reason to continue our efforts to develop risk scales for IPV is the high potential for psychological trauma, physical injury, and death from this crime (Campbell, Glass, Sharps, Laughon, & Bloom, 2007; Golding, 1999) and the significant impact of interparental violence on child witnesses (Kitzman, Gaylord, Holt & Kenny, 2003).

At least four IPV-specific risk scales are found in the literature with sufficient support for their validity to merit discussion here. The Spousal Assault Risk Assessment (SARA; Kropp, Hart, Webster, & Eaves, 1995) is a 20-item guide that includes both dynamic and static factors that are rated by a trained mental health clinician. Several studies have demonstrated the reliability and validity of the scale (Grann & Wedin, 2002; Hilton, Harris, Rice, Lang, Cormier, & Lines, 2004; Kropp & Hart, 2000; Williams & Houghton, 2004). The Ontario Domestic Violence Risk Assessment (ODARA; Hilton et al., 2004) consists of 13 dichotomous items that can be rated easily by law enforcement officers. In contrast to the SARA, whose items were identified from the literature, the ODARA was developed and cross-validated using purely statistical methods. The resulting actuarial scale has demonstrated strong concurrent and predictive validity. The third measure, the Domestic Violence Screening Instrument (DVSI; Williams & Houghton, 2004) consists of 12 items that are answered using criminal justice records available to most law enforcement and correctional agencies. While the scale's predictive validity may not be as good as the ODARA, some agencies may find the items on the DVSI easier to rate using existing data sources. Finally, the 15-item Danger Assessment (DA; Campbell, 1995) is perhaps the most widely used IPV risk scale.[1] In contrast to the other three measures, the DA is completed directly by victims. The reliability and validity of the scale has been independently verified in several studies (Goodman, Dutton, & Bennett, 1999; Heckert & Gondolf, 2004; Weisz et al., 2000).

While an exhaustive review of the strengths and weaknesses of these four scales is beyond the scope of this article, there are two limitations that are central to the current study. As in the case of treatment programs for this offense, much of the IPV risk assessment research and scale development has occurred in isolation, with minimal reference to the larger body of literature on general offenders. This pattern may be changing, however, with several recent studies raising the question of whether specialized scales are even required for IPV. Two studies have found that the LSI-R, a scale commonly used with general offenders, accurately predicts recidivism by IPV offenders (Girard & Wormith, 2004; Hanson & Wallace-Capretta, 2004). Hilton, Harris, and Rice (2001) observed a similar finding when they used the VRAG to predict recidivism in a sample of 88 men with a history of severe wife battering. Unfortunately, none of these studies focused specifically on IPV recidivism; instead, any type of subsequent violence was coded as reoffending. Additional research is needed to determine whether risk factors from the general offender literature might be useful in predicting IPV recidivism. The present study examined five such factors, including age, antisocial attitudes, delinquent peer associations, IQ, and childhood conduct problems (Bonta et al., 1998; Hanson & Bussiere, 1998).

A second limitation of the currently available IPV risk assessment scales is that all have been validated solely for use with male offenders. While research on female recidivism in general lags far behind that seen with males (Jones & Sims, 1997), there has been even less effort to study recidivism by

---

[1]   A more recent version of this scale that includes 20 items is now available (Campbell et. al., 2003).

female IPV offenders. This issue has become increasingly important over the past decade with the dramatic rise observed in female IPV arrests following the implementation of mandatory arrest laws (Chesney-Lind, 2002; Steffensmeier, Zhong, Ackerman, Schwartz, & Agha, 2006). Women now account for up to one in five arrests in some jurisdictions (Henning & Feder, 2004; Miller, 2001) and yet only three published studies have addressed their recidivism. Wooldredge and Thistlethwaite (2002) compared male and female IPV offenders and found that men were significantly more likely to recidivate. Renauer and Henning (2005) obtained similar findings: female suspects in samples from two demographically dissimilar cities were half as likely to recidivate compared to males. The women were twice as likely, however, to show up in subsequent reports as the victim of domestic violence. These two studies contrast with a third study by Muftic and Bouffard (2007), who observed similar rates of IPV recidivism across gender.

Whether the same factors that predict recidivism for male IPV offenders work with female offenders is examined in the present study. Two distinct possibilities regarding the results emerge from the broader literature on women's use of aggression in intimate relationships. First, it has been argued that women use aggression largely for defensive purposes and that the recent increase in IPV arrests has resulted from inadequate efforts on the part of police officers to properly identify the primary aggressor in domestic conflicts (Miller, 2001). If this were true, then women's prior criminal histories, psychological functioning, childhood conduct, etc., should not predict later offenses to the same degree observed with males. Another group of family violence scholars believes that women not only perpetrate violence in intimate relationships at the same rate as men, but that the factors contributing to their aggression are similar (Dutton & Corvo, 2006; Dutton & Nicholls, 2005; Ross & Babcock, 2009). Extrapolating from this position, it could be hypothesized that the risk factors predicting recidivism among male IPV offenders should work equally well for women. One factor complicating the testing of these alternative hypotheses is the potential for bias in IPV recidivism data. Dutton and Nicholls (2005) have argued that police officers are commonly trained to think of IPV as a male-perpetrated offense, resulting in higher arrest rates for men, even in situations in which the female partner was the primary aggressor. To address this potential bias, two forms of "recidivism" were examined in the present study: recidivism as a suspect and recidivism as a victim.

METHODS

Participants

The sample for the present study consisted of 2,854 men and 353 women convicted of an IPV offense involving a heterosexual intimate partner. These offenders ranged in age from 18 to 70, with an average age of 32.7

(*SD* = 9.3). The majority of the participants were African American (84.1%), followed by Caucasian (13.4%), Hispanic (1.8%), and "other" racial groups (.8%). Slightly more than one third of the participants (35.5%) never graduated from high school and 44.0% were either unemployed or working less than full time. A majority (63.5%) had been arrested for assaulting a dating partner as opposed to a spouse (36.5%).

Procedure

Cases included in the sample and data on all of the risk factors considered were extracted from a database maintained at a centralized Domestic Violence Assessment Center (DVAC) in a large southern city. The local domestic violence court requires individuals convicted of IPV and sentenced to probation to complete a comprehensive assessment through the DVAC. Court personnel schedule the offenders to attend an evaluation session, which begins with a brief reading screen and review of the center's informed consent. Participants are then escorted to a large group room where they complete paper-and-pencil tests under the supervision of DVAC staff. The offenders also participate in a 30- to 60-minute clinical interview with a counselor. The DVAC staff then score all of the measures used during the evaluation, enter the data into computer database, and generate a report for the court. The individuals included in the present sample were all evaluated between January 1999 and December 2001.

Recidivism data were obtained from a local police database containing all domestic violence reports for the region from January 1999 through December 2002. For each person in the sample, subsequent reports were located in which the individual was identified as the suspect (including dual arrest cases) in a new incident, regardless of whether an arrest was made or whether the victim was the same person from the index offense. The dichotomous recidivism variable created based on these searches was labeled *recidivated as a suspect*. A second dichotomous "recidivism" variable was created to reflect whether a subject *recidivated as a victim*. In these cases, the offender from the original index offense was listed as the victim in at least one subsequent DV police report. Follow-up times in the study ranged from 54 to 207 weeks and did not vary as a function of gender ($F[1, 3205] = .01$, *ns*).

Measures

A total of 17 risk factors previously linked to either IPV or general recidivism were examined in the present study. The factors were grouped into five distinct categories as described below.

Demographic

Available demographic factors collected at the time of the DVAC assessment included current age, education, and employment status. Age was considered a continuous variable in some analyses and dichotomized in others based on a median split (18–30 vs. 31+). The education variable contrasted those who earned a high school diploma or a GED with those who failed to complete high school. Current employment status was also dichotomized, with full-time employees compared to those who were unemployed or working just part time.

Relational

Two variables addressed characteristics of the relationship between the offenders and their victim from the index offense. The type of relationship with the victim was coded as either married or dating. A second dichotomous variable, prior IPV, indicated whether offenders had ever assaulted their intimate partner prior to the index offense. Local criminal records, victim reports, and the offenders' self-reported information were used to code this variable.

Childhood history

Two aspects of the participants' early history were considered as risk factors in the present study. A total family adversity score, ranging from 0 to 5, was calculated by combining five dichotomous items, including parental separation or divorce during childhood, parental incarceration, parental substance abuse, exposure to interparental violence, and child abuse. The first three items of the scale were based on single questions addressed to the participants during the intake assessment (e.g., "Did either of your parents or caregivers ever spend time in prison during your childhood [under age 16]?"). Childhood exposure to interparental violence was assessed using the 9-item Physical Aggression subscale of the Conflict Tactics Scale (CTS; Straus, 1990). Respondents indicated whether or not they had ever witnessed as a child their parents committing certain acts of violence toward each other. Childhood physical abuse was assessed using the child abuse version of the CTS (CTS-PC; Straus, Hamby, Finkelhor, Moore, & Runyan, 1998). Seven of the 13 items on this scale reflect severe actions that parents use in disciplining their children that are typically considered abusive (e.g., burning or scalding, grabbing by the neck and choking). Respondents who admitted having experienced any of these acts were considered to have been physically abused.

The second measure assessing the offenders' self-reported childhood history involved a conduct disorder scale. The total score for each offender was determined by summing eight dichotomously coded items characteristic of conduct disorder as defined in the *Diagnostic and Statistical Manual of Mental Disorders-IV* (*DSM-IV*; American Psychiatric Association [APA], 1994). This includes physical fighting (e.g., "Did you get into physical fights as a kid [under age 16]?"), suspension from school (e.g., "Were you ever suspended or expelled from school?"), stealing things, damaging or vandalizing property, breaking curfew, early alcohol and/or drug use, being arrested as a juvenile, and running away. The scale had moderate internal consistency (Cronbach's α = .68).

PSYCHOLOGICAL FUNCTIONING

Six measures of the offenders' psychological functioning were tested as predictors of recidivism. First, antisocial attitudes were assessed using a slightly modified version of the Criminal Sentiments Scale (CSS; Simourd, 1997).The CSS is a 41-item self-report scale that measures deviant attitudes in three general areas: (a) attitudes about the law, courts and police; (b) tolerance of law violations; and (c) identification with criminal others. For the present study, the original 5-point Likert scale was changed to include just three response choices, *Agree*, *Undecided*, and *Disagree*. Total scores on the CSS ranged from 0 to 82, and prior research suggests that the scale has good psychometric properties (Simourd, 1997; Simourd & van de Ven, 1999).

Four psychological characteristics were assessed using the Millon Clinical Multiaxial Inventory-III (MCMI-III; Millon, 1994). The MCMI-III is the most commonly used measure of personality and clinical functioning in recent studies with IPV offenders (Gondolf, 1999). It consists of 175 true-false questions that yield four validity scales, 14 personality scales (Axis II, *DSM-IV*), and 10 clinical syndrome scales (Axis I) that largely reflect the diagnostic criteria established for these disorders in the *DSM-IV* (APA, 1994). Scales assessing the two personality disorders most commonly linked to general criminal recidivism and domestic violence (Dutton, 2007), antisocial personality and borderline personality, were included in the present study. Two additional scales from the MCMI-III assessed for the presence of alcohol and drug dependence. It should also be noted that the MCMI-IIIs were only available on a subset of the larger sample (*n* = 1,391) as a consequence of the elimination of this scale in later DVAC evaluations due to time constraints. Profiles that were deemed invalid using the MCMI-III's validity scale (8.1%) were also excluded.

A final measure of psychological functioning assessed the offenders' current intellectual ability. The Shipley Institute for Living Scale (SILS; Zachary, 1986), a commonly used screening instrument consisting of 60 items, evaluates intellectual functioning across two dimensions: vocabulary and abstraction. Total SILS scores were converted to Wechsler Adult Intelligence

Scale-Revised (WAIS-R; Wechsler, 1981) full-scale IQ scores as directed in the scoring manual. Because the SILS is a self-administered paper-and-pencil measure that requires some degree of reading ability, it was not administered to clients who failed an initial reading screen (13.5%).

CRIMINAL HISTORY

Four dichotomous variables were available to describe the offenders' history of antisocial activity and peer relations. Each of the first three variables, extrafamilial violence, nonviolent offense, and probation/parole violation, was coded using a combination of self-report and county-level arrest records. If either source indicated a prior offense of that nature, the variable was coded affirmatively. The fourth variable, delinquent peer associations, was based solely on self-report in response to the following question: "Have any of your friends ever been arrested?"

RESULTS

Table 1 provides descriptive information for the risk factors coded in the present study and a comparison of these factors across gender. Male offenders, in comparison to their female counterparts, were significantly more likely to evidence a history of childhood conduct problems and adult antisocial behavior, including prior violence against intimate partners and nonfamily members. Female offenders were younger on average, less likely to be employed full time, and had experienced more family adversity during childhood. Table 1 also provides details on the recidivism of these men and women. Male IPV offenders were twice as likely to recidivate as a suspect in a new DV offense (28.2% vs. 15.3%, $\chi^2[1, N = 3,207] = 26.8$, $p < .001$), whereas female offenders were more than five times as likely to be the victim in a subsequent DV report (23.5% vs. 4.3%, $\chi^2[1, N = 3,207] = 192.7$, $p < .001$).

Correlations between the given risk factors and recidivism as a suspect are presented separately for each gender in Table 2. All of the risk factors were found to be significantly correlated ($p < .001$) with recidivism for the male IPV offenders and the direction of the correlations was as expected given the prior research in this area. The overall strength of the correlations was low, ranging from a low of $r = .07$ (prior IPV) to a high of $r = -.16$ (age); however, this is largely consistent with other studies attempting to predict DV recidivism (Hanson & Wallace-Capretta, 2004; Hilton et al., 2004; Williams & Houghton, 2004).

By contrast, only a few of the risk factors were significantly associated with recidivism as a suspect for the female offenders. Women with less education, those who were underemployed, and those with less childhood

TABLE 1 Gender Differences in Risk Factors and Recidivism of Male and Female Intimate Partner Violence (IPV) Offenders

Variables & N (men/women)	Men % or M (SD)	Women % or M (SD)	F or $\chi 2$
Demographic			
Age (2854/353)	32.8 (9.4)	31.6 (8.7)	5.4*
Did not complete high school (2852/351)	35.6%	35.0%	.0
Employed < full-time (2848/351)	42.2%	58.4%	33.1***
Relational			
Dating relationship (2851/353)	63.5%	63.7%	.0
Prior IPV (2012/227)	89.1%	81.1%	12.6***
Childhood history			
Family adversity (2854/353)	1.4 (1.2)	1.5 (1.2)	4.0*
Conduct disorder (1722/205)	1.8 (1.7)	1.3 (1.6)	18.8***
Psychological functioning			
Criminal sentiments (2061/267)	21.7 (11.9)	19.1 (10.1)	12.0***
MCMI-III antisocial (1262/122)	41.4 (22.8)	43.3 (23.1)	.8
MCMI-III borderline (1260/122)	32.6 (26.5)	32.9 (29.3)	.0
MCMI-III alcohol dependent (1262/122)	44.4 (26.0)	50.3 (23.0)	6.0*
MCMI-III drug dependent (1262/122)	40.9 (22.0)	44.7 (24.8)	3.2
Estimated WAIS-r IQ (2440/333)	84.5 (12.9)	86.0 (12.2)	3.7
Criminal history			
Extrafamilial violence (2534/309)	30.7%	15.5%	30.7***
Nonviolent offense (2661/319)	75.7%	44.2%	141.5***
Probation violation (2537/312)	35.4%	10.9%	75.8***
Delinquent peer association (1690/201)	62.3%	29.4%	80.5***
Recidivism			
As a suspect (2854/353)	28.2%	15.3%	26.8***
As a victim (2854/353)	4.3%	23.5%	192.7***

*$p < .05$, **$p < .01$, ***$p < .001$.

adversity were more likely to recidivate. While the lower number of significant correlations for women results in part from the difference in sample sizes, it is worth noting that the direction of the correlations was actually reversed on some variables. Men in dating relationships, as opposed to being married, were more likely to recidivate ($r = .08$), while women in dating relationships were less likely to recidivate ($r = -.09$). Men with more childhood family adversity were at greater risk to recidivate ($r = .08$), whereas women were more likely to recidivate when they had fewer family problems in childhood ($r = -.15$). Finally, men who scored higher on the MCMI-III Borderline Personality scale recidivated more frequently ($r = .09$), while women scoring higher on this scale were less likely to commit another DV offense ($r = -.09$).

Fisher's Z-test was used to determine whether the size of the correlations between the risk factors and recidivism differed as a function of gender. It should be noted that Fisher's Z-test is influenced by the overall magnitude of the correlations under examination. An absolute difference of .10 with weak correlations (e.g., men $r = .10$, women $r = .20$) is less

TABLE 2 Correlations Between Risk Factors and Recidivism by Gender of Suspect

Risk factors	Recidivated as suspect			Recidivated as victim		
	Men	Women	Z-test	Men	Women	Z-test
Demographic						
Age	−.16***	−.01	−2.65**	−.01	−.10	1.52
Did not complete high school	.10***	.12*	−.36	.01	.09	−1.41
Employed < full-time	.11***	.10*	.10	.01	−.01	.24
Relational						
Dating relationship	.08***	−.09	2.93**	.03	.11*	−1.56
Prior IPV	.07***	.10	−.43	.04	.05	−.09
Childhood history						
Family adversity	.08***	−.15**	4.00**	.02	−.01	.38
Conduct disorder	.12***	.10	.32	.03	.08	−.66
Psychological functioning						
Criminal sentiments	.12***	.01	1.74	−.01	.00	−.12
MCMI-III antisocial	.11***	.00	1.10	.00	.15	−1.51
MCMI-III borderline	.09***	−.09	1.84	.00	.08	−.86
MCMI-III alcohol dependent	.11***	.10	.07	.03	.19*	−1.79
MCMI-III drug dependent	.10***	.03	.79	.01	.19*	−1.91
Estimated WAIS-r IQ	−.09***	−.03	−1.00	.00	−.19***	3.25*
Criminal history						
Extrafamilial violence	.12***	.09	.50	.00	−.01	.17
Nonviolent offenses	.10***	.06	.68	−.01	.04	−.91
Probation/parole violations	.11***	.03	1.34	.00	.03	−.35
Delinquent peer association	.09***	.03	.72	.04	.08	−.47

*$p < .05$, **$p < .01$, ***$p < .001$.

Note: Sample sizes vary by comparison (see Table 1).

likely to exceed the critical value for the Z-statistic (≥ 1.96) than would a similar difference with stronger correlations (e.g., men $r = .70$, women $r = .80$). Despite this limitation, three correlations were found to significantly differ between the men and women: age, relationship type, and family adversity.

Additional analyses were conducted to assess the combined utility of the given risk factors in predicting the recidivism of these male and female offenders. The following steps were taken to create a total risk scale for use in these analyses. First, the four MCMI-III scales were excluded due to the significantly lower sample size resulting from the discontinuation of this scale in later assessments. Second, the five remaining continuous items were dichotomized based on either a median split (age [31+ vs. 18–30], childhood adversity [<2 events vs. 2+], conduct problems [<2 behaviors vs. 2+], and CSS [<20 vs. 20+]) or the scale's established breakpoint (estimated WAIS-r IQ [low average or above vs. borderline or below]). Third, the coding direction of the resulting 13 dichotomous items was determined based on the correlations observed with the male offenders. A "1" indicated the presence of the risk factor (i.e., increased risk of recidivism) and "0" was used to indicate its absence. Finally, a prorated total score was computed for all cases where at least 10 of the 13 risk factors were valid (2,311 men and 290 women).

Scores on the risk scale ranged from 0 to 13 for both males and females; however, men as a group scored higher on the scale than women ($M = 6.5$, $SD = 2.6$ vs. $M = 5.6$, $SD = 2.4$; $F[1, 2,599] = 35.8$, $p < .001$). The scale reliably predicted recidivism as a suspect for the men ($r = .23$, $p < .001$) but not for the women ($r = .03$, $p = ns$), and the resulting correlations differed significantly by gender (Fisher's Z = 3.25, $p < .01$). Gender-specific receiver operating curves (ROC) were also created to evaluate the predictive utility of the risk scale. ROC has become a standard analytic tool in the validation of risk assessment scales (Rice & Harris, 1995; Swets, Dawes, & Monahan, 2000; Williams & Houghton, 2004). It yields a statistic, the area under the curve (AUC), which measures the accuracy of prediction across all possible cutoff points. An AUC of .50 indicates that the scale does no better than chance in predicting the given outcome. Sample AUCs in the prediction of DV recidivism include .61 for the DVSI (Williams & Houghton, 2004), .72 for the ODARA (Hilton et al., 2004), and .70 for the DA (Heckert & Gondolf, 2004). The current scale produced an AUC for men of .65, which suggests a significant improvement in predicting recidivism as compared to chance alone ($p < .001$). By contrast, the scale was not a good predictor of recidivism for the women (AUC = .53, ns).

One limitation of the previous analyses is that police officers may be biased toward listing men as the suspect in DV reports involving intimate partners (e.g., Dutton & Corvo, 2006; Dutton & Nicholls, 2005). To test this hypothesis, we used the same analytic approach detailed above for recidivism as a suspect, only this time we sought to predict whether the offenders show up in later DV police reports as a victim. As previously noted, women were roughly five times more likely to recidivate as a victim as compared to males (23.5% vs. 4.3%).

Table 2 presents the results of bivariate correlations between recidivism as a victim and the 17 risk factors considered. Not a single factor was reliably correlated with this type of recidivism among men. Recidivism as a victim was more likely for women when they were in a dating relationship ($r = .11$, $p < .05$), when they scored higher on scales assessing alcohol ($r = .19$, $p < .05$) and drug problems ($r = .19$, $p < .05$), and when they had a lower estimated WAIS-r IQ ($r = -.19$, $p < .001$). Despite these four significant correlations, the utility of the combined risk scale in predicting women's recidivism as a victim was very poor ($r = .06$ and AUC = .56, $p = ns$). Similar results were found for the men ($r = .01$ and AUC = .51, $p = ns$).

DISCUSSION

Before discussing the findings from the present study, it may be useful to review the different perspectives that have emerged regarding the prevalence and nature of relationship violence committed by men and women that may result in their arrest. On one side of this debate are those who argue that women use violence less often than men in intimate relationships, and when they do act aggressively, it is primarily for defensive purposes (Miller, 2001; Saunders, 2002). Differentiating defensive from offensive actions may not always be easy for law enforcement officers, however, resulting in increasing numbers of women being arrested for IPV following the implementation of mandatory arrest laws (Chesney-Lind, 2002).

On the other side of the debate are those who believe that women perpetrate as much (or more) physical aggression in relationships as men. Additionally, the motivations for women's use of violence and the factors that contribute to their aggression are believed to be the same. Dutton and colleagues (Dutton & Corvo, 2006; Dutton & Nicholls, 2005) have provided considerable evidence regarding the equivalency of physical aggression rates in community samples. Dutton and Nicholls (2005) have also argued that the historical gender imbalance observed in criminal justice samples, namely higher numbers of men arrested, results from biases in the criminal justice system that lead to women's violence being disregarded. Presumably, the recent increases in female IPV arrests might be viewed as evidence that the system is becoming more neutral with respect to gender.

The results of the present study addressed three questions that are pertinent to this ongoing discussion. First, who is more likely to recidivate with a new domestic violence offense, male or female IPV offenders? Second, are there gender differences among IPV offenders in the prevalence of violence risk factors that have been identified in the literature? Third, are the factors that predict IPV recidivism the same for men and women? Starting with the first question, we found that women who had been convicted of IPV were half as likely to recidivate with a new domestic violence offense as compared to male offenders (15% vs. 28%). This finding is consistent with two other published studies addressing this issue (Renauer & Henning,[2] 2005; Wooldredge & Thistlethwaite, 2002). Similar to Renauer and Henning (2005), women in the present study were also significantly more likely than men to show up as the victim in subsequent domestic violence reports (24% vs. 4%).

Analyses addressing the second question, whether male and female IPV offenders differ on violence risk factors, also revealed clear gender differences. Women, as compared to the men, were younger, less likely to be employed full time, and came from family backgrounds marked by greater discord. Based on prior research with men at least, these factors would presumably increase their risk for recidivism (Quinsey et al., 1998).

---

[2]   It is possible that a small number of cases from Renauer and Henning's (2005) study were present in the current sample.

Male offenders, on the other hand, were significantly more likely to have previously assaulted an intimate partner, they had greater conduct problems during childhood, more extensive violent and nonviolent criminal histories, probation/parole violations, more deviant attitudes, and antisocial peer associations, all factors that could contribute to higher recidivism. Overall, these findings are consistent with those reported by Henning and Feder[3] (2004), who concluded that male IPV offenders as a group appear to have criminal histories and indices of psychological functioning that are more consistent with the use of violence.

To our knowledge, the present study is the first published report to evaluate the third question: are there gender differences in risk factors for IPV recidivism? In the broader offender literature, there seems to be some consensus that women are less likely to recidivate than men (Harer & Langan, 2001; Jones & Sims, 1997). There is less agreement as to whether the factors that predict general recidivism are the same for men and women. Several studies suggest female recidivism is best predicted by a distinct set of factors (Bonta, Pang, & Wallace-Capretta, 1995; de Vogel & de Ruiter, 2005) while other reports find that risk scales developed for use with men work equally well for women (Folsom & Atkinson, 2007; Harer & Langan, 2001). Analyses addressing this issue in the present study lend support to the former position. Very few of the risk factors that predicted recidivism for male offenders worked to predict recidivism for women, and in some cases the correlations were in the opposite direction (e.g., type of relationship to victim, childhood adversity). A second set of analyses addressed the possibility of bias on the part of police officers: perhaps many of the female offenders reoffended against their spouse/partner but officers listed them as the victim rather than offender. Once again, however, our ability to predict this type of recidivism for women was severely limited.

At least initially, these results appear to support those who argue that women use aggression for different reasons than men and that some women are being arrested for acts of self-defense. Female victims who are erroneously arrested would be less likely to recidivate as offenders and more likely to show up later as victims, they would be less likely to have criminal histories consistent with the use of violence, and their characteristics would be poor predictors of reoffending, all of which was observed in the present findings at the aggregate level. Nevertheless, some of the women in the sample did reoffend (15%) and some had a history of extrafamilial criminal involvement, including violence (16%), nonviolent offenses (44%), probation violations (11%), and delinquent peer associations (29%). It seems most likely, therefore, that the women arrested for IPV represent a

---

[3] Some of the cases used in Henning and Feder's (2004) study may also have been included in the present sample.

heterogeneous group. Some women are likely victims who are arrested for acts of self-defense. Other women may have responded to a situational conflict in a way that was largely inconsistent with their prior history and were arrested for it. As demonstrated in other studies (Conradi, Geffner, Hamberger, & Lawson, in press; Henning, Renauer, & Holdford, 2006; Ross & Babcock, 2009), a third subset of women are likely the primary aggressor in their relationship or equally aggressive as their spouse/partner. While the recidivism rates of these types of cases would conceivably differ, the factors that might account for this variation unfortunately were not clearly identified in the present study.

Several recommendations regarding IPV risk assessment with women result from these findings. Perhaps most important, these data raise serious concerns about the utility of using available risk scales with female IPV offenders (e.g., ODARA, DAS, SARA, DVSI). Many of the items on these scales were tested in the present study and were unrelated to recidivism by women, or in some cases they worked in the opposite direction compared to men. This could lead to an incorrect assessment of a woman's risk to reoffend and the actions taken, or not taken, to prevent this could be harmful (e.g., loss of custody over children, fines, incarceration). At the same time, failing to use validated measures in the case of female offenders is also problematic. In the absence of an objective guide, criminal justice agents tend to overpredict dangerousness, potentially leading to more severe sanctions for women than is warranted.

Efforts thus need to be taken to develop and validate tailored risk assessment scales for female IPV offenders. As for the items to include on these measures, the results of the present study suggest that new areas need to be considered. One direction to explore is the characteristics of these women's intimate partners (e.g., Swan & Snow, 2006). Women in relationships with men demonstrating a high-risk profile (e.g., younger, extensive criminal history, early conduct problems, personality disorder, antisocial peers and attitudes) may be at increased risk for later conflicts that lead to their arrest and/or victimization. Similarities between the women's characteristics and the men's might also be important, as in the case of when both partners are abusing substances. In the present study, women's alcohol and drug use were significant predictors of later victimization. Relationship conflicts may be further compounded when both partners are abusing substances, increasing the risk for both victimization and perpetration. Finally, a broader range of relationship factors needs to be examined, including indicators of instability (e.g., prior separations, infidelity, marital dissatisfaction), jealousy, communication skills deficits, and the presence of children. For example, Campbell et al. (2007) found that having stepchildren in the home raises the risk for lethal assaults against women. Perhaps there are other child-related issues that increase a woman's risk to reoffend against her spouse/partner.

In creating and applying new gender-specific scales, researchers and practitioners should be mindful of the results from the current and prior studies showing a reoffending base rate that is lower for women than men (Renauer & Henning, 2005; Wooldredge & Thistlethwaite, 2002). Among practitioners, this means that female clients as a group should be considered generally at lower risk than men. For researchers, this will present an additional statistical challenge to the development of valid scales for women and will necessitate larger sample sizes. The significantly higher risk for later victimization among female offenders also warrants efforts to predict this form of recidivism and intervene where necessary.

As for the second major research question addressed in the current study, the utility of factors from the broader risk assessment literature, our findings concur with other studies on this topic. Girard and Wormith (2004), Hanson and Wallace-Capretta (2004), and Hilton et al. (2001) all found that scales and items used in risk assessment with general offenders predicted recidivism by IPV offenders. Whereas these three studies examined any type of violent recidivism, the current study focused solely on IPV reoffending. Items considered that are not presently found in any of the four IPV scales reviewed herein (i.e., ODARA, DAS, SARA, and DVSI) include age, antisocial attitudes, deviant peer associations, IQ or cognitive functioning, and childhood conduct problems. All of these factors were significantly correlated with IPV recidivism for male offenders, as were the items currently found on most IPV scales.

These results lead to several recommendations regarding the next generation of risk assessment scales for male IPV offenders. First, there is strong support for including items that account for an offender's history of violent and nonviolent criminal activity outside the family. While the ODARA, DVSI, and SARA already address this area, the DA does not. The methodological design used to develop and validate the DA may account for this omission. Campbell et al. (2003) selected items based on their ability to differentiate lethal from nonlethal assaults rather than recidivism per se. Second, like the ODARA, SARA, and DVSI, new scales should include measures of noncompliance, including probation and parole violations. Once again, the DA does not assess this factor despite evidence for its utility. Third, the lack of attention to the offenders' age in all four of the current scales should be explored. Age is one of the most robust predictors in the general offender literature (Jones & Sims, 1997; Quinsey et al., 1998) and was shown in both the present study and prior research to be inversely related to IPV recidivism (e.g., Hanson & Wallace-Capretta, 2004; Renauer & Henning, 2005). Hilton et al. (2004) also reported that age was a significant correlate of recidivism in their bivariate analyses with the ODARA, but the item dropped out in multivariate regressions. Nevertheless, the ease with which this item is obtained certainly makes it worth consideration in subsequent scales. Fourth, the present study suggests that early conduct problems, a strong risk item for general offending, also predicts later IPV reoffenses with male offenders. Longitudinal research by Ehrensaft, Moffitt and Caspi (2004) similarly noted the importance of conduct disorder in the development of IPV for both men and women. While archival records for coding conduct problems may not always be accessible, it is worth recalling that the current study used a self-report scale and still found a significant correlation with recidivism. Fifth, the present study suggests that additional dynamic risk factors used in the general literature should be tested in new IPV scales, including measures of antisocial attitudes, cognitive functioning, and peer associations. Sixth, further research is needed to determine whether existing risk scales from the general offender literature (e.g., VRAG, LSI-R) do as well or better than IPV-specific measures in predicting reoffending by this population. It may be that we have minimal need for IPV-specific scales in the first place. Finally, future studies should evaluate the feasibility of implementing and the validity of using various risk scales at different stages in the criminal justice process (arrest, prosecution, sentencing, probation, treatment). Some of the items assessed in the present study (e.g., IQ, antisocial attitudes, and personality functioning) would be difficult to collect in law enforcement settings.

As for the limitations of the present study, one notable concern is that predictor variables were obtained from mandatory assessments that were later sent to the local domestic violence judge. The court may have acted on these evaluations and ordered individuals into treatment(s) that impacted recidivism in ways that cannot be easily controlled. Another limitation is that recidivism was coded using individuals' names and dates of birth rather than unique IDs based on fingerprints or other reliable means. Because women's names may be subject to greater change from subsequent marriage and divorce, it is possible that recidivism rates for females were underreported. Lower rates of reporting offenses to the police by male victims, as suggested by Dutton and Nicholls (2005), may also have contributed to lower recidivism rates for women. At the same time, research using the National Crime Victim Surveys (Rennison & Welchans, 2000) has not found significant differences in the reporting rates of men and women subject to abuse by an intimate partner. The generalizability of the present findings may also be limited based on the characteristics of the sample. The majority of the offenders were African American and all of the data were collected between 1999 and 2001. Similarly, the present study focused exclusively on convicted IPV offenders and the results may not generalize to the broader population of men and women who perpetrate relationship aggression. Finally, the recidivism data used in the present study were based solely on official records and may seriously underestimate the true prevalence of reoffending among both male and female offenders. It is possible that the utility of risk factors could vary from one type of recidivism measure to the next (e.g., official records vs. victim reported vs. offender reported).

These limitations notwithstanding, the present study represents a valuable contribution to the literature on gender and IPV. It is among the first published works to compare risk factors for men and women in this population and one of but a handful looking at IPV recidivism rates by gender. While the findings here cannot ultimately resolve the debate about similarities or differences in male- and female-initiated relationship violence, they do highlight important differences in criminal justice samples that need to be further explored. The findings also lend support to the idea that IPV recidivism is influenced by many of the same factors observed in the broader violent offender literature. Hilton and Harris (2005) summarized the research on IPV recidivism and came to the same conclusion: "The strongest predictors of wife assault recidivism identified by research are strikingly similar to the predictors of violent recidivism in general: young age, unemployment, prior criminal history, and other indices of an unstable, antisocial lifestyle" (p. 15). As such, those working in IPV risk assessment and treatment need to do a better job of incorporating some of the scales, practices, theories, and interventions that have proven to be successful in managing offenders in the general population.

REFERENCES

American Psychiatric Association. (1994). *Diagnostic and statistical manual of mental disorders* (4th ed.). Washington, DC: Author.

Andrews, D. A., & Bonta, J. (1995). *The Level of Service Inventory–Revised.* Toronto, Canada: Multi-Health Systems.

Andrews, D. A., Bonta, J., & Hoge, R. D. (1990). Classification for effective rehabilitation: Rediscovering psychology. *Criminal Justice and Behavior, 17,* 19–52.

Andrews, D. A., Bonta, J., & Wormith, J. S. (2006). The recent past and near future of risk and/or need assessment. *Crime & Delinquency, 52*(1), 7–27.

Andrews, D. A., & Dowden, C. (2006). Risk principle of case classification in correctional treatment: A meta-analytic investigation. *International Journal of Offender Therapy and Comparative Criminology, 50*(1), 88–100.

Bonta, J., Law, M., & Hanson, R. K. (1998). The prediction of criminal and violent recidivism among mentally disordered offenders: A meta-analysis. *Psychological Bulletin, 123,* 123–142.

Bonta, J., Pang, B., & Wallace-Capretta, S. (1995). Predictors of recidivism among incarcerated female offenders. *The Prison Journal, 75,* 277–294.

Campbell, J. C. (1995). *Assessing dangerousness: Violence by sexual offenders, batterers, and child abusers.* Thousand Oaks, CA: Sage.

Campbell, J. C., Glass, N., Sharps, P., Laughon, K., & Bloom, T. (2007). Intimate partner homicide: Review and implications of research and policy. *Trauma, Violence, & Abuse, 8*(3), 246–269.

Campbell, J. C., Webster, D., Koziol-McLain, J., Block, C., Campbell, D., Curry, M., et al. (2003). Risk factors for femicide in abusive relationships: Results from a multisite case control study. *American Journal of Public Health*, *93*(7), 1089–1097.

Cattaneo, L., Bell, M., Goodman, L., & Dutton, M. (2007). Intimate partner violence victims' accuracy in assessing their risk of re-abuse. *Journal of Family Violence*, *22*, 429–440.

Chesney-Lind, M. (2002). Criminalizing victimization: The unintended consequences of pro-arrest policies for girls and women. *Criminology & Public Policy*, *2*(1), 81–90.

Conradi, L. M., Geffner, R., Hamberger, L. K., & Lawson, G. (in press). An exploratory study of women as dominant aggressors of physical violence in their intimate relationships. *Journal of Aggression, Maltreatment, & Trauma*.

Corvo, K., & Johnson, P. (2003). Vilification of the "batterer": How blame shapes domestic violence policy and interventions. *Aggression and Violent Behavior*, *8*(3), 259–282.

Cunningham, M., & Reidy, T. (1999). Don't confuse me with the facts: Common errors in violence risk assessment at capital sentencing. *Criminal Justice and Behavior*, *26*(1), 20–43.

de Vogel, V. & de Ruiter, C. (2005). The HCR-20 in personality disordered female offenders: A comparison with a matched sample of males. *Clinical Psychology & Psychotherapy*, *12*(3), 226–240.

Dutton, D. (2007). *The abusive personality: Violence and control in intimate relationships* (2nd ed.). New York: Guilford Press.

Dutton, D., & Corvo, K. (2006). Transforming a flawed policy: A call to revive psychology and science in domestic violence research and practice. *Aggression and Violent Behavior*, *11*(5), 457–483.

Dutton, D., & Kropp, R. (2000). A review of domestic violence risk instruments. *Trauma, Violence, & Abuse*, *1*(2), 171–181.

Dutton, D., & Nicholls, T. (2005). The gender paradigm in domestic violence research and theory: Part 1--The conflict of theory and data. *Aggression and Violent Behavior*, *10*(6), 680–714.

Ehrensaft, M., Moffitt, T., & Caspi, A. (2004). Clinically abusive relationships in an unselected birth cohort: Men's and women's participation and developmental antecedents. *Journal of Abnormal Psychology*, *113*(2), 258–271.

Fagan, J. (1996). *The criminalization of domestic violence: Promises and limits* (NCJ 157641). Washington, DC: Office of Justice Programs.

Folsom, J., & Atkinson, J. L. (2007). The generalizability of the LSI-R and the CAT to the prediction of recidivism in female offenders. *Criminal Justice and Behavior*, *34*(8), 1044–1056.

Girard, L., & Wormith, J. (2004). The predictive validity of the Level of Service Inventory-Ontario Revision on general and violent recidivism among various offender groups. *Criminal Justice and Behavior*, *31*(2), 150–181.

Golding, J. M. (1999). Intimate partner violence as a risk factor for mental disorders: A meta-analysis. *Journal of Family Violence*, *14*, 99–133.

Gondolf, E. W. (1997). Patterns of reassault in batterer programs. *Violence and Victims*, *12*(4), 373–387.

Gondolf, E. W. (1999). MCMI-III results for batterer program participants in four cities: Less "pathological" than expected. *Journal of Family Violence*, *14*(1), 1–17.

Goodman, L., Dutton, M., & Bennett, M. (1999). Predicting repeat abuse among arrested batterers: Use of the danger assessment scale in the criminal justice system. *Journal of Interpersonal Violence, 15,* 63–74.

Grann, M., & Wedin, I. (2002). Risk factors for recidivism among spousal assault and spousal homicide offenders. *Psychology, Crime & Law, 8*(1), 5–23.

Grove, W. M., & Meehl, P. E. (1996). Comparative efficacy of informal (subjective, impressionistic) and formal (mechanical, algorithmic) prediction procedures: The clinical-statistical controversy. *Psychology, Public Policy, and Law, 2,* 293–323.

Hanson, K., & Wallace-Capretta, S. (2004). Predictors of criminal recidivism among male batterers. *Psychology, Crime & Law, 10*(4), 413–427.

Hanson, R. K., & Bussière, M. T. (1998). Predicting relapse: A meta-analysis of sexual offender recidivism studies. *Journal of Consulting and Clinical Psychology, 66,* 348–363.

Harer, M., & Langan, N. (2001). Gender differences in predictors of prison violence: Assessing the predictive validity of a risk classification system. *Crime and Delinquency, 47*(4), 513–536.

Heckert, A., & Gondolf, E. (2004). Battered women's perceptions of risk versus risk factors and instruments in predicting repeat reassault. *Journal of Interpersonal Violence, 19*(7), 778–800.

Henning, K., & Feder, L. (2004). A comparison between men and women arrested for domestic violence: Who presents the greater threat? *Journal of Family Violence, 19*(2), 69–80.

Henning, K., Renauer, B., & Holdford, R. (2006). Victim or offender? Heterogeneity among women arrested for intimate partner violence. *Journal of Family Violence, 21,* 351–368.

Hilton, N., & Harris, G. (2005). Predicting wife assault: A critical review and implications for policy and practice. *Trauma, Violence, & Abuse, 6*(1), 3–23.

Hilton, N., Harris, G., Rice, M., Lang, C., Cormier, C., & Lines, K. (2004). A brief actuarial assessment for the prediction of wife assault recidivism: The Ontario Domestic Assault Risk Assessment. *Psychological Assessment, 16*(3), 267–275.

Hilton, N. Z., Harris, G. T., & Rice, M. E. (2001). Predicting violence by serious wife assaulters. *Journal of Interpersonal Violence, 16*(5), 408–423.

Hirschel, D., & Buzawa, E. (2002). Understanding the context of dual arrest with directions for future research. *Violence Against Women, 8*(12), 1449–1473.

Holtzworth-Munroe, A. (2002). Standards for batterer treatment programs: How can research inform our decisions? *Journal of Aggression, Maltreatment & Trauma, 5*(2), 165–180.

Jones, M., & Sims, B. (1997). Recidivism of offenders released from prison in North Carolina: A gender comparison. *The Prison Journal, 77*(3), 335–348.

Kitzman, K., Gaylord, N., Holt, A., & Kenny, E. (2003). Child witnesses to domestic violence: A meta-analytic review. *Journal of Consulting and Clinical Psychology, 71*(2), 339–352.

Kropp, P. R (2004). Some questions regarding spousal assault risk assessment. *Violence Against Women, 10*(6), 676–697.

Kropp, P. R., & Hart, S. D. (2000). The Spousal Assault Risk Assessment (SARA) Guide: Reliability and validity in adult male offenders. *Law and Human Behavior, 24*(1), 101–118.

Kropp, P. R., Hart, S. D., Webster, C.W., & Eaves, D. (1995). *Manual for the Spousal Assault Risk Assessment Guide* (2nd ed.). Vancouver, Canada: B.C. Institute on Family Violence.

Miller, S. (2001). The paradox of women arrested for domestic violence: Criminal justice professionals and service providers respond. *Violence Against Women*, 7(12), 1339–1376.

Millon, T. (1994). *Manual for the MCMI-III*. Minneapolis, MN: National Computer Systems.

Muftic, L., & Bouffard, J. (2007). An evaluation of gender differences in the implementation and impact of a comprehensive approach to domestic violence. *Violence Against Women*, 13(1), 46–69.

Pence, E., & Paymar, M. (1993). *Education groups for men who batter: The Duluth model*. New York: Springer.

Quinsey, V. L., Harris, G. T., Rice, M. E., & Cormier, C. A. (1998). *Violent offenders: Appraising and managing risk*. Washington, DC: American Psychological Association.

Renauer, B., & Henning, K. (2005). Investigating intersections between gender and intimate partner violence recidivism. *Journal of Offender Rehabilitation*, 41(4), 99–124.

Rennison, C. M., & Welchans, S. (2000). *Intimate partner violence*. Washington, DC: US Department of Justice, Office of Justice Programs.

Rice, M., & Harris, G. (1995). Violent recidivism: Assessing predictive validity. *Journal of Consulting and Clinical Psychology*, 63, 737–748.

Roehl, J., & Guertin, K. (2000). Intimate partner violence: The current use of risk assessments in sentencing offenders. *The Justice System Journal*, 21, 171–198.

Ross, J. M., & Babcock, J. C. (2009). Gender differences in partner violence in context: Deconstructing Johnson's (2001) control-based typology of violent couples. *Journal of Aggression, Maltreatment, & Trauma*, 18(6), 604–622.

Saunders, D. (2002). Are physical assaults by wives and girlfriends a major social problem? *Violence Against Women*, 8(12), 1424–1448.

Sherman, L. (1992). *Policing domestic violence: Experiments and dilemmas*. New York: Free Press.

Simourd, D. J. (1997). The Criminal Sentiments Scale-Modified and Pride in Delinquency scale: Psychometric properties and construct validity of two measures of criminal attitudes. *Criminal Justice and Behavior*, 24(1), 52–70.

Simourd, D. J., & van de Ven, J. (1999). Assessment of criminal attitudes: Criterion-related validity of the Criminal Sentiments Scale—Modified and Pride in Delinquency Scale. *Criminal Justice and Behavior*, 26(1), 90–106.

Steffensmeier, D., & Demuth, S. (2000). Ethnicity and sentencing outcomes in U.S. federal courts: Who is punished more harshly? *American Sociological Review*, 65, 705–729.

Steffensmeier, D., Zhong, H., Ackerman, J., Schwartz, J., & Agha, S. (2006). Gender gap trends for violent crimes, 1980 to 2003: A UCR-NCVS comparison. *Feminist Criminology*, 1(1), 72–98.

Straus, M. (1990). The Conflict Tactics Scales and its critics: An evaluation and new data on validity and reliability. In M. A. Straus & R. J. Gelles (Eds.), *Physical violence in American families: Risk factors and adaptations to violence in 8,145 families* (pp. 49–73). New Brunswick, NJ: Transaction Publishers.

Straus, M., Hamby, S., Finkelhor, D., Moore, D., & Runyan, D. (1998). Identification of child maltreatment with the Parent-Child Conflict Tactics Scales: Development and psychometric data for a national sample of American parents. *Child Abuse and Neglect, 22,* 249–270.

Swan, S., & Snow, D. (2006). The development of a theory of women's use of violence in intimate relationships. *Violence Against Women, 12*(11), 1026–1045.

Swets, J., Dawes, R., & Monahan, J. (2000). Psychological science can improve diagnostic decisions. *Psychological Science in the Public Interest, 1,* 1–26.

Vigorita, M. S. (2003). Judicial risk assessment: The impact of risk, stakes, and jurisdiction. *Criminal Justice Policy Review, 14*(3), 361–376.

Webster, C. D., Douglas, K. S., Eaves, D., & Hart, S. D. (1997). *The HCR-20: Assessing risk for violence (Version 2).* Burnaby, Canada: Simon Fraser University.

Wechsler, D. (1981). *Wechsler Adult Intelligence Scale—Revised* [manual]. New York: Psychological Corporation.

Weisz, A., Tolman, R., & Saunders, D. G. (2000). Assessing the risk of severe domestic violence: The importance of survivors' predictions. *Journal of Interpersonal Violence, 15,* 75–90.

Williams, K., & Houghton, A. (2004). Assessing the risk of domestic violence reoffending: A validation study. *Law and Human Behavior, 28*(4), 437–455.

Wooldredge, J., & Thistlewaite, A. (2002). Reconsidering domestic violence recidivism: Conditioned effects of legal controls by individual and aggregate levels of stake in conformity. *Journal of Quantitative Criminology, 18*(1), 45–70.

Zachary, R. (1986). *Shipley Institute of Living Scale: Revised manual.* Los Angeles: Western Psychological Services.

Relationships Among Women's Use of Aggression, Their Victimization, and Substance Use Problems: A Test of the Moderating Effects of Race/Ethnicity

TAMI P. SULLIVAN and COURTENAY E. CAVANAUGH

Yale University School of Medicine, New Haven, Connecticut, USA

MICHELLE J. UFNER

Science Applications International Corporation, Arlington, Virginia, USA

SUZANNE C. SWAN

University of South Carolina, Columbia, South Carolina, USA

DAVID L. SNOW

Yale University School of Medicine, New Haven, Connecticut, USA

This study examined whether relationships among women's aggression, their victimization, and substance use problems were moderated by race/ethnicity. A total of 412 community women (150 African Americans, 150 Latinas, and 112 Whites) who recently were aggressive against a male partner completed a 2-hour computer-assisted interview. ANOVA and path analysis revealed that (a) for all women, victimization and aggression were strongly related; (b) race/ethnicity moderated the relationships between victimization and alcohol and drug use problems; and (c) no groups evidenced a relationship between alcohol or drug use problems and aggression. Findings suggest that it is essential to develop culturally relevant, gender-specific interventions to reduce both

women's aggression and victimization, as well as related negative
behaviors such as alcohol and drug use.

Physical intimate partner violence (IPV) is most often bidirectional such that women both experience victimization and act aggressively toward their partners (Caetano, Ramisetty-Mikler, & Field, 2005; Field & Caetano, 2005; Sullivan, Meese, Swan, Mazure, & Snow, 2005). Further, women's victimization and aggression often co-occur with their use of substances (for a review of the literature, see Schafer, Caetano, & Cunradi, 2004). Evidence regarding the co-occurrence suggests that women use alcohol and drugs to cope with victimization (Kaysen et al., 2007; Martino, Collins, & Ellickson, 2005) and that women's alcohol and drug use is a risk factor for their aggressive behavior (Conradi, Geffner, Hamberger, & Lawson, in press; Schafer et al., 2004; Stuart, Meehan et al., 2006). The notion of using alcohol and drugs to cope with victimization is consistent with tension reduction theory (Conger, 1956) and the more contemporary self-medication hypothesis (Khantzian, 1997), which posit that individuals use alcohol or drugs to manage negative affective and mood states such as those resulting from IPV (e.g., anxiety and fear; Foa, Cascardi, Zoellner, & Feeny, 2000; Swan & Snow, 2003). The concept of alcohol and drug use as a risk factor for aggression is consistent with the proximal effects model, which encompasses both psychopharmacological and expectancy theories (Chermack & Taylor, 1995; Critchlow, 1983; Hoaken & Stewart, 2003; Leonard & Quigley, 1999). Psychopharmacological theory posits that a substance's psychopharmacological properties facilitate aggressive behavior, whereas expectancy theory posits that aggression following substance use is a learned behavior. Further, relationships among women's physical victimization, their use of aggression, and substance use problems appear to vary by race/ethnicity (Field & Caetano, 2004; U.S. Department of Health and Human Services, 2003).

Although theory suggests and studies consistently find that women who are victimized are more likely to use substances and that women's substance use is a risk factor for their aggression, few studies have integrated this information to examine the complex relationships among all of these variables. To date, most studies have analyzed relationships between pairs of variables separately. Analyzing victimization and aggression separately in relation to their precursors and correlates, such as women's substance use, may lead to erroneous conclusions about their relative associations. For example, Sullivan and colleagues (2005) demonstrated that when women's aggression and victimization were analyzed simultaneously in relation to psychological symptoms, aggression was unrelated to symptoms; however, when victimization was deleted from the analysis, it was concluded in error that women's aggression was directly related to psychological symptoms. Similarly, Anderson (2002) found that after accounting for the relationships between victimization and alcohol/drug problems, the once significant relationships between women's alcohol/drug problems and aggression became nonsignificant. Finally, there is a dearth of information about how these relationships may operate differently for African American, Latina, and White women. An investigation such as this is needed if culturally relevant programs are to be developed that address domestic violence and/or alcohol and drug use problems.

CO-OCCURRING AGGRESSION AND VICTIMIZATION

Although women recruited from community settings use physical aggression in intimate relationships at rates equal to or greater than men (Archer, 2000; Dutton, Nicholls, & Spidel, 2005), women who use aggression but who are not victimized are the exception rather than the rule (Sullivan et al., 2005). Findings from a meta-analytic study indicated a large effect size between women's victimization and their use of aggression (Stith, Smith, Penn, Ward, & Tritt, 2004). This finding is concerning since bidirectional physical IPV has been found to be more severe than male-to-female or female-to-male physical IPV alone and may be more difficult to prevent and treat (Caetano et al., 2005). Further, while the temporal order between women's victimization and aggression has not been clearly established and no single theory can explain women's use of aggression (Graham-Kevan & Archer, 2005), there is increasing evidence that women are aggressive in response to men's aggression (Downs, Rindels, & Atkinson, 2007; Swan & Snow, 2002) to defend themselves against intimates, out of fear of physical victimization, to protect their children, to establish control (Caldwell, Swan, Allen, Sullivan, & Snow, in press; Leisring, in press), and for retribution (Babcock, Miller, & Siard, 2003; Stuart, Moore et al., 2006; Swan & Snow, 2003, 2006).

SUBSTANCE USE CORRELATES

A substantial body of literature has linked women's victimization and use of aggression with their drinking, use of drugs, and related substance use disorders (Bonomi et al., 2006; Caetano et al., 2005; Chermack, Walton, Fuller, & Blow, 2001; Cunradi, Caetano, Clark, & Schafer, 1999; Martino et al., 2005; Schafer et al., 2004; Stith et al., 2004; Stuart, Meehan et al., 2006). However, the majority of these studies have examined women's substance use in relation to victimization and aggression in separate analyses. As previously mentioned, results of analyses that separately examine the relationship between substance use and victimization or substance use and aggression may be confounded by the strong intercorrelation between victimization and aggression. What appears to be a correlation between aggression and substance use may, in fact, be a function of the relationship between victimization and substance use (Anderson, 2002; Sullivan et al., 2005).

To date, only four studies have investigated women's victimization and use of aggression simultaneously with their substance use (Anderson, 2002; Martino et al., 2005; Schafer et al., 2004; Stuart, Meehan et al., 2006). Two of these studies (Anderson, 2002; Martino et al., 2005) suggest that women's substance use problems are related to their victimization but not to their use of aggression. After controlling for the significant relationships of victimization to substance use problems, Anderson (2002) found that the relationships between women's substance use problems and aggression disappeared. Results of a longitudinal study by Martino et al. (2005) found women's victimization to be associated with their subsequent heavy drinking (but not recreational drug use); neither women's alcohol use nor their drug use were associated with women's subsequent use of aggression. These studies, along with others of victimized women, provide support for the tension reduction theory (Conger, 1956) and the self-medication hypothesis (Khantzian, 1997), which suggest that women use alcohol and drugs to cope with the adverse consequences of victimization (Hien, Cohen, & Campbell, 2005; Kaysen et al., 2007; Khantzian, 1997).

There are several theories that can explain the relationship between substance use and aggression, many of which are consistent with the proximal effects model (Leonard & Quigley, 1999), which has received the most empirical support (Klostermann & Fals-Stewart, 2006). The proximal effects model posits that alcohol intoxication facilitates aggression and, further, that the alcohol-aggression relationship may be mediated by a person's expectancies about alcohol (Critchlow, 1983) and/or the pharmacological effects of alcohol, which impair cognitive processing (Chermack & Taylor, 1995). Many studies have provided empirical support for the proximal effects model among men (e.g., Fals-Stewart, 2003; Fals-Stewart, Golden, & Schumacher, 2003; Fals-Stewart, Leonard, & Birchler, 2005). Few studies have provided support for this model among women (Schafer et al., 2004; Stuart, Meehan et al., 2006).

Of the four aforementioned studies that examined women's victimization and their use of aggression simultaneously with substance use, the final two studies to note found women's alcohol use problems to be a risk factor for their use of aggression (Schafer et al., 2004; Stuart, Meehan et al., 2006); however, the strength of this relationship was small in one study (Stuart, Meehan et al., 2006) and not reported in another (Schafer et al., 2004). Therefore, while the proximal effects model and some research suggest that women's substance use and use of aggression are related, we contend that it is unlikely that the proximal effects model would be supported among women. It is not clear that women's substance use serves the same function as it does for men; consequently, women's substance use may not be related to their use of aggression—that is, women often use aggression in response to men's aggression against them (Downs et al., 2007; Hamberger & Guse, 2005), therefore, we reason that substance use problems may not be related to women's use of aggression but rather may be related exclusively to their victimization.

RACE/ETHNICITY AS A MODERATOR OF VICTIMIZATION, SUBSTANCE USE, AND AGGRESSION

Accumulating research by Caetano, Schafer, Cunradi, Field, and colleagues suggests that the relationships between women's (a) victimization and use of aggression, (b) victimization and substance use problems, and (c) substance use problems and use of aggression vary by race/ethnicity (Caetano et al., 2005; Field & Caetano, 2005; Schafer et al., 2004). For example, in a cross-sectional study, African Americans were found to have higher rates of bidirectional physical partner aggression than Hispanics or Whites (Caetano et al., 2005). Findings from a longitudinal study suggest that African Americans and Hispanics have comparable and higher rates of bidirectional physical aggression than Whites. However, only African American ethnicity was an independent predictor of bidirectional aggression above and beyond education, income, employment status, alcohol problems, and history of aggression in one's family of origin (Caetano et al., 2005). For African American couples, consistent evidence links women's alcohol use problems to their victimization. For White couples, the literature is contradictory. For Hispanic couples, there is no evidence for the relationship between alcohol use problems and victimization. Findings are not entirely consistent regarding the relationships among specific groups.

To our knowledge, only one study has examined whether race/ethnicity moderated the relationships among women's victimization, aggression, and alcohol use problems (Schafer et al., 2004). Specifically, Schafer et al. showed that for African American women, alcohol use problems were significantly associated with their victimization and use of aggression in intimate relationships. No such relationships emerged for White or Hispanic women. While the Schafer et al. study permitted an examination of the relationship between alcohol use problems and victimization/aggression by racial/ethnic group, it did not investigate the co-occurrence of victimization and aggression or the relationship of these variables to drug use problems.

Based on these considerations, the current study aimed to test the extent to which the relationships among women's victimization, alcohol and drug use problems, and use of aggression are moderated by racial/ethnic group. The hypotheses to be tested are as follows. First, women's victimization will be positively related to their use of aggression. Second, women's victimization will be positively related to alcohol and drug use problems. Third, given the lack of evidence, no prediction is made regarding the relationship between alcohol and drug use problems and use of aggression. Fourth, it is hypothesized that race/ethnicity will moderate the relationships among women's victimization, alcohol and drug use problems, and use of aggression.

METHOD

Sample

Recruitment flyers advertising the Women's Relationship Study were posted in four urban-area primary care clinics and emergency departments. Recruitment materials also were posted in local businesses such as grocery stores, laundromats, and shops, as well as selected state offices such as the Department of Employment. Eligibility was determined via a phone screen and was based on the following inclusion criteria: (a) female sex, (b) current involvement in a heterosexual intimate relationship of at least six months' duration, (c) a woman's commission of at least one act of physical aggression against her male partner within the past six months, (d) age 18 to 64, (e) residency in the greater urban area, and (f) household income of less than $50,000 (determined a priori to methodologically control for the differential resources associated with higher income). The sample of 412 women was stratified by racial/ethnic group (150 women of African American descent, 150 Latina women, and 112 non-Latina White women).

Overall, the sample was largely comprised of high school–educated ($n = 284$; 69%), unemployed ($n = 171$; 66%) women with low levels of annual income (mode < $10,000; 43%). The majority of women lived with their partners ($n = 259$; 63%) and had been in their relationships for 1–5 years ($n = 171$; 42%); an additional 22% had been with their partners for 5–10 years and 23% for 10–20 years. Regarding the Latina subsample, 96% were born outside of the United States, with the mean number of years living in the United States being 15.3 ($SD = 12.08$). Over half (53%) were Puerto Rican, followed by 11% Mexican, 7% Colombian, 5% Venezuelan, with the remaining 24% from various other nations. Over three quarters of the Latina sample (85%) reported that their partners also were Latino.

Procedures

To screen specifically for women's use of physical aggression, items from the Conflict Tactics Scale-2 (CTS2; Straus, Hamby, Boney-McCoy, & Sugarman,

1996) were used. In order not to reveal the specific interest in women's use of physical aggression as the main inclusion criterion, both victimization and aggression items from the negotiation, psychological aggression, and physical assault scales were included.

Eligible participants met with a trained female interviewer of the same race/ethnicity who administered one 2-hour protocol via computer-assisted interviewing (NOVA Research Company, 2003) conducted in English or Spanish. Approximately half of the Latina participants (i.e., 49%) elected to have the protocol administered in Spanish. All study materials were translated into Spanish. If an established Spanish version of a measure did not exist, a bilingual member of the research team translated the instrument. The translated version was reviewed by a bilingual consultant and back-translated into English to ensure accurate translation (Brislin, 1970). All data were self-reported by the participant. At the conclusion of the interview, participants were debriefed, remunerated $50, and provided with a list of community resources for food, employment, housing and benefits assistance, mental health and substance use treatment, and IPV-related services.

Measures

PHYSICAL AGGRESSION AND PHYSICAL VICTIMIZATION

Women's aggression and their victimization were assessed on three dimensions: physical, sexual, and psychological IPV. Only the 12 items from the CTS2 (Straus et al., 1996) physical assault scales were the focus of the present study. A referent time period of six months was used to assess a participant's commission of an aggressive behavior toward her partner and the partner's commission of each behavior toward her. The response scale ranged from *never, once, twice, 3–5 times, 6–10 times,* to *more than 10 times in the past six months.* The two response categories presented as a range were recoded so that the midpoint of each range was the variable's value (i.e., 3–5 = 4; 6–10 = 8); more than 10 times was conservatively recoded to a value of 11. Two scores, women's physical aggression and their physical victimization, were created by summing the 12 items for each of these subscales. The reliability of the items for women's physical aggression was $\alpha = .87$ and for women's physical victimization was $\alpha = .91$.

ALCOHOL USE PROBLEMS

The Alcohol Use Disorder Identification Test (AUDIT; Babor & Grant, 1989) is a 10-item measure used to screen for those at high risk for alcohol use problems within the past 6 months. The measure has been used internationally and has high and well-established sensitivity and specificity (Allen, Litten, Fertig, & Babor, 1997) and test-retest reliability (Selin, 2003). By summing participants' responses to questions about the frequency and quantity of drinking behaviors, as well as problems related to their drinking, the AUDIT produces a total score that is used to determine if an individual screens positively for problematic alcohol use. The total score is used in the analytic models. Typically, a cutoff score ≥ 8 is used to classify individuals as problem drinkers (Babor & Grant, 1989). However, a more recent study of the general population (Selin, 2003) showed that the optimal cutoff for women is 6. Based on this gender-specific cutoff of 6, 26% of the sample was classified as having a drinking problem. Internal consistency in the current sample was α = .89.

Drug use problems

The Drug Abuse Screening Test (DAST; Skinner, 1982) is a measure widely used to screen for drug use problems over the past 6 months. The DAST yields a quantitative index of the degree of drug use problems or consequences by summing participants' responses (*no = 0, yes* = 1). The 20-item version (Skinner, 1982) was used in this study. Both a total score and a score that classifies participants with drug use problems akin to the *Diagnostic and Statistical Manual of Mental Disorders-IV* (American Psychiatric Association, 1994) substance abuse or dependence can be calculated. A score of 0 indicates no drug-related problems or consequences (55% of the total sample), 1 to 5 indicates low levels of problems or consequences (25% of the total sample), and a score ≥ 6 indicates that the paticipant likely meets the criteria for a drug use problem (29% of the total sample). For the purposes of the analyses, the drug use problems variable was a total score created by summing all 20 items. Internal consistency in the current sample was α = .86.

Data Analysis

The first step in data analysis was to examine data for skew. All four variables (physical victimization, alcohol use problems, drug use problems, and use of physical aggression) demonstrated skew for at least one of the three racial/ethnic groups. Transformations were based on recommendations of Tabachnick and Fidell (2007). The log10 transformation was the best method for normalizing data for the four variables across groups.

The rationale for multigroup path analysis is to determine if the relationships among variables in a given model vary across groups (Kline, 2005); in other words, does the grouping variable (racial/ethnic group) serve to moderate relationships among model variables? In order to determine if path coefficients differ among groups for any given relationship between two variables, critical ratios of the differences between parameters are inspected. If the path coefficients are not significantly different between any two groups or across all three groups, the relevant parameters are constrained to be equal (i.e., a cross-group equality constraint is imposed for that path).

The AMOS 7.0 statistical program (SPSS Inc., 2006), which uses Full Information Maximum Likelihood to deal with missing data, was employed to analyze the path models, obtain maximum-likelihood estimates of model parameters, and provide goodness-of-fit indices. The percentage of missing data for each variable in any group was less than 1%. To obtain the most parsimonious model, (a) the initial model, with no cross-group equality constraints imposed, was modified by a one-by-one addition of cross-group equality constraints; (b) then, this alternative model was compared to the previous model (initial model or model with an additional constraint imposed) using the chi-square difference statistic (χ^2_D) to determine if there was a decrement in model fit. If the chi-square difference statistic showed that there was not a decrement in fit of the alternative model (i.e., the alternative model was not "worse"), this model was accepted. Because the dispersion of variables differs across groups, the unstandardized estimates should be used to compare parameter estimates (path coefficients) across groups. Standardized estimates can be viewed to compare parameters within a group; these estimates are reported in the text (Kline, 2005).

RESULTS

Mean Racial/Ethnic Group Differences

Intercorrelations, means, standard deviations, and ranges for each group are included in Table 1. For all groups, the strongest correlations were evidenced between victimization and aggression and between alcohol and drug use problems.

ANOVA tests revealed statistically significant differences for victimization, alcohol and drug use problems, and use of aggression scores among the three racial/ethnic groups: $F(2,409) = 3.82$, $p < .05$; $F(2,403) = 34.44$, $p < .001$; $F(2,408) = 25.28$, p $< .001$; and $F(2,409) = 14.87$, $p < .001$, respectively (see Table 2). Post hoc comparisons (see Figure 1) using the Tukey HSD test, and the Games Howell test when the homogeneity of variances assumption was violated, indicated that alcohol use problems was the only variable to differ significantly among all three groups. African Americans reported the highest alcohol use problems scores and Latinas the lowest. For drug use problems, both White and African American women's mean scores were significantly higher than Latinas' but not different from each other's. Regarding experiences of victimization, the only significant difference was between African American and Latina women's means scores, with African

TABLE 1 Intercorrelations, Means, Standard Deviations, and Ranges of Study Variables ($N = 412$)

Variable	1	2	3	4	M	SD	Range
African American ($n = 150$)							
Physical victimization	—				22.63	26.40	0–111
Alcohol use problems	.23**	—			6.98	7.78	0–36
Drug use problems	.27**	.46**	—		3.46	4.28	0–16
Physical aggression	.45**	.24**	.20*	—	23.75	22.08	1–104
Latina ($n = 150$)							
Physical victimization	—				15.20	20.42	0–95
Alcohol use problems	.18*	—			2.01	3.83	0–28
Drug use problems	.19*	.33**	—		.85	2.46	0–18
Physical aggression	.46**	.12	.16†	—	16.67	16.96	1–87
White ($n = 112$)							
Physical victimization	—				15.68	20.34	0–108
Alcohol use problems	−.10	—			4.58	4.05	0–32
Drug use problems	−.05	.35**	—		3.23	4.67	0–16
Physical aggression	.44**	−.07	.09	—	12.50	15.65	1–103

Note: Means, standard deviations, and ranges are for untransformed scores. Correlations are based on transformed scores.

*$p < .05$; **$p < .001$.

TABLE 2 Analysis of Variance for Victimization, Alcohol and Drug Use Problems, and Use of Aggression by Racial/Ethnic Group

Source	df	SS	MS	F
Victimization				
Between groups	2	2.24	1.12	3.82*
Within group	409	120.14	.29	
Total	411	122.39		
Alcohol Use Problems				
Between groups	2	10.75	5.38	31.44***
Within group	403	68.92	.17	
Total	405	79.68		
Drug Use Problems				
Between groups	2	7.52	3.76	25.28***
Within group	408	60.71	..15	
Total	410	68.23		
Use of Aggression				
Between groups	2	4.06	2.30	14.87***
Within group	409	63.28	.16	
Total	411	67.89		

Note: ANOVAs were performed with transformed scores.

$p < .05$; **$p < .01$; ***$p < .001$.

Americans reporting more victimization. Regarding women's use of aggression, African American and Latina women's mean scores did not differ from each other, but each group had significantly higher scores than White women.

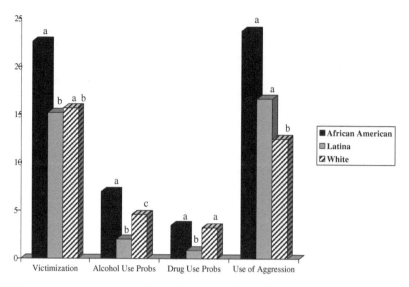

FIGURE 1 Post goc comparisons for victimization, alcohol and drug problems, and use of aggression.

Note. Bars with the same superscripts denote that means between the two groups for each variable are not significantly different according to Tukey HSD or Games-Howell PostHoc tests.

Path Models

In order to test for moderation, the data first must have good fit to the initial model (Kline, 2005). A preliminary model included a test of the path between drug use problems and aggression since bivariate correlations showed a significant relationship between these variables for African American women. Results of this preliminary model showed that this path was nonsignificant for all groups. To avoid a saturated model whereby fit statistics are not provided, the path between drug use problems and aggression was dropped from the model. The unconstrained, initial model provided excellent fit to the data, with a nonsignificant chi-square, χ^2 (3, N = 412) = 2.71, p = .44, a χ^2/df = .91, and an RMSEA = .00, a confidence interval of .00 to .08, and a p for test of close fit of .77. None of the groups significantly differed from one another regarding the paths between victimization and aggression and between alcohol use problems and aggression. As a result, cross-group equality constraints were imposed across all three groups for each of these parameters. A constraint also was imposed for the path between victimization and alcohol use problems for African Americans and Latinas because the relationship between these variables did not differ for these groups. However, the path between victimization and alcohol use problems for African Americans and Latinas each differed from the path for White women. Therefore, the parameters between African American and White women and between Latinas and White women were free to vary.

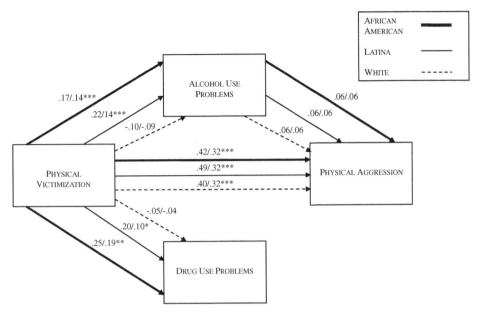

FIGURE 2 Path model for African American, Latina, and white women's use of aggression.

$^*p < .05, ^{**}p < .01, ^{***}p < .001, ^{\dagger}p < .10.$

Standardized estimates should be used to compare parameters within groups (and are noted preceding the virgule) while unstandardized estimates should be used to compare parameters across groups (and are noted following the virgule).

With the constraints imposed as described above, the final model provided an excellent fit to the data, with a nonsignificant chi-square, χ^2 (8, $N = 412) = 6.61$, $p = .58$, a $\chi^2/df = .83$, and an RMSEA = .00, a confidence interval of .00 to .05, and a p for test of close fit of .95 (see Figure 2). The nonsignificant chi-square difference, $\chi^2_D = .73$ ($p = .39$), indicated that the more parsimonious model, with cross-group equality constraints imposed, did not show a decrement in fit compared to previous models and therefore is preferred as the final model. Each model explained a sizable amount of variance in women's use of aggression, ranging from 16% for White women and 19% for African American women to 25% for Latinas. Standardized and substandardized parameter estimates for the final models are shown in Table 3.

As hypothesized, victimization was strongly and positively related to women's aggression for African American ($\beta = .42$, $p < .001$), Latina ($\beta = .49$, $p < .001$), and White ($\beta = .40$, $p < .001$) women. This was the only path that was significant across all groups. For African Americans and Latinas, findings supported the hypothesis that victimization was related to substance use problems: higher levels of victimization were related to greater alcohol use problems ($\beta = .17$, $p < .001$ and $\beta = .22$, $p < .001$, respectively) and drug use problems ($\beta = .25$, $p < .001$ and $\beta = .20$, $p < .05$, respectively). This hypothesis was not supported among White women. No groups evidenced a

TABLE 3 Maximum Likelihood Parameter Estimates for Analysis of a Path Model of Victimization, Substance Use, and Aggression Across Samples of African American, Latina, and White Women

Parameter	African American			Latina			White		
	Unstandard	SE	Standard	Unstandard	SE	Standard	Unstandard	SE	Standard
Unconstrained estimates Parameter									
Direct effects									
PhysVic → DrgProbs	.19	.06	.25***	.10	.04	.20*	−.04	.09	−.05
AlcProbs → PhysAggrs	.06	.04	.06	.06	.04	.06	.06	.04	.06
Disturbance variances									
D$_{AlcProbs}$	.20	.02	.97	.12	.01	.95	.19	.03	.99
D$_{DrgProbs}$	.17	.02	.94	.07	.01	.96	.20	.03	100
D$_{PhysAggrs}$	.15	.02	.81	.09	.01	.75	.13	.02	.84
Equality-constrained estimates Parameter									
Direct effects									
PhysVic → PhysAggrs	.32	.03	.42***	.32	.03	.49***	.32	.03	.40***
PhysVic → AlcProbs[a]	.14	.04	.17***	.14	.04	.22**	−.09	.08	−.10

Note. Standardized estimates for disturbances are proportions of unexplained variance.

[a]Equality constraint imposed between African Americans and Latinas only.

*p < .10, **p < .01, ***p < .001.

relationship between alcohol use problems and women's aggression. In summary, race/ethnicity was shown to moderate the relationships between victimization and both alcohol and drug use problems. However, race/ethnicity did not moderate the relationships between victimization and aggression or between alcohol use problems and aggression.

DISCUSSION

Among women who recently were aggressive against their intimate partners, important differences among racial/ethnic groups emerged regarding level of victimization, number of alcohol and drug use problems, and use of aggressive behavior. Furthermore, race/ethnicity moderated relationships between victimization and both alcohol and drug use problems.

Racial/ethnic groups differed in their use of aggression as well as in their experiences of victimization. African American and White women had comparable and higher levels of victimization than Latina women, while African American and Latina women had comparable and higher levels of aggression than White women. Furthermore, differences were evident regarding substance use problems, with African American women having the greatest number of alcohol use problems, while African American and White women had comparable and higher numbers of drug use problems than Latina women. Regarding model findings, only one significant relationship between variables existed for all groups—women's victimization was strongly related to their use of aggression, a finding that is in line with previous research (Stith et al., 2004; Sullivan et al., 2005). The relationships between victimization and substance use problems were moderated by racial/ethnic group: African American and Latina women's victimization was related to both their alcohol and drug use problems, while White women's victimization was unrelated to either their alcohol or drug use problems.

Culturally specific norms and attitudes may elucidate some of the study findings. Swan and Snow (2006), in their development of a theory of women's use of aggression, suggested that cultural norms may make it more acceptable for women from some racial/ethnic groups to use aggression compared to other groups. For example, these authors noted that African American women are expected to be strong, able to manage adversity independently, and to be involved in egalitarian relationships—expectations that may influence African American women's use of aggressive behavior, particularly in the context of their victimization. For Latinas, acculturation to a more egalitarian and "socially progressive environment that supports [Latinas'] opinions and encourages them...to challenge their partners and families" (Adames & Campbell, 2005, p. 1359) might help to explain their higher rates of aggressive behavior. Further, the higher rates of aggression demonstrated by African American and Latina women may be due, in part, to the fact that they are less likely to use community resources and interventions (Department of Health and Human Services: U.S. Public Health Service, 2001; Wells, Klap, Koike, & Sherbourne, 2001). Similarly, cultural factors—including norms and attitudes about alcohol use—may account for racial/ethnic differences in alcohol use problems (Galvan & Caetano, 2003); factors that may account for the higher numbers of drug use problems for African American and White women are not clear.

Contrary to expectations, tension reduction theory (Conger, 1956) and the self-medication hypothesis (Khantzian, 1997) do not seem to apply universally—they seem only to be supported among African American and Latina women. Women from both groups with greater experiences of victimization exhibited a higher number of alcohol and drug use problems. However, none of these relationships was significant for White women. These findings are consistent with the results of Schafer et al. (2004), but the reason for the findings is not entirely clear. Some scholars (Collins & McNair, 2002; Schafer & Caetano, 2002) suggested that the lower rates of treatment utilization among ethnic-minorities may contribute to the differential patterns of substance use and related problems. While this may offer a partial explanation, it is highly likely that each group has different mechanisms of action operating on the relationship between victimization and substance use problems. For example, Collins and McNair (2002) found that with respect to alcohol use patterns, religiosity is more relevant for African American women while acculturation is more influential for Latinas. In summary, attempting to explain the findings between victimization and substance use problems for each racial/ethnic group with the same theory is likely too simplistic.

Finally, for all women, alcohol and drug use problems were unrelated to their use of aggression. These results are contrary to findings of studies of men whereby men's substance use is related to their aggressive behavior (Fals-Stewart, 2003; Fals-Stewart et al., 2003; Snow, Sullivan, Swan, Tate, & Klein, 2006). These results also are contrary to Schafer et al.'s (2004) findings that the relationship between women's alcohol problems and their use of aggression against intimate partners varied by racial/ethnic group. It is possible that other studies have erroneously concluded that women's aggression is related to their substance use because those studies did not simultaneously examine women's victimization. Perhaps the current study's findings are the result of including victimization as a predictor of women's use of aggression and therefore reflect that after accounting for the relationship of victimization to aggression, no relationship exists between substance use and aggression. The current study's nonsignificant findings call into question whether or not the proximal effects model, whereby substance use precedes the use of aggression, applies to women as it does to men. One plausible explanation for this gender difference is that women may not have learned to expect that their substance use will lead to their use of aggression.

Limitations

A number of limitations are worth noting. First, data collection relied on self-report. It is possible that women's partners might have reported different frequencies of women's experiences of victimization or use of aggression. However, research shows that women's self-reports of victimization and aggression are reliable (Magdol, Moffitt, Caspi, & Silva, 1998). Second, the data were cross-sectional in nature. Therefore, alternative models whereby women's aggression contributes to their victimization or women's substance use problems contribute to their victimization are plausible. Third, the sample size limited the number of variables that could be included in the model. Examining variables such as childhood abuse, coping strategies, and motivations for substance use—as well as motivations for, meaning of, and impact of aggression—might shed more light on the relationships among variables. Additionally, covarying for key demographic differences such as income, level of education, and age is needed to determine whether or not they affect the relationships investigated here. Fourth, the generalizability of findings are limited to African American, Latina, and White urban women with low levels of income who are able to attend and complete study interviews; therefore, it is highly likely that the most severely abused women are not represented in this sample. Fifth, Latinas were examined as a homogenous group and, as such, findings should be interpreted with caution since there may be differences among subgroups of Latinas. Finally, the coding scheme for the CTS2 (Straus et al., 1996) may have allowed for the under- or overrepresentation of the frequencies of physical victimization and aggression.

Directions for Future Research and Implications

Findings have direct implications for research on women's IPV and substance use. Given that the majority of research on women's victimization and their substance use supports tension reduction theory (Conger, 1956) and the self-medication hypothesis (Khantzian, 1997), the current study's lack of support for these theories among White women is unexpected and thus warrants further research. Similarly, the lack of support for the proximal effects model warrants further research given the inconsistent findings in the extant literature among women (Martino et al., 2005; Schafer et al., 2004; Stuart, Meehan et al., 2006). To determine the temporal relationships of victimization, aggression, and substance use among women, longitudinal studies are needed to examine event-level data that would allow for the identification of patterns of relationships among these variables both within events as well as within women over time. Finally, the complex relationships among victimization, aggression, and substance use can be further elucidated by the examination of potential correlates that may be specific to a given racial/ethnic group, such as religiosity among African Americans or level of acculturation among Latinas.

Findings from the current study can inform the development and/or refinement of programs that address women's aggression, victimization, or substance use. Based on study findings, it is essential to develop culturally relevant, gender-specific interventions to reduce both women's aggressive behavior and their experiences of victimization, as well as related negative behaviors such as substance use. Programs developed to reduce women's aggression in intimate relationships need to attend to co-occurring victimization regardless of women's race/ethnicity. In victimization-focused services, there needs to be greater attention to substance use problems in general and among minority women in particular. In substance use programs, it is especially important to attend to victimization for African American and Latina women. Further, within a substance abuse prevention framework, it could be productive to inform African American and Latina women of the resources available to address potential substance use problems and, as necessary, to develop and provide services that are culturally relevant.

In summary, this study concluded that regardless of race/ethnicity, women's victimization was strongly related to their use of aggression in intimate relationships. Further, race/ethnicity was identified as an important moderator of the relationships between victimization and both alcohol and drug use problems, which underscores the need to understand what factors contribute to these important subgroup differences. Findings of future research aimed at elucidating the relationships between women's victimization and their aggression as well as the relationships between victimization and substance use problems have the potential to significantly impact the prevention and treatment of both IPV and substance abuse or dependence.

REFERENCES

Adames, S. B., & Campbell, R. (2005). Immigrant Latinas' conceptualizations of intimate partner violence. *Violence Against Women, 11*(10), 1341–1364.

Allen, J. P., Litten, R. Z., Fertig, J. B., & Babor, T. (1997). A review of research on the Alcohol Use Disorders Identification Test (AUDIT). *Alcoholism: Clinical & Experimental Research, 21*(4), 613–619.

American Psychiatric Association. (1994). *Diagnostic and statistical manual of mental disorders* (4th ed.). Washington, DC: American Psychiatric Publishing, Inc.

Anderson, K. L. (2002). Perpetrator or victim? Relationships between intimate partner violence and well-being. *Journal of Marriage and Family, 64*(4), 851–863.

Archer, J. (2000). Sex differences in aggression between heterosexual partners: A meta-analytic review. *Psychological Bulletin, 126*(5), 651–680.

Babcock, J. C., Miller, S. A., & Siard, C. (2003). Toward a typology of abusive women: Differences between partner-only and generally violent women in the use of violence. *Psychology of Women Quarterly, 27*(2), 153–161.

Babor, T. F., & Grant, M. (1989). From clinical research to secondary prevention: International collaboration in the development of the Alcohol Use Disorders Identification Test (AUDIT). *International Perspectives, 13*, 371–374.

Bonomi, A. E., Thompson, R. S., Anderson, M., Reid, R. J., Carrell, D., Dimer, J. A., et al. (2006). Intimate partner violence and women's physical, mental, and social functioning. *American Journal of Preventive Medicine, 30*(6), 458–466.

Brislin, R. (1970). Back-translation for cross-cultural research. *Journal of Cross-Cultural Psychology, 1*(3), 185–216.

Caetano, R., Ramisetty-Mikler, S., & Field, C. A. (2005). Unidirectional and bidirectional intimate partner violence among White, Black, and Hispanic couples in the United States. *Violence & Victims, 20*(4), 393–406.

Caldwell, J. E., Swan, S. C., Allen, C. T., Sullivan, T. P., & Snow, D. L. (in press). Why I hit him: Women's reasons for intimate partner violence. *Journal of Aggression, Maltreatment, & Trauma.*

Chermack, S. T., & Taylor, S. P. (1995). Alcohol and human physical aggression: Pharmacological versus expectancy effects. *Journal of Studies on Alcohol, 56*(4), 449–456.

Chermack, S. T., Walton, M. A., Fuller, B. E., & Blow, F. C. (2001). Correlates of expressed and received violence across relationship types among men and women substance abusers. *Psychology of Addictive Behaviors, 15*(2), 140–151.

Collins, R., & McNair, L. D. (2002). Minority women and alcohol use. *Alcohol Research & Health, 26*(4), 251–256.

Conger, J. J. (1956). Alcoholism: Theory, problem and challenge. *Quarterly Journal of Studies on Alcohol, 13*, 296–305.

Conradi, L. M., Geffner, R., Hamberger, L. K., & Lawson, G. (in press). An exploratory study of women as dominant aggressors of physical violence in their intimate relationships. *Journal of Aggression, Maltreatment, & Trauma.*

Critchlow, B. (1983). Blaming the booze: The attribution of responsibility for drunken behavior. *Personality and Social Psychology Bulletin, 9*(3), 451–473.

Cunradi, C. B., Caetano, R., Clark, C. L., & Schafer, J. (1999). Alcohol-related problems and intimate partner violence among white, black, and Hispanic couples in the U.S. *Alcoholism: Clinical & Experimental Research, 23*(9), 1492–1501.

Department of Health and Human Services: U.S. Public Health Service. (2001). *Mental health: Culture, race, and ethnicity: A supplement to mental health: A report of the Surgeon General.* Retrieved September 14, 2007, from http://www.surgeongeneral.gov/library/mentalhealth/cre/sma-01-3613.pdf

Downs, W. R., Rindels, B., & Atkinson, C. (2007). Women's use of physical and non-physical self-defense strategies during incidents of partner violence. *Violence Against Women, 13*(1), 28–45.

Dutton, D. G., Nicholls, T. L., & Spidel, A. (2005). Female perpetrators of intimate abuse. *Journal of Offender Rehabilitation, 41*(4), 1–31.

Fals-Stewart, W. (2003). The occurrence of partner physical aggression on days of alcohol consumption: a longitudinal diary study. *Journal of Consulting & Clinical Psychology, 71*(1), 41–52.

Fals-Stewart, W., Golden, J., & Schumacher, J. A. (2003). Intimate partner violence and substance use: A longitudinal day-to-day examination. *Addictive Behaviors, 28*(9), 1555–1574.

Fals-Stewart, W., Leonard, K. E., & Birchler, G. R. (2005). The occurrence of male-to-female intimate partner violence on days of men's drinking: The moderating effects of antisocial personality disorder. *Journal of Consulting and Clinical Psychology, 73*(2), 239–248.

Field, C. A., & Caetano, R. (2004). Ethnic differences in intimate partner violence in the U.S. general population: The role of alcohol use and socioeconomic status. *Trauma, Violence, & Abuse, 5*(4), 303–317.

Field, C. A., & Caetano, R. (2005). Longitudinal model predicting mutual partner violence among White, Black, and Hispanic couples in the United States general population. *Violence and Victims, 20*(5), 499–511.

Foa, E. B., Cascardi, M., Zoellner, L. A., & Feeny, N. C. (2000). Psychological and environmental factors associated with partner violence. *Trauma Violence & Abuse, 1*(1), 67–91.

Galvan, F. H., & Caetano, R. (2003). *Alcohol use and related problems among ethnic minorities in the United States* [Electronic version]. Retrieved September 10, 2007, from http://pubs.niaaa.nih.gov/publications/arh27-1/87-94.htm

Graham-Kevan, N., & Archer, J. (2005). Investigating three explanations of women's relationship aggression. *Psychology of Women Quarterly, 29*(3), 270–277.

Hamberger, L. K., & Guse, C. (2005). Typology of reactions to intimate partner violence among men and women arrested for partner violence. *Violence & Victims, 20*(3), 303–317.

Hien, D., Cohen, L., & Campbell, A. (2005). Is traumatic stress a vulnerability factor for women with substance use disorders? *Clinical Psychology Review, 25*(6), 813–823.

Hoaken, P. N., & Stewart, S. H. (2003). Drugs of abuse and the elicitation of human aggressive behavior. *Addictive Behaviors, 28*(9), 1533–1554.

Kaysen, D., Dillworth, T. M., Simpson, T., Waldrop, A., Larimer, M. E., & Resick, P. A. (2007). Domestic violence and alcohol use: Trauma-related symptoms and motives for drinking. *Addictive Behaviors, 32*(6), 1272–1283.

Khantzian, E. J. (1997). The self-medication hypothesis of substance use disorders: A reconsideration and recent applications. *Harvard Review of Psychiatry, 4*(5), 231–244.

Kline, R. B. (2005). *Principles and practices of structural equation modeling* (2nd ed.). New York: Guilford Press.

Klostermann, K. C., & Fals-Stewart, W. (2006). Intimate partner violence and alcohol use: Exploring the role of drinking in partner violence and its implications for intervention. *Aggression and Violent Behavior, 11*(6), 587–597.

Leisring, P. A. (in press). What will happen if I punch him? Expected consequences of female violence against male dating partners. *Journal of Aggression, Maltreatment, & Trauma.*

Leonard, K. E., & Quigley, B. M. (1999). Drinking and marital aggression in newlyweds: An event-based analysis of drinking and the occurrence of husband marital aggression. *Journal of Studies on Alcohol, 60*(4), 537–545.

Magdol, L., Moffitt, T. E., Caspi, A., & Silva, P. A. (1998). Developmental antecedents of partner abuse: A prospective-longitudinal study. *Journal of Abnormal Psychology, 107*(3), 375–389.

Martino, S. C., Collins, R. L., & Ellickson, P. L. (2005). Cross-lagged relationships between substance use and intimate partner violence among a sample of young adult women. *Journal of Studies on Alcohol, 66*(1), 139–148.

NOVA Research Company (2003). *Questionnaire Development System*^{TM} *user's manual*. Bethesda, MD: Author.

Schafer, J., & Caetano, R. (2002). Violence and alcohol: Cultural issues and barriers to treatment. In C. Wekerle & A. Wall (Eds.), *The violence and addiction equation: Theoretical and clinical issues in substance abuse and relationship violence* (pp. 2239–2253). New York: Brunner-Routledge.

Schafer, J., Caetano, R., & Cunradi, C. B. (2004). A path model of risk factors for intimate partner violence among couples in the United States. *Journal of Interpersonal Violence, 19*(2), 127–142.

Selin, K. H. (2003). Test-retest reliability of the Alcohol Use Disorder Identification Test in a general population sample. *Alcoholism: Clinical & Experimental Research, 27*(9), 1428–1435.

Skinner, H. A. (1982). The Drug Abuse Screening Test. *Addictive Behaviors, 7*(4), 363–371.

Snow, D. L., Sullivan, T. P., Swan, S. C., Tate, D. C., & Klein, I. (2006). The role of coping and problem drinking in men's abuse of female partners: Test of a path model. *Violence and Victims, 21*(3), 267–285.

SPSS Inc. (2006). AMOS 7 (Version 6.0) [Computer software]. Spring House, PA: AMOS Development Corporation.

Stith, S. M., Smith, D. B., Penn, C. E., Ward, D. B., & Tritt, D. (2004). Intimate partner physical abuse perpetration and victimization risk factors: A meta-analytic review. *Aggression and Violent Behavior, 10*(1), 65–98.

Straus, M. A., Hamby, S. L., Boney-McCoy, S., & Sugarman, D. B. (1996). The revised Conflict Tactics Scales (CTS2): Development and preliminary psychometric data. *Journal of Family Issues, 17*(3), 283–316.

Stuart, G. L., Meehan, J. C., Moore, T. M., Morean, M., Hellmuth, J., & Follansbee, K. (2006). Examining a conceptual framework of intimate partner violence in men and women arrested for domestic violence. *Journal of Studies on Alcohol, 67*(1), 102–112.

Stuart, G. L., Moore, T. M., Gordon, K. C., Hellmuth, J. C., Ramsey, S. E., & Kahler, C. W. (2006). Reasons for intimate partner violence perpetration among arrested women. *Violence Against Women, 12*(7), 609–621.

Sullivan, T. P., Meese, K. J., Swan, S. C., Mazure, C. M., & Snow, D. L. (2005). Precursors and correlates of women's violence: Childhood abuse traumatization, victimization of women, avoidance coping and psychological symptoms. *Psychology of Women Quarterly, 29*(3), 290–301.

Swan, S. C., & Snow, D. L. (2002). A typology of women's use of violence in intimate relationships. *Violence Against Women, 8*(3), 286–319.

Swan, S. C., & Snow, D. L. (2003). Behavioral and psychological differences among abused women who use violence in intimate relationships. *Violence Against Women, 9*(1), 75–109.

Swan, S. C., & Snow, D. L. (2006). The development of a theory of women's use of violence in intimate relationships. *Violence Against Women, 12*(11), 1026–1045.

Tabachnick, B. G., & Fidell, L. S. (2007). *Using multivariate statistics* (5th ed.). Boston: Allyn & Bacon/Pearson Education.

U.S. Department of Health and Human Services. (2003). *Drug use among racial/ ethnic minorities* (No. NIH Publication No. 03-3888, revised September 2003). Bethesda, MD: Author.

Wells, K., Klap, R., Koike, A., & Sherbourne, C. (2001). Ethnic disparities in unmet need for alcoholism, drug abuse, and mental health care. *American Journal of Psychiatry, 158*(12), 2027–2032.

Introduction to Part II

LISA CONRADI

Chadwick Center for Children and Families, Rady Children's Hospital, San Diego, San Diego, California, USA

ROBERT GEFFNER

Institute on Violence, Abuse and Trauma, Alliant International University, San Diego, California, USA

The literature on female offenders of intimate partner violence (IPV) continues to stress the importance of assessing the context and motivation of women's use of violence and the need to adapt interventions to meet the needs of these women. This special issue is the second of a two-part issue that critically examines the prevalence of female offenders of IPV and addresses the gaps in current research. The six articles contained in this issue provide updated research on the context and motivation of women's use of violence in intimate relationships and present examples of current treatment strategies for this population.

There has been considerable controversy about women's use of violence in intimate relationships. While a review of the issues has been provided elsewhere (see Graham-Kevan, 2009; Hines & Douglas, 2009; Straus, 2009), there continues to be significant debate regarding the context and motivation for women's use of violence in their intimate relationships. On the one hand, it has been suggested that female-perpetrated intimate partner violence (IPV) is a genuine problem that has been uncovered by the rigorous use of representative samples and quantitative methods of data collection (Straus, 2009). On the other hand, it has been suggested that the use of methods that simply measure acts of physical aggression and ignore the context and meaning of any violence results in the failure to demonstrate very obvious differences between male- versus female-perpetrated IPV (Hamberger, Lohr, Bonge, & Tolin, 1997).

MOTIVATION

While many national surveys have suggested that males and females are equally aggressive in domestic relationships (Straus & Gelles, 1986), they have not examined the motivation for this aggression across genders. Hamberger et al. (1997) found that motivations common to both male and female perpetrators included control, anger expression, and coercive communication. On the other hand, motivations specific to male perpetrators were alcohol abuse and the imposition of coercive emotional control, while motivations specific to female perpetrators were response to verbal abuse and retaliation or self-defense. Therefore, while men and women may commit acts of aggression in intimate relationships at an equivalent rate, their acts appear to be differentially motivated. In addition, there is an important distinction between aggression and abuse. While aggression includes the intent to cause physical or psychological injury or harm, abuse serves as a mechanism to assert power and control over another person. In comparison to aggression, abuse produces different prevalence rates and different levels of violence severity and subsequent injuries across genders.

CONTEXT

When examining female crime and offenses, it is important to understand the context in which they occur. "Context" refers to the characteristics of a particular offense, including both the circumstances surrounding and the nature of the act (Steffensmeier, 1996). Contextual characteristics include the location where the offense occurred, the characteristics of the offender, the type of victim, the victim–offender relationship, whether a weapon was used, the extent of any injuries, and the purpose of the offense (Steffensmeier, 1996). The context of a crime is often neglected or minimized by quantitative studies, particularly those examining the differences between male and female offending rates in IPV. Context is particularly important when examining female violence in intimate relationships, because although the aggressive act may be the same, the reasons why a woman uses violence may be very different from the reasons why a man uses violence. In his examination of the context in which female offenders of IPV used violence with their partners, Hamberger (1997) found that two-thirds of the women had been battered and used violence to protect themselves or to retaliate for previous violence against them.

TREATMENT IMPLICATIONS

Since 1979, most domestic violence offenders have been channeled out of the criminal justice system into counseling or psychoeducational programs. Following the advent of mandatory and proarrest laws for domestic violence offenders, the number of women mandated to treatment for domestic violence has increased significantly (Hamberger & Arnold, 1990). The preferred mode of treatment for women arrested for IPV has consistently been group treatment with other women arrested for domestic violence. The mode of group treatment presents unique challenges to group facilitators since the women arrested for IPV have often used physical aggression and violence for many different reasons. Recent research has emerged suggesting that women who are arrested for IPV often fall into three distinct groups: violence as a form of self-defense, women involved in bidirectionally violent relationships, and women who are classified as dominant aggressors of IPV (Swan & Snow, 2002, 2003). Women involved in bidirectionally violent relationships may be primarily the victim in their relationships or primarily the aggressor. Therefore, like men, the treatment needs of women arrested for IPV are as varied as the women themselves, especially depending on their motivations for violence, criminal history, trauma history, and personal characteristics. Very few curricula designed specifically for women who have been arrested for IPV exist (for an example, see Koonin, Cabarcas, & Geffner, 2002). Many of the programs for these women are usually slightly modified versions of programs that were designed for and utilized by male offenders. It appears, however, that this approach may not be appropriate for many women. Therefore research on existing curricula and the development of new curricula designed specifically for women is warranted.

OVERVIEW OF THE ARTICLES IN THIS SPECIAL ISSUE

The present collection of articles attempts to address the large gap in the literature that exists regarding the role of context and motivation in women's use of violence in their intimate relationships and treatment implications for this population. In the opening article, Caldwell, Swan, Allen, Sullivan, and Snow explore the relationship between women's motives for

IPV and their perpetration of physical, psychological, and sexual aggression toward partners. In their article, Walley-Jean and Swan describe a study focusing on the motivations and justifications for hypothetical partner aggression in a sample of African American women, a largely underrepresented group. The article by Conradi, Geffner, Hamberger, and Lawson describes a qualitative study that focused on the unique characteristics and motivations that can be attributed to women who are classified as the dominant aggressors of physical violence in their intimate relationships. Leisring examines expected consequences for using physical aggression against dating partners among aggressive and nonaggressive college women.

The final set of articles focuses on treatment implications for working with women who have been violent in their intimate relationships. Goldenson, Spidel, Greaves, and Dutton provide a review of research on the subject, including psychopathology, and discuss current treatment options with recommendations for the future. Tutty, Babins-Wagner, and Rothery describe recent research on mandated versus nonmandated women in a treatment program called Responsible Choices for Women.

With this second of two special issues devoted to female-perpetrated violence in intimate relationships, it is our hope that readers will critically examine the research regarding the context and motivation of women's use of violence in intimate relationships and design and evaluate interventions that have been specifically developed to meet the unique needs of this population.

REFERENCES

Graham-Kevan, N. (2009). The psychology of women's partner violence: Characteristics and cautions. *Journal of Aggression, Maltreatment & Trauma, 18*(6), 587–603.

Hamberger, L. K. (1997). Female offenders in domestic violence: A look at actions in their context. *Journal of Aggression, Maltreatment & Trauma, 1*(1), 117–129.

Hamberger, L. K., & Arnold, J. (1990). The impact of mandatory arrest on domestic violence perpetrator counseling services. *Family Violence & Sexual Assault Bulletin, 6*(1), 11–12.

Hamberger, L. K., Lohr, J. M., Bonge, D., & Tolin, D. F. (1997). An empirical classification of motivations for domestic violence. *Violence Against Women, 3*, 401–423.

Hines, D. A., & Douglas, E. M. (2009). Women's use of intimate partner violence against men: Prevalence, implications, and consequences. *Journal of Aggression, Maltreatment & Trauma, 18*(6), 572–586.

Koonin, M., Cabarcas, A., & Geffner, R. (2002). *Treatment of women arrested for domestic violence: Women ending abusive/violent episodes respectfully (W.E.A.V.E.R.) manual.* San Diego, CA: Family Violence & Sexual Assault Institute.

Steffensmeier, D. (1996). Gender and crime: Toward a gendered theory of female offending. *Annual Review of Sociology, 22*, 459–487.

Straus, M. A. (2009). Why the overwhelming evidence on partner physical violence by women has not been perceived and is often denied. *Journal of Aggression, Maltreatment & Trauma, 18*(6), 552–571.

Straus, M. A., & Gelles, R. J. (1986). Societal change and change in family violence from 1975 to 1985 as revealed by two national surveys. *Journal of Marriage and the Family, 48*(August), 465–479.

Swan, S. C., & Snow, D. L. (2002). A typology of women's use of violence in intimate relationships. *Violence Against Women, 8*(3), 286–319.

Swan, S. C., & Snow, D. L. (2003). Behavioral and psychological differences among abused women who use violence in intimate relationships. *Violence Against Women, 9*(1), 75–109.

RESEARCH EXAMINING THE MOTIVATION OF WOMEN'S USE OF INTIMATE PARTNER VIOLENCE

Why I Hit Him: Women's Reasons for Intimate Partner Violence

JENNIFER E. CALDWELL, SUZANNE C. SWAN, and
CHRISTOPHER T. ALLEN

University of South Carolina, Columbia, South Carolina, USA

TAMI P. SULLIVAN and DAVID L. SNOW

Yale University, New Haven, Connecticut, USA

This study examines motives for intimate partner violence (IPV) among a community sample of 412 women who used IPV against male partners. A "Motives and Reasons for IPV Scale" is proposed, and exploratory factor analyses identified five factors: expression of negative emotions, self-defense, control, jealousy, and tough guise. To our knowledge, the study is the first to investigate the relationship between women's motives for IPV and their perpetration of physical, psychological, and sexual aggression, as well as coercive control, toward partners. Hierarchical regression analyses revealed participants' aggression was driven by complex, multiple motives. All five motives were related to a greater frequency of perpetrating IPV. Treatment programs focusing on women's IPV perpetration should address both defensive and proactive motives.

Increased arrest rates of women for domestic violence offenses (Swan & Snow, 2002; Henning, Martinsson, & Holdford, 2009) highlight the importance of understanding the reasons that women, as well as men, use intimate partner violence (IPV; Stuart et al., 2006). To develop effective interventions, researchers and service providers working with individuals who use IPV need to understand what the individuals themselves see as their reasons for committing aggressive behaviors. However, knowledge of these reasons for IPV, particularly for women, is hampered by a lack of empirical data (Hettrich & O'Leary, 2007; Stuart et al., 2006). The purpose of this study is to examine reasons and motives for IPV among a community sample of women who used IPV against male intimate partners. A "Motives and Reasons for IPV Scale" is proposed, and exploratory factor analyses are conducted to identify the factor structure of the scale. The relationships between scale factors and women's IPV is examined, controlling for victimization the women received from their partners. The study is the first, to our knowledge, to investigate the relationship between a comprehensive measure of women's reasons and motives for IPV and their perpetration of physical, psychological, and sexual aggression, as well as coercive control, toward their partners.

WOMEN'S MOTIVES FOR IPV

Motives are defined as "underlying psychological processes that impel people's thinking, feeling, and behaving" (Fiske, 2004, p. 14). Motives for aggressive behavior in general have been conceptualized as reactive (responding to a perceived threat, such as defending oneself when attacked) versus proactive (aggression that is initiated with the goal of dominating, controlling, threatening, or bullying someone else; Dodge & Coie, 1987). Similarly, women's motivations for aggression against intimate partners have been organized into two types: defensive or reactive motives (i.e., self-protective violence) and active motives, or those that are goal oriented, such as retaliation and attempts to control the partner (Swan & Snow, 2006).

The following section provides an overview of research on women's defensive and active motives and reasons for IPV. While reviewing these research findings, it is helpful to keep in mind that aggressors typically have multiple motives for their behavior (Fiske, 2004). Some motives, such as self-defense and control, may be proximally related to the psychological processes impelling the person's aggressive behavior at that moment. Other reasons for aggression, such as previous abusive relationships, likely are more distally related. Henceforth the term "motives" refers to proximal psychological processes that impel behavior, while "reasons" is used as a more general term that refers to motives or to more distal contributors to aggression.

Expression of Negative Emotions

One of the primary functions of aggression in general, and IPV in particular, is to express strongly felt negative emotions, such as anger and frustration (Fiske, 2004; Kimmel, 2002). Women who were arrested for IPV indicated that showing anger was a motive for their violence 39% of the time (Stuart et al., 2006); Babcock, Miller, and Siard (2003) found similar results. In several studies of college women who completed a motives measure and then identified which motive was the "main cause" of their aggression toward partners, "to show anger" was the most frequently identified primary motive (Hettrich & O'Leary, 2007; Walley-Jean & Swan, 2009).

Self-Defense

Women who engage in IPV commonly report using violence to defend themselves from their partners (Babcock et al., 2003). That self-defense is a frequent motive is not surprising given that the majority of women who use IPV also experience violence from their partners (Orcutt, Garcia, & Pickett, 2005; Straus & Gelles, 1990; Stuart et al., 2006; Swan & Snow, 2002; Temple, Weston, & Marshall, 2005). Among a sample of women who used IPV, 75% of participants indicated that self-defense was a motive for their violence; it was also the most frequently endorsed motive (Swan & Snow, 2003).

We expect that women in our sample who report that self-defense is never a motive for their violence may be primary aggressors who commit more violence against partners than they receive. These women likely have other, nondefensive motives for their violence, such as expressing negative emotions or control. They may commit higher levels of aggression relative to women who do have self-defensive motives for their violence. In contrast, women who score high on the self-defense motive (i.e., most of the time when they are aggressive, they are defending themselves) may be primarily victims. In response to their high levels of victimization, these women may commit more aggression than other groups.

Thus we anticipate that the relationship between self-defense motives and women's perpetration of physical aggression might be curvilinear, with higher aggression being committed by women whose aggression is *never* motivated by self-defense, and by women whose aggression is *very often* motivated by self-defense. Women in between these two extremes may use aggression less than the other two groups. These women may be in more mutually aggressive relationships, in which both partners may become aggressive but neither has dominance or control over the other. These relationships may be similar to Johnson's (2006) "situational couple violence," in which IPV is usually mutual, infrequent, not severe, and not part of a general pattern of control and domination. Mutually aggressive relationships tend to be less violent than relationships in which one partner is much more violent than the other (Swan & Snow, 2003).

Control

Some women use IPV in an attempt to control their partners. Swan and Snow (2003) found that 38% of women who used IPV stated that they had threatened to use violence to make their partners do the things they wanted them to do. Stuart et al.'s (2006) sample of women arrested for IPV indicated that "to feel more powerful" was a motive 26% of the time; other control-related motives included "to get control over your partner," 22%; "to get your partner to do something or stop doing something," 22%; and "to make your partner agree with you," 17%. Similarly, Follingstad Wright, Lloyd, and Sebastian (1991) found that 22% of college women said they used violence to get control over their partner, while 12% agreed that "I feel personally empowered when I behave aggressively against my partner."

While some individuals use aggression to increase their feelings of control or power, others attribute their aggression to a lack of control over their emotions and themselves (Thomas, 2005). For example, women who were arrested for IPV in Stuart et al.'s (2006) study endorsed reasons for aggression related to losing self-control, including "because your partner provoked you or pushed you over the edge" and "because you didn't know what to do with your feelings" (reported 39% and 35% of the time, respectively).

Jealousy

Jealousy is another common motive for women's IPV. Follingstad et al.'s (1991) college population indicated that 9% of women attributed their aggression toward their partners to jealousy, and Bookwala, Frieze, Smith, and Ryan's (1992) study of college women found that jealousy was a significant predictor of women's IPV. Women who were arrested for IPV indicated that "because you were jealous," "because your partner cheated on you," and "to prove you love your partner" motivated their violence 25%, 25%, and 27% of the time, respectively (Stuart et al., 2006).

Tough Guise

Most women who use IPV are also victims of aggression from their partners (Swan, Gambone, Caldwell, Sullivan, & Snow, 2008), and this is true for participants in the current study. In the current sample, 90% of participants experienced physical aggression from partners, 95% experienced coercive control, and 53% were sexually victimized. In a relationship characterized by IPV, a woman may use aggression to convey the message to her partner that she is not to be trifled with and that he had better take her seriously— there will be violent consequences if he tries to hurt her (Thomas, 2005). Hettrich and O'Leary's (2007) study of college women's reasons for their physical aggression in dating relationships illustrates this point with participants' open-ended explanations of what led up to their aggression, including the response, "to show seriousness" (p. 1138). Similarly, studies have found that a relatively small number of women used IPV for purposes of intimidation. Stuart et al. (2006) found that women used IPV "to make your partner scared or afraid" 11% of the time.

HYPOTHESES

An exploratory factor analysis (described in the results section) indicated that the Motives and Reasons for IPV Scale has five factors: expression of negative emotions, self-defense, control, jealousy, and tough guise. We developed the following hypotheses: (a) all motive factors, except self-defense, will be positively related to the perpetration of physical aggression; (b) the self-defense motive factor will display a curvilinear relationship to the perpetration of physical aggression; (c) all five motive factors will be positively related to the perpetration of psychological aggression; and (d) the motive factors of control and jealousy will be positively related to the perpetration of coercive control.

Sexual aggression is likely a qualitatively different form of aggression than physical or psychological aggression (Frieze, 2005). Because so little is known about women's perpetration of sexual aggression, no predictions are made regarding the motives and reasons that may be related to this form of aggression.

METHOD

Participants

A community sample of 150 African American, 112 White, and 150 Latina women participated in the study (N = 412). Participants were recruited from a northeastern city by placing English and Spanish-language brochures and posters in various locations, including medical clinics, stores, churches, libraries, restaurants, and laundromats throughout the city. Many (43%) of the participants had family incomes of less than $10,000 per year, 28% earned $10,000 to $20,000 per year, 17% earned $20,000 to $30,000 per year, and 12% earned more than $30,000 per year. Most (64%) of the participants were unemployed, 20% worked part time, and 14% worked full time. Twenty-eight percent of participants had not completed high school, 41% had graduated from high school or obtained a GED, 23% had some education beyond high school, and 8% had earned a college or advanced degree. The average age of participants was 36.6 years (SD = 8.9), with a range of 18 to 65 years. Somewhat less than half (43%) of the sample was unmarried and cohabitating with their partners, 24% were married, 26% were in a dating relationship but lived apart, and 7% had ended their relationships (although they still saw their former partners at least once a week). The length of time that the participants had been with their partners ranged from 4 months to more than 20 years; 9.3% of the participants had been with their partner for 1 year or less, 41.6% had been with their partner for more than 1 year up to 5 years, 36.1% had been with their partner more than 5 years up to 15 years, and 13.2% had been with their partner for more than 15 years. The majority (77%) of the women were mothers with an average of 2 children.

Procedure

A short telephone screening was conducted with participants to assess if they met criteria for inclusion in the study. Participants had to self-identify as African American, White, or Latina, have a yearly family income of no more than $50,000 (to reduce income disparities between racial/ethnic groups), and committed at least one act of physical violence against a male significant other in the last 6 months. Participants who met study criteria were invited to participate in face-to-face interviews. A female interviewer of the same race/ethnicity as the participant conducted the 2-hour semis-tructured interview. Latina participants were interviewed by a bilingual/bicultural interviewer and had the option of being interviewed in Spanish. A bilingual/bicultural research associate translated the survey instruments and recruiting materials as necessary. Seventy-four of the 150 Latina partici-pants completed the interview in Spanish. The measures were administered on notebook computers using Questionnaire Development System software (NOVA Research Company, 2003). Participants were compensated $50 for their time.

Measures

PERPETRATION AND VICTIMIZATION

Perpetration and victimization were assessed with three measures: the Revised Conflict Tactics Scale (CTS2; Straus, Hamby, Boney-McCoy, & Sugarman, 1996), the short Psychological Maltreatment of Women Inven-tory (PMWI; Tolman, 1999), and the Sexual Experiences Survey (SES; Koss, Gidycz, & Wisniewski, 1987). All CTS2, PMWI, and SES items were worded to assess the participants' own aggressive behavior (perpetration) and the aggressive behavior of their partners toward them (victimization) during the past six months. The response scale for all items was never (0), once in the past six months (1), twice in the past six months (2), three to five times in the past six months (3), six to ten times in the past six months (4), more than ten times in the past six months (5), or not in the past six months but it happened before (6). The sixth option was recoded to zero, since this study specifically examined aggression committed in the past six months.

Physical aggression was assessed using the CTS2, the most frequently used survey of aggression in the IPV field (Straus et al., 1996). The CTS2 has demonstrated adequate reliability and validity for female samples (Straus, Hamby, & Warren, 2003). The physical aggression perpetration and victimization scales each included 12 items. The reliability alphas for physical aggression perpetration and victimization in this study were .87 and .91, respectively. A sample item representing physical aggression is, "Did you throw something at your partner that could hurt?" (perpetration); "Did your partner throw something at you that could hurt?" (victimization).

Psychological aggression was assessed by using both the psychological aggression subscale of the CTS2 (Straus et al., 2003) and the emotional/verbal abuse subscale of the PMWI (Tolman, 1999) for a total of 13 perpetration and 13 victimization items. The PMWI has demonstrated adequate reliability and validity, and has discriminated between abused and non-abused women (Tolman, 1999). The combined psychological aggression measure using items from both scales was more reliable than either the CTS2 or the PMWI psychological aggression subscales. Psychological perpetration and victimization in this study had reliability alphas of .76 and .83, respectively. An example of an item representing psychological aggression is, "Did you insult or swear at your partner?" (perpetration); "Did your partner insult or swear at you?" (victimization).

Coercive control was measured using the dominance/isolation subscale of the PMWI (Tolman, 1999). The coercive control perpetration and victimization scales each included seven items. In this study, coercive control perpetration and victimization had reliability alphas of .61 and .75, respectively. An example of an item representing coercive control is, "Did you monitor your partner's time and make him account for where he was?" (perpetration); "Did your partner monitor your time and make you account for where you were?" (victimization).

Sexual aggression was examined with the SES (Koss et al., 1987), which assessed unwanted sexual contact, sexual coercion, attempted rape, and rape. The sexual victimization scale included 10 items. The victimization scale was developed with college populations (Koss et al., 1987) and has been found to be valid and reliable with a sample of community women (Testa, VanZile-Tamsen, Livingston, & Koss, 2004). Because high-level reading skills are necessary to understand the items (Testa et al., 2004), item wording was simplified for the present study. Ten items parallel in wording to the victimization items were added to assess women's perpetration of sexually aggressive behaviors. The reliability alphas for sexual aggression perpetration and victimization in this study were .92 and .90, respectively. An example of an item representing sexual coercion is, "Have you tried to make your partner have sex by using force, like twisting an arm or holding them down, or by threatening to use force?" (perpetration); "Has your partner tried to make you have sex by using force, like twisting your arm or holding you down, or by threatening to use force?" (victimization).

MOTIVES

The Motives and Reasons for IPV Scale was developed for this study (Swan & Sullivan, 2002). Participants were asked, "How often did you use violence, such as slapping, hitting, etc. for the following reasons?" The original measure consisted of 35 motives or reasons with possible responses of never (0), sometimes (1), often (2), and almost always (3). An exploratory factor analysis (see below) was conducted and indicated that a five-factor solution was the best fit. The factors and associated reliability coefficients are expression of negative emotions (five items, α = .82), self-defense (five items, α = .86), control (six items, α = .78), jealousy (two items, α = .73), and tough guise (eight items, α = .82). The items representing each of these factors are listed in Table 1. The final Motives and Reasons for IPV Scale had a total of 26 items and an overall reliability alpha of .92. As explained in more detail below, nine items were deleted from the measure after conducting the exploratory factor analysis.

SOCIAL DESIRABILITY

Participants completed a 10-item social desirability measure based on the widely used Marlowe–Crowne Scale, containing items such as "No matter who I'm talking to, I'm always a good listener" and "There have been occasions when I took advantage of someone" (reverse-coded; Greenwald & Satow, 1970). The response scale ranged from strongly disagree (1) to strongly agree (5). The reliability of the measure in the present study was α = .76.

Data Analyses

EXPLORATORY FACTOR ANALYSIS

An exploratory factor analysis (EFA) was performed with the 35 items from the Motives and Reasons for IPV Scale. EFA was chosen over confirmatory factor analysis (CFA) because CFA requires "clear predictions as to which factors exist, how they relate to the variables, and how they relate to each other" (Gorsuch, 1997, p. 534), which were not evident for the Motives and Reasons for IPV Scale based on the literature. To identify the underlying factor structure, an EFA was performed in Mplus 5 (Muthén & Muthén, 2007) using the mean- and variance-adjusted weighted least square (WLSMV) estimator (due to use of ordinal data) and Promax oblique rotation (due to assumed correlation between factors). EFA is used to identify latent constructs

TABLE 1 Descriptive Statistics for Motives, Perpetration, Victimization, and Social Desirability

Motives

How often did you use violence. . .	% endorsed	M	SD
Expression of negative emotions	95	1.09	0.65
Because your partner said something that hurt you	77	1.07	0.81
Because he made you angry	87	1.28	0.81
Because you wanted to let him know he couldn't get away with mistreating you	74	1.12	0.91
Because you were frustrated	72	1.01	0.83
Because you were fed up with his behavior	67	0.98	0.89
Control	89	0.74	0.55
To make your partner do the things you wanted him to do	67	0.85	0.76
Because you wanted him to give you something, like money, or something for your children	36	0.48	0.75
Because you wanted him to do something	57	0.70	0.74
Because you couldn't stop yourself	57	0.78	0.82
To feel in control	50	0.66	0.79
Because he tried to control you	68	0.98	0.88
Tough guise	84	0.45	0.46
To harm your partner	44	0.56	0.74
To intimidate your partner	39	0.53	0.77
Because you feel better after a fight	18	0.24	0.56
To scare him	35	0.45	0.71
Because you were drinking or using drugs	33	0.47	0.79
To physically hurt him	35	0.45	0.71
To get "turned on" sexually	5	0.07	0.33
To get him to take you seriously	63	0.81	0.77
Self-defense	83	0.84	0.74
To defend yourself from your partner	77	1.28	0.99
To get your partner to stop hitting or hurting you	65	1.07	1.03
Because you knew a beating was coming and you wanted to get it over with	28	0.39	0.71
Because he became abusive when he drank	45	0.75	1.00
To get away as he was beating you	46	0.68	0.33
Jealousy	67	0.71	0.68
Because you thought your partner was unfaithful	54	0.69	0.75
Because you were jealous	58	0.74	0.78
Perpetration and victimization			
Physical aggression perpetration	100	1.00	0.80
Psychological aggression perpetration	100	2.19	0.83
Coercive control perpetration	88	1.16	0.84
Sexual aggression perpetration	32	0.18	0.56
Physical aggression victimization	90	0.97	0.98
Psychological aggression victimization	100	2.26	1.03
Coercive control victimization	95	1.73	1.16
Sexual aggression victimization	53	0.50	0.93
Social desirability		3.55	0.64

Note: Responses for motive items were never (0), sometimes (1), often (2), and almost always (3). Responses for perpetration and victimization items were never (0), once in the past 6 months (1), twice in the past 6 months (2), 3 to 5 times in the past 6 months (3), 6 to 10 times in the past 6 months (4), and more than 10 times in the past 6 months (5). Responses for social desirability items were strongly disagree (1), disagree (2), undecided or unsure (3), agree (4), and strongly agree (5).

(i.e., factors), with the goal of understanding the structure of correlations among the observed variables. Specifically EFA models the structure of correlations among observed variables by estimating the pattern of relations between the common factor(s) and each of the measured variables (as indexed by factor loadings; Fabrigar, Wegener, MacCallum, & Strahan, 1999). The final solution (i.e., factor model) was selected through evaluation of the following model fit criteria. A model that is generally interpreted as providing a good fit to the data is one that has a root mean square of approximation (RMSEA) value $\leq .05$, a root mean square residual (SRMR) $\leq .08$ (Hu & Bentler, 1999), and a comparative fit index (CFI) value close to 1 (Bentler, 1990).

REGRESSION ANALYSES

Because only 3.4% of the data were missing, listwise deletion was used to address missing values (Schafer, 1999). Hierarchical regression analyses were conducted to examine the relationship between the factors in the Motives and Reasons for IPV measure and participants' perpetration of physical, psychological, and sexual aggression and coercive control toward partners. The covariates of women's physical, psychological, and sexual victimization, coercive control, and social desirability were entered in the first step of each regression analysis. Victimization was controlled for in the analyses because a strong relationship between victimization from partners and female perpetration of IPV has been found in several studies (Graves, Sechrist, White, & Paradise, 2005; Magdol et al., 1997; Sullivan, Meese, Swan, Mazure, & Snow, 2005; Swan, Gambone, Fields, Sullivan, & Snow, 2005). Similarly, as social desirability concerns may impact women's reports of motives, social desirability was entered as a covariate. The five factors (i.e., expression of negative emotions, self-defense, control, jealousy, and tough guise) were entered in the second step.

In order to test for a nonlinear relationship between self-defense and physical perpetration, we used a polynomial regression approach (Cohen, Cohen, West, & Aiken, 2003). Polynomial equations relate X to Y by using transformed variables (X^2, X^3, etc.) that possess a known nonlinear relationship to the original variables. By structuring nonlinear relationships in this way, it is possible to determine whether the relationship between X and Y is nonlinear, as well as the form of the relationship.

In the current analyses, we tested for a curvilinear relationship between the self-defense motive factor and physical perpetration by centering the self-defense motive (i.e., subtracting the overall self-defense mean from each score) variable and then creating a polynomial term (X^2) from the centered variable. Centering of predictors in this manner renders all regression coefficients in a polynomial regression equation meaningful by reflecting the regression function at the mean of the predictor. Centering also eliminates the extreme multicollinearity resulting from using powers of predictors in a single equation (Cohen et al., 2003). To properly test for the presence of a curvilinear relationship, the highest-order term (which determines the overall shape of the regression function) is entered with all lower-order terms (Aiken & West, 1991; Cohen et al., 2003). The centered linear and polynomial forms of the self-defense variable were used as predictors in the regression analysis to test for the presence of a curvilinear relationship.

RESULTS

Exploratory Factor Analysis: Determining the Number of Factors

To determine the number of factors on the Motives and Reasons for IPV Scale, we first examined the eigenvalues for the correlation matrix based on all 35 items. The Kaiser (1960) criterion, which recommends that the number of factors be equivalent to the number of eigenvalues greater than 1, suggested seven factors. Based on research that suggested the Kaiser criterion tends to overestimate the number of factors as the number of variables approaches 40 (Stevens, 2002), the value of seven was regarded as the upper limit for the number of factors.

Next, we examined the scree plot as proposed by Cattel (1966) as a graphical method for determining the number of factors. Cattel (1966) recommended retaining all eigenvalues in the sharp descent before the point at which the plot begins to level off. The plot suggested that a model containing one to six factors was most appropriate for consideration.

Third, we conducted an EFA with the 35 items from the Motives and Reasons for IPV Scale. After estimating a model with the number of factors ranging from one to six, we considered interpretability of the results suggested by the EFA by examining the item pattern and structure coefficients (commonly called "factor loadings"). In EFA, the contribution of a variable to a given factor is indicated by both factor pattern and structure coefficients. Thompson and Daniel (1996) noted that structure coefficients, or correlations between observed and latent variables, "are usually essential to interpretation" (p. 199).

In factor analysis, the factor structure matrix gives the correlations between all observed variables and all extracted (latent) factors. When factors are orthogonally rotated, they remain uncorrelated, and the factor structure matrix will be an identity matrix, exactly matching the factor pattern matrix (Gorsuch, 1983). However, when an oblique rotation is used, as in the current study, the factors are allowed to correlate with each other. In such cases, the factor correlation matrix will not be an identity matrix, and the structure matrix will not equal the pattern matrix. Appropriate interpretation, then, must invoke both the factor pattern and factor structure matrices (Courville & Thompson, 2001; Thompson & Borrello, 1985). To decide which items were significant indicators of a factor (i.e., "loaded on a factor"), we used a cutoff of .40, which exceeds the .30 criteria suggested by Briggs and MacCallum (2003). After examining the matrices, the five-factor model was considered best among other alternatives with regard to interpretability and other decision criteria. The fit indices for the five-factor model with 35 items indicated a good fit of the model to the data: $\chi^2(117, N = 412) = 310.60$, $p \leq .0001$; RMSEA = 0.06; SRMR = .05. (In large samples, a significant chi square is not necessarily indicative of poor model fit; see Barrett, 2007.) Pattern and structure matrices for the final model are shown in Tables 2 and 3, respectively.

EFA IN A CONFIRMATORY FACTOR ANALYSIS FRAMEWORK

In order to make sure that the large values of the factor loadings found in EFA were in fact all statistically significant, to see if the low value of the factor loadings was statistically nonsignificant, and to identify the items that were unrelated to any of the factors in a statistically significant way, we ran a confirmatory factor model equivalent to the above exploratory factor model with five factors (Jöreskog, 1969; Skrondal & Rabe-Hesketh, 2004) to obtain standard errors for item loadings. To fit the EFA model in a CFA framework, one must use the same number of restrictions as in an EFA model, where the number of restrictions is equal to the number of factors squared. For our model we imposed 25 (5^2) restrictions by (a) fixing factor variances to a value of 1 for all five factors; (b) choosing an anchor item for each factor (i.e., an item with a large loading for a given factor and small loadings for the other factors) and fixing the factor loading for the "anchored" factor to 1; (c) fixing the factor loadings for anchor items on all other factors to 0; and (d) allowing all other factor loadings to be free. For our data, items 4, 6, 9, 11, and 14 were selected as anchors for their respective factors. These restrictions resulted in the same number of restrictions as the traditional EFA model and thus gave the same chi square and p values, $\chi^2(117, N = 412) = 310.60$, $p \leq .0001$; RMSEA = 0.06; SRMR = .05; CFI = .93, suggesting a very good model fit.

To decide which items were significant indicators of a factor (i.e., "loaded on a factor"), we considered both statistical and substantive significance. For the statistical significance, we used a t value ≥ 1.96. This value was chosen so that the individual Type I error rate was approximately .01 when the family-wise Type I error rate was set to .025 for Bonferroni adjustment of about 175 (35 × 5) simultaneous tests on the factor loadings. The conservative Type I error rate protected against finding statistically significant factor loadings simply by chance. To assess substantive significance, we used the cutoff value of .40 for the factor loading. Items not meeting these statistical and substantive significance criteria or that significantly loaded on multiple factors were dropped.

TABLE 2 Exploratory Factor Analysis Pattern Coefficient Matrix

	Control	Tough guise	Self-defense	Express negative emotions	Jealousy
Control subscale (α = .78)					
1. To make your partner do the things you wanted him to do	**.79**	−.11	−.01	−.02	.10
13. Because you wanted him to give you something, like money, or something for your children	**.64**	.27	.02	−.11	−.07
14. Because you wanted him to do something	**.86**	−.01	−.06	−.05	.01
15. Because you couldn't stop yourself	**.56**	−.01	−.11	.29	−.04
25. To feel in control	**.51**	.25	−.15	.03	.15
29. Because he tried to control you	**.47**	−.22	.37	.22	.04
Tough guise subscale (α = .82)					
9. To harm your partner	−.09	**.89**	.12	−.12	.02
10. To intimidate your partner	.09	**.68**	−.08	.16	.11
19. Because you feel better after a fight	.11	**.67**	−.09	.13	.03
20. To scare him	.34	**.59**	−.06	−.03	.05
26. Because you were drinking or using drugs	.03	**.59**	.13	−.09	−.10
32. To physically hurt him	−.05	**.79**	.25	−.15	.02
34. To get "turned on" sexually	−.01	**.74**	.02	−.08	.02
36. To get him to take you seriously	.21	**.40**	−.01	.31	−.07
Self-defense subscale (α = .86)					
3. To defend yourself from your partner	−.05	−.05	**.84**	.17	.09
4. To get your partner to stop hitting or hurting you	−.23	.01	**.97**	.05	.13
16. Because you knew a beating was coming and you wanted to get it over with	.39	.03	**.63**	−.03	−.06
17. Because he became abusive when he drank	.18	.04	**.61**	.07	−.07
33. To get away as he was beating you	−.05	.16	**.89**	−.14	.09
Express negative emotions subscale (α = .82)					
8. Because your partner said something that hurt you	.28	−.16	.16	**.52**	.11
11. Because he made you angry	.34	−.19	−.04	**.66**	.09
12. Because you wanted to let him know he couldn't get away with mistreating you	−.16	.27	.25	**.55**	.02
18. Because you were frustrated	.47	−.11	−.03	**.54**	−.02
23. Because you were fed up with his behavior	.11	.22	.26	**.49**	−.04
Jealousy subscale (α = .73; r = .57)					
6. Because you thought your partner was unfaithful	.10	.01	.21	−.03	**.79**
27. Because you were jealous	.02	.14	.00	.12	**.69**

(*Continued*)

TABLE 2 (*Continued*)

	Control	Tough guise	Self-defense	Express negative emotions	Jealousy
Dropped items					
2. To get even with your partner for something he had done	.16	.33	−.03	.14	.29
7. To prevent your partner from leaving or going out	.16	.33	.11	−.01	.33
21. To stop the argument	.33	.25	.12	.17	−.13
22. As a joke or just playing around	−.26	.49	−.18	.15	.04
24. Because he was being mean to you	.02	.10	.41	.50	−.09
28. To get your point across	.19	.32	−.11	.42	.04
30. Because you have a bad temper	.30	.22	−.22	.35	.04
31. Because of your past abusive relationships	.25	.30	−.01	.16	−.10
35. To get him to leave you alone	.00	.37	.39	.17	−.17

Note: Factor loadings in bold represent items that were retained for that factor.

Considering significance according to the cutoff values stated above, eight items (2, 7, 21, 24, 28, 30, 31, and 35) were unrelated to any factor and were dropped. One item (22) reduced scale reliability and therefore was dropped. The final measure retained 26 of the original 35 items with excellent reliability (α = .92). We conducted an additional EFA using only the items that comprised the five-factor structure. Refitting these remaining 26 items resulted in very good model fit, superior to the fit of the 35 items, $\chi^2(117, N = 412) = 215.55$, $p \leq .0001$; RMSEA = 0.06; SRMR = .04.

Descriptive Analyses

All five of the motive factors assessed were commonly viewed by the participants as motives for their aggression toward partners (see Table 1 for descriptive statistics on the motive factors and individual items). The participants most frequently endorsed motives relating to the expression of negative emotions: almost 95% of the women indicated that negative emotions were a cause of their aggression, with "because he made you angry" being the most frequently endorsed item. More than 89% endorsed motives relating to control. Interestingly, motives relating both to women reacting against being controlled by their partners and to the women's attempts to control their partners loaded onto this factor: 68% of women stated that they used aggression "because he tried to control you" and 67% used aggression "to make your partner do the things you wanted him to do." Eighty-four percent indicated they used aggression to be taken seriously or to intimidate or harm their partner. This factor is primarily driven by wanting their partner to take them seriously (63%); fewer women actually wanted to harm

TABLE 3 Exploratory Factor Analysis Structure Coefficient Matrix

	Control	Tough guise	Self-defense	Express negative emotions	Jealousy
Control subscale (α = .78)					
1. To make your partner do the things you wanted him to do	**.76**	.27	.16	.38	.31
13. Because you wanted him to give you something, like money, or something for your children	**.69**	.49	.26	.36	.18
14. Because you wanted him to do something	**.82**	.35	.14	.54	.23
15. Because you couldn't stop yourself	**.67**	.36	.14	.54	.23
25. To feel in control	**.65**	.49	.09	.44	.40
29. Because he tried to control you	**.60**	.27	.50	.50	.20
Tough guise subscale (α = .82)					
9. To harm your partner	.29	**.83**	.37	.35	.23
10. To intimidate your partner	.50	**.81**	.24	.58	.39
19. Because you feel better after a fight	.47	**.77**	.23	.53	.31
20. To scare him	.59	**.72**	.24	.46	.32
26. Because you were drinking or using drugs	.26	**.58**	.33	.26	.06
32. To physically hurt him	.31	**.79**	.48	.35	.20
34. To get "turned on" sexually	.30	**.70**	.26	.32	.21
36. To get him to take you seriously	.29	**.83**	.37	.35	.23
Self-defense subscale (α = .86)					
3. To defend yourself from your partner	.27	.34	**.86**	.42	.12
4. To get your partner to stop hitting or hurting you	.10	.32	**.93**	.30	.09
16. Because you knew a beating was coming and you wanted to get it over with	.54	.41	**.74**	.40	.07
17. Because he became abusive when he drank	.38	.37	**.70**	.38	.03
33. To get away as he was beating you	.22	.41	**.89**	.25	.09
Express negative emotions subscale (α = .82)					
8. Because your partner said something that hurt you	.57	.35	.36	**.68**	.32
11. Because he made you angry	.62	.33	.21	**.75**	.35
12. Because you wanted to let him know he couldn't get away with mistreating you	.33	.59	.50	**.70**	.22
18. Because you were frustrated	.69	.38	.24	**.71**	.27
23. Because you were fed up with his behavior	.54	.62	.53	**.75**	.22
Jealousy subscale (α = .73; r = .57)					
6. Because you thought your partner was unfaithful	.39	.35	.24	.35	**.81**
27. Because you were jealous	.37	.43	.10	.43	**.78**

(*Continued*)

TABLE 3 (*Continued*)

	Control	Tough guise	Self-defense	Express negative emotions	Jealousy
Dropped items					
2. To get even with your partner for something he had done	.48	..56	.18	..49	.49
7. To prevent your partner from leaving or going out	.44	.53	.27	.39	.48
21. To stop the argument	.53	.50	.36	.48,	10
22. As a joke or just playing around	.01	.40	−.02	.22	.15
24. Because he was being mean to you	.41	.50	.62	.67	.11
28. To get your point across	.55	.60	.20	.67	.33
30. Because you have a bad temper	.54	.48	.06	.57	.31
31. Because of your past abusive Relationships	.45	.48	.23	.43	.13
35. To get him to leave you alone	.32	.55	.58	.45	.00

Note: Factor loadings in bold represent items that were retained for that factor.

their partner (44%). Eighty-three percent of women indicated that self-defense was a motive for their aggression, and approximately two-thirds stated their aggression was motivated by jealousy. It is clear that many participants indicated multiple motives for their perpetration of partner aggression. The participants endorsed an average of 14 of the 26 motive items in the final scale.

Table 1 also provides descriptive statistics for women's perpetration of and victimization by IPV, as well as social desirability. Paired sample t tests were conducted to compare mean perpetration and victimization frequencies. Physical IPV perpetration and victimization means for the participants were not significantly different ($t = 0.79$, $p > .05$), and neither were psychological aggression perpetration and victimization means, $t = −1.58$, $p > .05$. Sexual perpetration and victimization means ($t[411] = −7.24$, $p < .001$) and coercive control perpetration and victimization means ($t[411] = −9.21$, $p < .001$) were significantly different. Women reported that they were victims of sexual aggression and coercive control significantly more than they perpetrated these types of aggression.

Regression Analyses

Hypothesis 1, that all motive factors except self-defense would be positively related to the perpetration of physical aggression, received support (see Table 4). The motive factors—expression of negative emotions, control, jealousy, and tough guise—were significantly and positively related to the perpetration of physical aggression, after controlling for previous victimization from partners and social desirability, and added predictive utility to the model.

Hypothesis 2, that the self-defense motive factor would display a curvilinear relationship to the perpetration of physical aggression, received partial support (see Table 4 and Figure 1). The quadratic self-defense term, which tested for a curvilinear relationship, did approach significance ($p = .069$), after controlling for previous victimization from partners and social desirability.

To further assess the relationship between the self-defense motive and physical aggression perpetration as well as physical victimization, analyses of covariance (ANCOVAs) were conducted. Participants were divided into four categories, based on their scores on the self-defense scale: participants who never endorsed self-defense as a motive (0); those who had low scores on the self-defense scale (1); those who had moderate scores on the self-defense scale (2); and those who had the highest scores on the self-defense

TABLE 4 Regression Analysis for Female Perpetration of Physical Aggression ($N = 412$)

Variable	B	SEB	β	R^2	ΔR^2
Step 1				.310***	.310***
Social desirability	−.04	.05	−.03		
Physical victimization	.45	.04	.55***		
Psychological victimization	.02	.04	.03		
Coercive control victimization	−.08	.05	−.07		
Sexual victimization	−.06	.04	−.06		
Step 2				.555***	.245***
Expression of negative emotions	.72	.16	.24***		
Self-defense (centered)	−.75	.15	−.29***		
Control	.34	.14	.12*		
Jealousy	.68	.28	.10*		
Tough guise	.66	.12	.25***		
Self-defense (quadratic)	.04	.02	.08[A]		

*$p < .05$; **$p < .01$; ***$p < .001$; [A]$p < .07$.

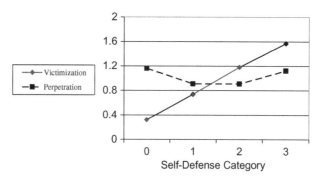

FIGURE 1 Mean Physical Victimization and Perpetration for Participants by Level of Self-Defense Category.

Note: For the self-defense categories, 0 = participants who never endorsed self-defense as a motive; 1 = participants who had low scores on the self-defense scale; 2 = participants who had moderate scores on the self-defense scale; and 3 = participants who had high scores on the self-defense motive scale.

scale (3). First, this variable was used to predict physical aggression, with physical victimization as a covariate. Physical aggression perpetration did differ significantly by self-defense category, $F(3, 407) = 3.91$, $p < .01$ (see Figure 1). Post hoc tests revealed the predicted curvilinear pattern: Participants who never endorsed self-defense as a motive, and those with high scores on the self-defense scale, had significantly higher frequencies of physical aggression perpetration than participants in the low and moderate categories. Second, the four-category self-defense motive was used to examine the relationship between self-defense motives and physical victimization, while controlling for physical perpetration. Physical victimization also differed significantly by self-defense category, $F(3, 407) = 45.50$, $p < .001$ (see Figure 1). Taken together, these results indicate that participants who never use aggression in self-defense are highly aggressive and experience low levels of victimization. Participants with the highest scores on self-defense are highly aggressive, but also are very highly victimized; their aggression appears to be in self-defense. Individuals in the middle two groups use aggression and are victimized at similar rates, and are less aggressive than those with the highest or lowest scores on self-defense.

Hypothesis 3, that all five motive factors would be positively related to the perpetration of psychological aggression, also received partial support (see Table 5). Expression of negative emotions, control, and tough guise were significantly and positively related to the perpetration of psychological aggression after controlling for previous victimization from partners and social desirability, and added predictive utility to the model. Contrary to our prediction, the jealousy motive was unrelated, and the self-defense motive was significantly and negatively related to perpetrating psychological aggression toward partners.

Hypothesis 4 was supported by the data (see Table 6). The motive factors of control and jealousy were significantly and positively related to the

TABLE 5 Regression Analysis for Female Perpetration of Psychological Aggression ($N = 412$)

Variable	B	SEB	β	R^2	ΔR^2
Step 1				.332***	.332***
Social desirability	−.11	.06	−.07		
Physical victimization	.003	.05	.003		
Psychological victimization	.46	.04	.56***		
Coercive control victimization	−.001	.06	−.001		
Sexual victimization	−.05	.05	−.04		
Step 2				.482***	.150***
Expression of negative emotions	.72	.19	.22***		
Self-defense	−.72	.15	−.25***		
Control	.53	.17	.16**		
Jealousy	.12	.33	.01		
Tough guise	.44	.14	.15**		

*$p < .05$; **$p < .01$; ***$p < .001$.

TABLE 6 Regression Analysis for Female Perpetration of Coercive Control ($N = 412$)

Variable	B	SEB	β	R^2	ΔR^2
Step 1				.088***	.088***
Social desirability	−.05	.04	−.05		
Physical victimization	.00	.03	.00		
Psychological victimization	.08	.03	.19*		
Coercive control victimization	.14	.04	.19**		
Sexual victimization	−.06	.03	−.10*		
Step 2				.304***	.216***
Expression of negative emotions	−.21	.12	−.12		
Self-defense	−.07	.09	−.05		
Control	.24	.11	.13*		
Jealousy	2.11	.21	.49***		
Tough guise	−.08	.09	−.05		

*$p < .05$; **$p < .01$; ***$p < .001$.

TABLE 7 Regression Analysis for Female Perpetration of Sexual Aggression ($N = 412$)

Variable	B	SEB	β	R^2	ΔR^2
Step 1				.180***	.180***
Social desirability	−.05	.04	−.06		
Physical victimization	−.03	.03	−.06		
Psychological victimization	.004	.03	.01		
Coercive control victimization	−.06	.04	−.09		
Sexual victimization	.25	.03	.41***		
Step 2				.248***	.068***
Expression of negative emotions	−.15	.12	−.09		
Self-defense	−.07	.09	−.05		
Control	.05	.11	.03		
Jealousy	.39	.21	.09		
Tough guise	.41	.09	.27***		

*$p < .05$; **$p < .01$; ***$p < .001$.

perpetration of coercive control after controlling for previous victimization from partners and social desirability, and added predictive utility to the model.

Table 7 provides a summary of the regression findings for sexual aggression perpetration. The tough guise motive factor was significantly and positively related to the perpetration of sexual aggression after controlling for previous victimization from partners and social desirability, and added predictive utility to the model.

DISCUSSION

Participants in the present study perceived their aggressive behavior toward their partners as driven by both proactive and defensive motives. On average, women indicated that 14 of the motives and reasons for using aggression against their male intimate partners applied to them at least some of the time. The EFA resulted in the Motives and Reasons for IPV scale with excellent model fit and five theoretically meaningful factors: expression of negative emotions, self-defense, control, jealousy, and tough guise.

Expressing negative emotions is clearly an important motive for women's perpetration of IPV, consistent with other studies (Babcock et al., 2003; Stuart et al., 2006). The top four most frequently endorsed items ("he made you angry," "he said something that hurt you," "you wanted to let him know he couldn't get away with mistreating you," and "you were frustrated") were components of this factor. Furthermore, participants who scored highly on the expressing negative emotions factor committed more frequent physical and psychological aggression, even when controlling for victimization and social desirability.

Self-defense is also an important motive for women's aggression. The second most frequently endorsed item ("to defend yourself from your partner") was in the self-defense factor. As predicted, evidence was found for a curvilinear relationship between the self-defense motive and women's physical aggression. Although the quadratic term in the regression analysis only approached significance, the relationship between the self-defense motive and aggression was statistically significant in the ANCOVA and did show the curvilinear pattern. Women who never endorsed the self-defense motive appeared to be primary aggressors. These women reported high levels of aggression and experienced low victimization. In contrast, women who endorsed high levels of self-defense also used high levels of aggression, but their victimization was even greater. These findings suggest that these women's aggression is often in self-defense. The two middle groups endorsed moderate levels of self-defense motives, and the frequency of aggression they used was more similar to the frequency of victimization they experienced relative to the high and no self-defense groups. Their relationships may resemble situational couple violence, in which IPV is usually mutual, less frequent, not severe, and not part of a general pattern of control and domination (Johnson, 2006).

An unexpected negative relationship emerged between the self-defense motive and psychological aggression. This may be because at high levels of self-defense, women seldom use psychological aggression because they do not want to further escalate their partner's violence. In contrast, at low levels of self-defense, women may not be concerned about violent retaliation from partners and so use psychological aggression freely.

The control motive factor was an interesting combination of items relating to women's efforts to control their partners' behavior (e.g., "to make him do the things you wanted him to do") and items relating to women's lack of control (e.g., "because he tried to control you"). The positive relationship between control motives and physical, psychological, and coercive control aggression suggests that at times women used aggression in a calculated attempt to get their partners to behave in a particular way, but some women also appeared to have used aggression to respond to their partners' attempts to control them. Still other women indicated their aggression was due to an inability to control themselves (e.g., "because you couldn't stop yourself").

The jealousy motive factor only had two items; however, the subscale was reliable and showed a strong positive relationship with coercive control perpetration, as well as a significant but small relationship with physical aggression. These findings are consistent with other literature, including a previous study that found jealousy was a significant predictor of women's IPV (Bookwala et al., 1992).

The tough guise motive factor contains motives to appear tough, intimidating, and willing to harm one's partner if necessary. By far the most frequently endorsed item in this factor was "to get him to take you seriously." This tough guise may, in part, be in response to the high levels of victimization experienced by most of the women in the sample; women endorsing these motives may adopt a tough guise as a strategy to protect them from further harm by their partners. Furthermore, many of the women in the sample were very poor and lived in inner-city neighborhoods with frequent community violence. Appearing tough may be a way to cope with these difficult living conditions. The item "because you were drinking or using drugs" indicates that substance use plays a role as well, perhaps by reducing inhibitions toward aggressive behavior. The tough guise factor was related to greater physical and psychological aggression.

Sexual aggression appears to be a distinct form of IPV. It is relatively unusual for women to perpetrate sexual aggression. Women were significantly more likely to be victims of sexual aggression than to perpetrate this behavior. Nevertheless, 32% of women did use some form of sexual aggression against their partners in the past 6 months. The only motive factor that was related to women's perpetration of sexual aggression was tough guise. This is likely driven in part by the "to get 'turned on' sexually" item that loaded on this factor. These results suggest that some women may use sexual aggression to frighten and intimidate their partners. Given the unique, negative effects of sexual victimization (Frieze, 2005) and the paucity of information on women's sexually aggressive behavior, this is a critical area for future study.

Limitations

We were surprised that a retaliation factor did not emerge from the factor analysis, as several previous studies have found that retaliation is a motive for women's IPV (see Swan et al., 2008). However, the Motives and Reasons for IPV scale had only one item assessing retaliation ("to get even with your partner for something he had done"), and this item failed to load on any factor. Thus there is room for revising the instrument, including adding retaliation items to determine whether such a factor might emerge in future analyses. Another avenue for future research would be to add additional jealousy items to improve the reliability of this factor.

A further limitation of the study is its reliance on self-report measures. Although self-report data are common within the IPV field, it does not take into account the other partner's viewpoint and also could be influenced by the reporter's memory or goal to appear socially desirable to the interviewer. For this reason, social desirability was controlled for in the regression analyses, and findings revealed that it was unrelated to women's reports of their aggression. A second limitation is that the participants were questioned regarding their motives or reasons for engaging in IPV weeks or months after the incidents occurred. Again, this is the typical method used in studies of IPV motives, but one cannot be sure how closely the retrospective report relates to the psychological processes motivating people's behavior when they are actually in the moment and how conscious they are of their motives (Stuart et al., 2006). Participants may have difficulty remembering or identifying their reasons for committing IPV, especially given the highly distressing nature of these incidents.

The dual perpetrator and victim status of most participants meant that it was essential to control for victimization when examining the relationships between motives and aggression. Therefore building these controls into the regression models is viewed as a strength of the study. Without controlling for victimization, what appears to be a relationship between motives and aggression could actually be a function of the relationship between victimization and aggression.

Implications

This study has a number of implications for intervention programs for domestically violent women. We concur with Stuart et al. (2006) and Hettrich and O'Leary (2007) that addressing the motives that women themselves see as underlying their use of violence is a promising approach. Obviously, for most women who use IPV, victimization issues need to be addressed through safety planning and access to community resources that can help provide protection from their partner's violence. It is very unlikely that women's aggression will end unless their partners' violence against them is stopped. Victimization is an especially important topic to address given the large number of women who used violence in self-defense, which may ultimately increase women's vulnerability to further victimization (Stuart et al., 2006).

While victimization and defensive motives are essential components of women's IPV, they are clearly not the whole story. Proactive motives also were frequently endorsed, and importantly, were predictive of women's perpetration of IPV. Expressing anger or frustration—characteristic of poor emotion regulation (Stuart et al., 2006)—was related to physical aggression and represents an important area of intervention. Building positive coping skills to assist domestically violent women in regulating and expressing their emotions in healthier ways may lead to less perpetration of aggression (see Goldenson, Spidel, Greaves, & Dutton, 2009, for a review). Trying to control the partner, jealousy, and attempting to harm or scare the partner to appear tough also were related to women's aggression. Findings from this study suggest that interventions for domestically violent women should not minimize the impact of women's own tendencies to act aggressively. Interventions that help participants understand what a healthy relationship is, with a focus on building coping strategies that include participants' use of assertive and effective communication, problem-solving skills, and social support, rather than aggression, will lead to more healthy relationships and are essential approaches to both the prevention and treatment of IPV perpetration.

REFERENCES

Aiken, L. S., & West. S. G. (1991). *Multiple regression: Testing and interpreting interactions.* Beverly Hills, CA: Sage.

Babcock, J. C., Miller, S. A., & Siard, C. (2003). Toward a typology of abusive women: Differences between partner-only and generally violent women in the use of violence. *Psychology of Women Quarterly, 27,* 153–161.

Barrett, P. (2007). Structural equation modeling: Adjusting model fit. *Personality and Individual Differences, 42,* 815–824.

Bentler, P. M. (1990). Comparative fit indexes in structural models. *Psychological Bulletin, 107,* 238–246.

Bookwala, J., Frieze, I. H., Smith, C., & Ryan, K. (1992). Predictors of dating violence: A multivariate analysis. *Violence and Victims, 7,* 297–311.

Briggs, N. E., & MacCallum, R. C. (2003). Recovery of weak common factors by maximum likelihood and ordinary least squares estimation. *Multivariate Behavioral Research, 38,* 25–56.

Cattel, R. B. (1966). The meaning and strategic use of factor analysis. In R. B. Cattel (Ed.), *Handbook of multivariate experimental psychology* (pp. 174–243). Chicago: Rand McNally.

Cohen, J., Cohen, P., West, S. G., & Aiken, L. S. (2003). *Applied multiple regression/ correlation analysis for the behavioral sciences.* Mahwah, NJ: Lawrence Erlbaum.

Courville, T., & Thompson, B. (2001). Use of structure coefficients in published multiple regression articles: β is not enough. *Educational and Psychological Measurement, 61,* 229–248.

Dodge, K. A., & Coie, J. D. (1987). Social-information-processing factors in reactive and proactive aggression in children's peer groups. *Journal of Personality and Social Psychology, 53,* 1146–1158.

Fabrigar, L., Wegener, D., MacCallum, R., & Strahan, E. (1999). Evaluating the use of exploratory factor analysis in psychological research. *Psychological Methods, 4,* 272–299.

Fiske, S. T. (2004). *Social beings: A core motives approach to social psychology* (1st ed.). Hoboken, NJ: John Wiley & Sons.

Follingstad, D. R., Wright, S., Lloyd, S., & Sebastian, J. A. (1991). Sex differences in motivations and effects in dating violence. *Family Relations, 40*, 51–57.

Frieze, I. H. (2005). *Hurting the one you love: Violence in relationships*. Belmont, CA: Thompson Wadsworth.

Goldenson, J., Spidel, A., Greaves, C., & Dutton, D. (2009). Female perpetrators of intimate partner violence: Within-group heterogeneity, related psychopathology, and a review of current treatment with recommendations for the future. *Journal of Aggression, Maltreatment & Trauma, 18*(7), 752–769.

Gorsuch, R. L. (1983). *Factor analysis* (2nd ed.). Hillsdale, NJ: Lawrence Erlbaum.

Gorsuch, R. L. (1997). Exploratory factor analysis: Its role in item analysis. *Journal of Personality Assessment, 68*, 532–560.

Graves, K. N., Sechrist, S. M., White, J. W., & Paradise, M. J. (2005). Intimate partner violence perpetrated by college women within the context of a history of victimization. *Psychology of Women Quarterly, 29*, 278–289.

Greenwald, H. J., & Satow, Y. (1970). A short social desirability scale. *Psychological Reports, 27*, 131–135.

Henning, K., Martinsson, R., & Holdford, R. (2009). Gender differences in risk factors for intimate partner violence recidivism. *Journal of Aggression, Maltreatment & Trauma, 18*(6), 623–645.

Hettrich, E. L., & O'Leary, K. D. (2007). Females' reasons for their physical aggression in dating relationships. *Journal of Interpersonal Violence, 22*, 1131–1143.

Hu, L. T., & Bentler, P. M. (1999). Cutoff criteria for fit indexes in covariance structure analysis: Conventional criteria versus new alternatives. *Structural Equation Modeling, 6*, 1–55.

Johnson, M. P. (2006). Conflict and control: Gender symmetry and asymmetry in domestic violence. *Violence Against Women, 12*, 1003–1018.

Jöreskog, K. G. (1969). A general approach to confirmatory maximum likelihood factor analysis. *Psychometrika, 34*, 183–202.

Kaiser, H. F. (1960). The application of electronic computers to factor analysis. *Educational and Psychological Measurement, 20*, 141–151.

Kimmel, M. S. (2002). "Gender symmetry" in domestic violence. *Violence Against Women, 8*, 1332–1363.

Koss, M. P., Gidycz, C. A., & Wisniewski, N. (1987). The scope of rape: Incidence and prevalence of sexual aggression and victimization in a national sample of higher education students. *Journal of Consulting and Clinical Psychology, 55*, 162–170.

Magdol, L., Moffitt, T. E., Caspi, A., Newman, D. L., Fagan, J., & Silva, P. A. (1997). Gender differences in partner violence in a birth cohort of 21-year-olds: Bridging the gap between clinical and epidemiological approaches. *Journal of Consulting and Clinical Psychology, 65*, 68–78.

Muthén, L. K., & Muthén, B. O. (2007). *Mplus user's guide* (5th ed.). Los Angeles, CA: Authors.

NOVA Research Company. (2003). *Questionnaire Development System* [computer software]. Bethesda, MD: Author.

Orcutt, H. K., Garcia, M., & Pickett, S. M. (2005). Female-perpetrated intimate partner violence and romantic attachment style in a college student sample. *Violence & Victims, 20,* 287–302.

Schafer, J. L. (1999). Multiple imputation: A primer. *Statistical Methods in Medical Research, 8,* 3–15.

Skrondal, A., & Rabe-Hesketh, S. (2004). *Generalized latent variable modeling: Multilevel, longitudinal, and structural equation models.* Boca Raton, FL: Chapman & Hall/CRC.

Stevens, J. (2002). *Applied multivariate statistics for the social sciences* (4th ed.). Mahwah, NJ: Lawrence Erlbaum.

Straus, M. A., & Gelles, R. J. (1990). *Physical violence in American families: Risk factors and adaptations to violence in 8,145 families.* New Brunswick, NJ: Transaction.

Straus, M. A., Hamby, S. L., Boney-McCoy, S., & Sugarman, D. B. (1996). The Revised Conflict Tactics Scale (CTS2). *Journal of Family Issues, 17,* 283–316.

Straus, M. A., Hamby, S. L., & Warren, W. L. (2003). *The Conflict Tactics Scales handbook.* Los Angeles: Western Psychological Services.

Stuart, G. L., Moore, T. M., Gordon, K. C., Hellmuth, J. C., Ramsey, S. E., & Kahler, C. W. (2006). Reasons for intimate partner violence perpetration among arrested women. *Violence Against Women, 12,* 609–621.

Sullivan, T. P., Meese, K. J., Swan, S. C., Mazure, C. M., & Snow, D. L. (2005). Precursors and correlates of women's violence: Child abuse traumatization, victimization of women, avoidance coping, and psychological symptoms. *Psychology of Women Quarterly, 29,* 290–301.

Swan, S. C., Gambone, L. J., Caldwell, J. E., Sullivan, T. P., & Snow, D. L. (2008). A review of research on women's use of violence with male intimate partners. *Violence and Victims, 23,* 301–314.

Swan, S. C., Gambone, L. J., Fields, A. M., Sullivan, T. P., & Snow, D. L. (2005). Women who use violence in intimate relationships: The role of anger, victimization, and symptoms of posttraumatic stress and depression. *Violence and Victims, 20,* 267–285.

Swan, S. C., & Snow, D. L. (2002). A typology of women's use of violence in intimate relationships. *Violence Against Women, 8,* 286–319.

Swan, S. C., & Snow, D. L. (2003). Behavioral and psychological differences among abused women who use violence in intimate relationships. *Violence Against Women, 9,* 75–109.

Swan, S. C., & Snow, D. L. (2006). The development of a theory of women's use of violence in intimate relationships. *Violence Against Women, 12,* 1026–1045.

Swan, S. C., & Sullivan, T. P. (2002). *The Motivations for Violence Scale.* Unpublished measure, Yale University, New Haven, Connecticut.

Temple, J. R., Weston, R., & Marshall, L. L. (2005). Physical and mental health outcomes of women in nonviolent, unilaterally violent, and mutually violent relationships. *Violence & Victims, 20,* 335–359.

Testa, M., VanZile-Tamsen, C., Livingston, J. A., & Koss, M. P. (2004). Assessing women's experiences of sexual aggression using the Sexual Experiences Survey: Evidence for validity and implications for research. *Psychology of Women Quarterly, 28,* 256–265.

Thomas, S. P. (2005). Women's anger, aggression, and violence. *Health Care for Women International, 26*, 504–522.

Thompson, B., & Borrello, G. M. (1985). The importance of structure coefficients in regression research. *Educational and Psychological Measurement, 45*, 203–209.

Thompson, B., & Daniel, L. G. (1996). Factor analytic evidence for the construct validity of scores: A historical overview and some guidelines. *Educational and Psychological Measurement, 56*, 197–208.

Tolman, R. M. (1999). The validation of the psychological maltreatment of women inventory. *Violence and Victims, 14*, 25–35.

Walley-Jean, J. C., & Swan, S. C. (2009). Motivations and justifications for partner aggression in a sample of African American college women. *Journal of Aggression, Maltreatment & Trauma, 18*(7), 698–717.

Motivations and Justifications for Partner Aggression in a Sample of African American College Women

J. CELESTE WALLEY-JEAN

Clayton State University, Morrow, Georgia, USA

SUZANNE SWAN

University of South Carolina, Columbia, South Carolina, USA

Little is known about African American college women's use, experience, and conceptualizations of intimate partner violence (IPV). The current study addresses this gap in the literature by investigating a sample of African American college women's motivations for perpetration of psychological and physical IPV and justifications for hypothetical aggressive behavior. Using factors derived from a factor analysis of the Motivations and Effects Questionnaire (Follingstad, Wright, Lloyd, & Sebastian, 1991), results revealed that African American women in the current sample were using IPV primarily as a destructive method of communication. Furthermore, justifications for aggression, in general, were significantly related to the perpetration of minor physical aggression. Implications of the study for the prevention of dating violence among college women are discussed.

Research on women's perpetration of intimate partner violence (IPV) is an area that has slowly but steadily grown in the last decade. Generally research has strongly supported that women are engaging in physical IPV at rates similar to and in some instances greater than men (for a review, see

Archer, 2000). There have, however, been consistent findings that women's use of IPV almost always occurs in the context of their own victimization (Cercone, Beach, & Arias, 2005; Hamberger & Potente, 1994; Swan & Snow, 2003; Temple, Weston, & Marshall, 2005). Moreover, several studies have found that male aggression is a strong predictor of women's use of aggressive behavior (e.g., Graham-Kevan & Archer, 2005; Graves, Sechrist, White, & Paradise, 2005). Critics have pointed out that men's aggression toward women is typically more severe and injurious than women's aggression toward men (e.g., Cascardi, Langhinrichsen, & Vivian, 1992) and worry that investigations of women's aggression may be inadvertently regarded as an excuse for men's aggression (Kurtz, 1993). Collectively, these concerns may have slowed of our understanding of women's use of aggression.

A major criticism of the research suggesting that women are equally as aggressive as men has focused on possible differences in women's motivations for engaging in partner aggression. There is, however, a lack of consensus in the literature regarding women's motivations for IPV. Some researchers have argued that, even if aggressive, women typically are acting in self-defense (e.g., DeKeseredy & Schwartz, 1998; Osthoff, 2002). Indeed, studies that have investigated women's motivations for IPV generally support this claim, finding that women, when compared to men, are more likely to use IPV in self-defense or in retaliation for previous physical and emotional assaults against them (e.g., Barnett, Lee, & Thelen, 1997; Hamberger, Lohr, & Bonge, 1994). Although studies indicate that self-defense is a primary motivation for women's aggressive behavior, it is not the only motivation reported by women. For example, Caldwell, Swan, Allen, Sullivan, and Snow (2009), Hamberger (2005), Kernsmith (2005), and Stuart et al. (2006) reported that some women use violence to dominate and control their partner because of anger toward their partner, to get their partner's attention, or because the women believed their partner provoked violence. Moreover, Follingstad, Wright, Lloyd, and Sebastian (1991) reported that men and women were equally likely to identify not knowing how to express themselves verbally and needing to protect themselves (i.e., self-defense) as reasons for their use of IPV. Furthermore, Follingstad et al. (1991) reported that both male and female perpetrators of IPV identified retaliation for emotional hurt or expression of anger as the strongest motivation for their physical aggression. Thus motivations for women's use of IPV appear to be more varied than previously presumed. Furthermore, previous studies of women's motivations have been descriptive in nature. In fact, to date, only one study (DeKeseredy, Saunders, Schwartz, & Alvi, 1997) has specifically investigated the relationship of motivations to actual perpetration. Thus the continued investigation of women's motivations and their relationship to perpetration of IPV is essential.

In addition to the need to broaden understanding of women's motivations for IPV, studies point to the likely importance of considering women's general attitudes toward violence. For example, previous research has supported that acceptance of the use of violence was an important determinant for males' use of aggressive behavior (e.g., Stets & Pirog-Good, 1987). Furthermore, in a sample of college students, Cauffman, Feldman, Jensen, and Arnett (2000) found that college students who were more accepting of violence were more likely to engage in violent behavior, and that dating violence was perceived as more acceptable when females were the aggressors than when males were the aggressors, regardless of the sex of the respondent. Cauffman et al. (2000) also reported that justifications of aggressive behavior that could be classified as reactive (i.e., defense and response to provocation) were perceived as more acceptable. Furthermore, Archer and Graham-Kevan's study (as cited in Nabors, Dietz, & Jasinski, 2006) found that beliefs supportive of domestic violence are more predictive of abuse in intimate relationships among college students than among either women in domestic violence shelters or men in prison convicted of physically abusing their partners. Thus the investigation of college women's views on aggression against a partner, in general, may be vital to not only understanding their use of IPV but also in predicting future aggressive behavior.

A limitation of the generalizability of some studies investigating women's use of aggression as well as their motivations is that most have examined samples of women who are in long-term relationships and experiencing severe, long-term violence (i.e., primarily battered women or women court ordered to domestic violence treatment; e.g., see Barnett et al., 1997; Cascardi & Vivian, 1995; Saunders, 1986). While some studies have evaluated motivations for aggressive behavior in college-age populations (e.g., DeKeseredy et al., 1997; Follingstad et al., 1991; Leisring, 2009), in general this area of the literature is limited. Research examining dating violence is critical, as aggression in young people's dating relationships is often the foundation of future violence in marital relationships (Roscoe & Benaske, 1985). Moreover, studies that have focused on IPV in college-age populations indicate that dating couples are more likely to be aggressive than married couples (e.g., Sugarman & Hotaling, 1989) and that IPV is widespread on college campuses (Straus, 2004).

Although current studies have indicated that the prevalence of dating aggression is high, one limitation of U.S. studies in particular is that the samples have consisted primarily of White, middle-class, college and university students (for a review, see Lewis & Fremouw, 2001). As a result, relatively little is known about the prevalence and nature of dating aggression among minority populations (Jackson, 1999; Sugarman & Hotaling, 1989; West & Rose, 2000). Nevertheless, what is known about IPV in minority samples strongly suggests a need for greater attention from researchers. For example, West (2002) suggested that African American women are at higher risk for IPV; indeed, a recent study reported that the leading cause of death among young African American women between the ages of 15 and 45 years is murder by an intimate partner (West, 2004). West (2004) further noted that in a nationally representative sample from the United States, when compared to their European American counterparts African American women consistently reported higher rates of partner abuse. This research, however, has focused largely on African Americans of lower socioeconomic status. Few studies, with the exception of Clark, Beckett, Wells, and Dungee-Anderson (1994) and DeMaris (1990), have investigated college-age, African Americans' perpetration and experience of aggression in dating relationships, and these studies did not specifically investigate women's use of aggression. Furthermore, only one study (Swan & Snow, 2003) specifically investigated women's motivations for IPV in a sample in which the majority were African American, with results suggesting patterns of motivation similar to those found in nonminority samples (e.g., Barnet et al., 1997; Hamberger et al., 1994). That is, the majority (75%) of participants reported using violence in self-defense at least some of the time, while 45% reported using violence for purposes of retribution. In addition, 38% reported using violence to control their partners. This sample, however, was largely limited to older (25 to 40 years old), lower income (69% of the sample earned less than $10,000 per year) women. To date, there are no studies specifically investigating motivations for aggressive behavior in African American college-age women.

The current study contributes to the literature by assessing associations between motivations for partner aggression, global attitudes toward partner aggression (i.e., justifications), and perpetration of and victimization from partner aggression. This study extended the use of Follingstad et al.'s (1991) Motivations and Effects Questionnaire (MEQ) with a sample of African American college-age women who had engaged in some form of aggressive behavior in the past year. Moreover, the current study performed an exploratory factor analysis, utilizing principal component analysis, to determine the simpler factor structure of the MEQ's 13 motivations for aggression. These factors are briefly described here to provide the basis for the study hypotheses. The Expression of Negative Emotions factor refers to motivations to use aggression to convey negative emotional states, such as jealousy and anger. The second factor, Aggression as Response, is comprised of motives related to retaliation, self-defense, and punishment. The final two components were Communication, in which aggression is used to get the partner's attention or because the aggressor cannot express herself verbally, and Expression of Positive Emotions, which included motivations linked to using aggression as a way of communicating affection or becoming sexually aroused.

HYPOTHESES

The following hypotheses are based on previous research indicating that women's primary motivations for aggression are often self-defensive or retaliatory (e.g., DeKeseredy & Schwartz, 1998; Osthoff, 2002), although women have also reported other motives, such as domination and control, anger, and to get their partner's attention (e.g., Hamberger, 2005; Kernsmith, 2005). Research also supports the predictive value of justifications for aggression for perpetration of aggressive behavior (e.g., Archer & Graham-Kevan, 2003, as cited in Nabors et al., 2006).

1. As a replication of previous findings, it is hypothesized that there will be a significant positive correlation between participants' reported perpetration of partner-specific aggression and their experience of partner-specific aggression.
2. There will be a significant positive relationship between the Aggression as Response and Expression of Negative Emotions motivation factors.
3. The Aggression as Response and Expression of Negative Emotions factors will be positively related to the perpetration of aggressive behavior.
4. The more justifications women have for aggression against a partner in general, the more motives they will have for their own perpetration of aggressive behavior.
5. There will be a positive relationship between justifications for aggressive behavior and perpetration of aggressive behavior.

METHOD

Procedures

Participants were recruited through flyers posted around the three campuses soliciting volunteers for a paid research study on aggressive behavior, or through solicitation in psychology courses in which extra credit in the course was offered. Interested participants contacted the research laboratory and either underwent a telephone screen or completed a paper questionnaire screening of their behavior in the past year. Because the current study was focused on women who use aggression, in order to be included in the study participants had to report one physical or verbal act of aggression (victim unspecified) in the past year. One hundred forty-two potential participants were screened, and 88% of those screened ($n = 125$) met the criteria for participation in the study. Of those who met the criteria for participation, 57% ($n = 81$) committed one or more acts of verbal aggression only in the past year, while the remainder committed one or more acts of verbal and physical aggression in the past year. Of the screened respondents, 66% ($n = 82$) agreed to participate in the current study.

Following completion of the study measures, participants, if warranted, were provided with a list of referrals for psychological intervention (i.e., campus counseling centers, community agencies) and the primary investigator's phone numbers to call in case they had any questions or were upset.

Participants were either monetarily compensated or received extra course credit for their participation.

Participants

The sample consisted of 82 female African American college students recruited from three urban institutions. The majority of the sample (74%) was recruited from a small, historically Black women's college, while the remainder of the participants (26%) were recruited from two large, coeducational universities, all in the southeastern United States. Participants' ages ranged from 18 to 32 years (M = 20.13, SD = 2.09). Participants were primarily heterosexual (96.3%) and single (96.4%). Approximately 94% (n = 77) of the sample reported having no children, while two participants reported having one child, two additional participants reported having two children, and one participant reported having three children.

Measures

USE AND EXPERIENCE OF PARTNER-SPECIFIC AGGRESSIVE BEHAVIOR

The Conflict Tactics Scale Revised (CTS2; Straus, Hamby, Boney-McCoy, & Sugarman, 1996) was used to assess participants' reported use and experience of partner-specific aggressive behavior. The CTS2 is a 78-item scale used to assess physical and psychological aggression and victimization, sexual coercion and victimization, injury (inflicted and sustained), and negotiation behaviors within the context of intimate relationships. The current study reports participants' use and experience of psychological and physical aggression. The CTS2 also divides the behavior into two categories: "minor" and "severe."

To complete the measure, participants indicated how many times they engaged in (perpetration) or experienced (victimization) psychological and physical aggression in the past year on a scale ranging from 0 (never) to 6 (more than 20 times), with a score of 7 indicating that perpetration or victimization had not occurred in the past year but had happened before. Items for minor psychological aggression included: "I insulted or swore at my partner," "I shouted or yelled at my partner," "I stomped out of the room or house or yard during a disagreement," and "I did something to spite my partner." Items for severe psychological aggression included: "I called my partner fat or ugly," "I destroyed something belonging to my partner," "I accused my partner of being a lousy lover," and "I threatened to hit or throw something at my partner." Items for minor physical aggression included: "I threw something at my partner that could hurt," "I twisted my partner's arm or hair," "I pushed or shoved my partner," "I grabbed my partner," and "I slapped my partner." Items for severe physical aggression included: "I used a knife or gun on my partner," "I punched or hit my partner with something that could hurt," "I choked my partner," "I slammed my partner against a wall," "I beat up my partner," "I burned or scalded my partner on purpose," and "I kicked my partner." All items assessing victimization were worded identically except "I" was changed to "My partner." The CTS2 is a widely used measure of self-reported interpersonal psychological and physical aggressive behavior with high internal consistency and adequate construct and discriminant validity (Straus et al., 1996). Alpha coefficients of the psychological and physical aggression perpetration subscales in the present study were .64 and .70, respectively, while the psychological and physical aggression victimization subscales were .44 and .69, respectively.

Responses on the CTS2 were scored in two ways. Consistent with the scoring recommendations of Straus et al. (1996), responses were assigned a value corresponding to the midpoint value (never = 0; once = 1; twice = 2; 3–5 times = 4; 6–10 times = 8; 11–20 times = 15; more than 20 times = 25; not in the past year, but it has happened before = 0) of each frequency category and then summed to provide subscale scores of the frequency of aggressive behavior over the past year. In addition to this typical manner of scoring, responses were dummy-coded to indicate whether a behavior had occurred in the past year or not and the percentage of participants who had engaged in the subscale behaviors was calculated.

WOMEN'S MOTIVATIONS AND EFFECTS OF AGGRESSIVE BEHAVIOR

To assess participants' motivations for their use of physical aggression toward their partners, as well as their perceptions of their partners' motivations for using physical aggression against them, the MEQ (Follingstad et al., 1991) was used. This measure also assessed self-reported effects of physical aggression on self and partners. The MEQ is a 13-item checklist assessing motives for and effects of physical force in a romantic relationship. Participants indicate whether they have "ever used physical force in a romantic relationship" and whether they have "ever been the victim of physical force in a romantic relationship."

Participants who reported the use of physical force were instructed to "check the reason you used physical force against your partner." Participants then checked all motives that applied to their use of physical force and left blank those motives that did not apply. In addition, of all the identified motivations for their physical aggression participants were asked to identify the "strongest" motivation for their aggression. The MEQ includes "motives" such as using physical violence "to show anger," "due to jealousy," "self-defense," and "to control the other person." All items are shown in Table 1. Likewise, if participants answered "yes" to the question of experiencing

TABLE 1 Frequencies of Own and Perceived Partner "Strongest" Motivations for Aggressive Behavior

	Own motivations (n = 42)	Percent	Partner's motivations (n = 34)	Percent
Show anger	11	26.2	3	8.8
Inability to express self verbally	6	14.3	6	18
In retaliation for emotional hurt	5	11.9	4	12
To get attention	5	11.9	1	2.9
To protect self	4	9.5	1	2.9
Anger displaced onto partner	3	7.1	2	5.9
In retaliation for being hit first	2	4.8	5	15
Because it was sexually arousing	2	4.8	3	8.8
More power	1	2.4	2	5.9
To get control over other person	1	2.4	3	8.8
Because of jealousy	1	2.4	2	5.9
Punishment for wrong behavior	1	2.4	1	2.9
To prove love	0	0	1	2.9

Note: Motives shown here are those identified by participants as the "strongest" motivations for their/their partner's aggression. Forty participants did not complete the MEQ measure; 5 had missing data and 35 neither used nor experienced physical aggression against/from an intimate partner.

"physical force" from their partners, they were asked to "check the reason you think the person used physical force against you" and "the strongest motivation for your partner's aggressive behavior." Participants' identified motivations and perceived partner motivations were coded as yes ("1") if endorsed and no ("0") if the item was left blank; furthermore, participants' strongest motivation and the strongest perceived motivation for their partners' aggressive behavior were tallied. The internal consistency of the MEQ (participants' motivations) was $\alpha = .58$.

WOMEN'S JUSTIFICATIONS FOR AGGRESSIVE BEHAVIOR

To assess participants' perception of justifiable reasons for the use of hypothetical physical aggression, the Justification for Physical Aggression Scale (JUST; Follingstad, Rutledge, Polek, & McNeill-Harkins, 1988) was used. The JUST is different from the MEQ in that, on the JUST scale, participants are rating their agreement/disagreement with *possible* reasons to use physical aggression rather than identifying their own justifications for their own aggression.

The JUST contains 24 possible reasons why someone might use physical force against a boyfriend/girlfriend. Participants rate whether each item is a justifiable reason for the use of physical force on a 4-point Likert-type scale from 1 (strongly disagree) to 4 (strongly agree). Participants rated justifications such as "loss of temper," "mental illness," "hate," "need for control," "as a reaction to verbal provocation," "love," and "in response for being hit first." The JUST showed very strong internal consistency in the present study ($\alpha = .95$).

RESULTS

Factor Structure of the MEQ

In order to investigate factor structure of the motivations associated with women's use of aggression, the 13 motivations of the MEQ were subjected to principal components analysis (PCA). Prior to performing PCA, the suitability of data for factor analysis was assessed. Inspection of the correlation matrix revealed the presence of many coefficients of .3 or greater. The Kaiser–Meyer–Oklin value was .61, exceeding the recommended value of .6 (Kaiser, 1970, 1974), and the Bartlett's Test of Sphericity (Bartlett, 1954) reached statistical significance, supporting the factorability of the correlation matrix.

A factor analysis performed in previous research (Kernsmith, 2005) revealed three factors (striking back for abuse, disciplining partner, and exerting power). The current PCA revealed the presence of four components with eigenvalues exceeding 1, explaining 33%, 18%, 12%, and 10% of the variance, respectively (see Table 2). A decision was made to retain all four components for further investigation. To aid in the interpretation of this component, Varimax rotation was performed. The rotated solution revealed the presence of a simple structure, with the components showing all variables loading substantially on the four components. All items loaded above .50 on each factor.

Perpetration and Victimization of Aggression: Descriptive Findings

In order to be considered for inclusion in the present study, participants had to have perpetrated at least one act of physical or verbal aggression in the

TABLE 2 Motivations Factor Analysis (Variance Explained)

Expression of negative emotions (33%)	Factor loadings
Because of jealousy	.853
To get control over other person	.821
Anger displaced onto partner	.789
In retaliation for emotional hurt	.526
Aggression as Response (18%)	
In retaliation for being hit first	.884
To protect self	.870
Punishment for wrong behavior	.708
Show anger	.512
Communication (12%)	
Unable to express self verbally	.833
More power	.783
To get attention	.684
Expression of Positive Emotions (9.8%)	
Because it was sexually arousing	.883
To prove love	.738

past year; however, the victim was not specified. The frequency of women's perpetration (and victimization) of psychological and physical aggression specifically against (and from) a romantic partner was assessed using the CTS2. The majority of the sample (87%, $n = 71$) reported both perpetrating and being the victim of psychological or physical aggression from an intimate partner in the past year (both perpetrator/victim), while 11% denied either perpetrating or being the victim of either type of aggressive behavior from an intimate partner ($n = 9$). One participant reported perpetrating only and one reported victimization only.

Fifty-seven percent of the sample reported perpetrating both physical and psychological aggression against a romantic partner in the past year ($n = 47$), while approximately 31% of the sample reported using psychological aggression only ($n = 25$). Furthermore, 51% of the sample ($n = 42$) reported being the victim of both psychological and physical aggression from a romantic partner, while 37% ($n = 30$) reported being the victim of psychological aggression only.

Information pertaining to participants' perpetration (and victimization) of physical aggression against (and from) a romantic partner at any point in their lives was also obtained using the MEQ. More than half (51%, $n = 42$) reported the use of physical aggression against a romantic partner, while 41.5% ($n = 34$) reported being the victim of physical aggression from a romantic partner. From this point forward, the term "aggression" will denote "physical or psychological aggression against (or sustained from) a romantic partner."

Paired sample t tests revealed that participants reported perpetrating significantly more minor psychological [$t(78) = 3.70$, $p < .001$], severe psychological [$t(79) = 2.13$, $p < .05$], and minor physical aggression [$t(80) = 2.51$, $p < .05$] than they received. There was no significant difference in perpetrating and receiving severe physical aggression, $t = .31$, ns.

Motivations and Justifications for Violence: Descriptive Findings

Although 47 participants reported using both psychological and physical aggression against an intimate partner, 89% ($n = 42$) completed the MEQ to indicate their motives for use of physical aggression against their partners. Participants endorsed an average of 2.07 motivations ($SD = 2.56$, range: 0–10). "To show anger" (26.2%, $n = 11$) was the most frequently endorsed "strongest" motivation for the perpetration of aggression. Furthermore, "inability to express [your] self verbally" (14.3%, $n = 7$) and "in retaliation for emotional hurt" (11.9%, $n = 5$) and "get attention" (11.9%, $n = 5$) were the second and third, respectively, most frequently endorsed strongest motivations for their aggression. Notably, only 9.4% of the sample ($n = 4$) identified "protect self" as the strongest motive for aggression, and only 4.8% ($n = 2$) said their aggression was "in retaliation for being hit first." Frequencies for all other identified strongest motivations are presented in Table 1. Participants also endorsed an average of 1.81 (SD = 2.57, range: 0–8) perceived motivations for their partners' aggression against them. The strongest perceived motivation for their partner's aggression was an "inability to express [self] verbally" (18%, n = 6), while the second and third most frequently identified strongest perceived motivations, respectively, were "in retaliation for being hit first" (15%; n = 5) and "in retaliation for emotional hurt" (12%, n = 4; see Table 1).

To explore general attitudes toward physical aggression against a partner, participants reported their agreement or disagreement with 24 potential justifications for the use of aggression. Binomial tests indicated that of the 24 rated justifications, the majority of participants (72%, n = 58) significantly agreed with only one as a justifiable reason for the use of physical force, "in response for being hit first" (p < .001).

Hypothesis Testing

To test the hypothesis that participants' use of partner-specific aggression would be associated with their experience of partner-specific aggression, correlations between perpetration and victimization from minor and severe forms of both psychological and physical aggression were calculated. Results largely supported this hypothesis (see Table 3). Almost all forms of perpetration were significantly and positively correlated with all forms of victimization, with the exception of two correlations (between minor psychological perpetration and severe psychological victimization, and between minor psychological perpetration and severe physical victimization).

TABLE 3 Means, Standard Deviations, and Correlations Among Perpetration (P)/Victimization (V) on CTS2 Subscales

		M	SD	1	2	3	4	5	6	7	8
1. Minor Psy. (P)		25.73	25.61	—	.42**	.44**	.29*	.81**	.16	.38**	.16
	n				79	79	76	79	79	79	78
2. Severe Psy. (P)		5.69	8.93	—	—	.65**	.68**	.52**	.38**	.41**	.35**
	n					80	77	79	80	80	79
3. Minor Phys. (P)		8.29	13.96	—	—	—	.70**	.53**	.31**	.77**	.52**
	n						77	80	81	81	80
4. Severe Phys. (P)		1.83	4.54	—	—	—	—	.31**	.23*	.38**	.55**
	n							76	77	77	77
5. Minor Psy. (V)		19.45	20.05	—	—	—	—	—	.32**	.56**	.30**
	n								80	80	79
6. Severe Psy. (V)		3.49	7.47	—	—	—	—	—	—	.53**	.63**
	n									81	80
7. Minor Phys. (V)		5.80	11.46	—	—	—	—	—	—	—	.74**
	n										80
8. Severe Phys. (V)		1.68	4.34	—	—	—	—	—	—	—	—

*p < .05; **p < .01.

The second hypothesis, that there would be a significant positive relationship between the Aggression as Response and Expression of Negative Emotions MEQ factors, was supported. Correlations between the four factors revealed that the Aggression as Response factor was significantly associated with Expression of Negative Emotions, $r = .47$, $p < .01$. Although it was not hypothesized, Aggression as Response was also correlated with Communication, $r = .46$, $p < .01$. The Communication and Expression of Positive Emotions factors were also correlated, $r = .28$, $p < .05$. All other correlations were not significant (r ranged from .02 to .10).

The third hypothesis, that Aggression as Response and Expression of Negative Emotions would be positively related to the perpetration of aggressive behavior, was partially supported. Multiple regression analyses were performed with perpetration of aggression (i.e., minor and severe psychological and physical aggression) as the dependent variables and the four motivation factors (i.e., Expression of Negative Emotions, Communication, Aggression as Response, and Expression of Positive Emotions factors) as independent variables (see Tables 4 and 5). Given the strong correlation between perpetration and victimization, victimization (i.e., experience of minor and severe psychological and physical aggression) was a covariate in all the regression analyses. The final regression models for minor physical aggression [$R^2 = .71$, $F(5, 80) = 36.36$, $p < .001$], severe psychological [$R^2 = .35$, $F(5, 79) = 7.81$, $p < .001$], and severe physical aggression [$R^2 = .43$, $F(5, 76) = 10.85$, $p < .001$] were significant (see Tables 4 and 5). The final model for minor psychological aggression was not significant, $R^2 = .67$, $F(5, 78) = 29.58$, ns. Specifically, the Expression of Negative Emotions factor significantly predicted minor physical aggression ($\beta = .36$, $p < .001$), severe psychological aggression ($\beta = .52$, $p < .001$), and severe physical aggression ($\beta = .43$, $p < .001$). None of the final models for the remaining three motives—Aggression as Response, Communication, and Expression of Positive Emotions—were significant (Tables 4 and 5).

The fourth hypothesis, that the more justifications women had for aggression against a partner in general, the more motives they would have for their own perpetration of aggressive behavior, was supported. The correlation between the summed total for motivations (MEQ) and summed totals for justifications (JUST) revealed a significant positive relationship, $r = .40$, $p < .01$. That is, as the number of justifications for hypothetical aggressive behavior increased, the number of motivations for participants' specific aggressive behavior also increased.

The final hypothesis, that there would be a positive relationship between justifications and perpetration of aggressive behavior, was partially supported. Summed justifications were significantly positively correlated with minor physical aggression, $r = .36$, $p < .01$. There were no other significant correlations.

TABLE 4 Summary of Regression Analysis for Motivation Factors and Perpetration of Psychological Aggression

Predictor variable	Minor psychological aggression				Severe psychological aggression			
	β	B	SE	CI	β	B	SE	CI
Expression of Negative Emotions	.10	2.34	1.77	−1.19 to 5.87	.52**	4.05	.85	2.36 to 5.75
Aggression as Response	−.05	−1.48	2.71	−6.88 to 3.92	−.24	−2.65	1.34	−5.32 to .03
Communication	−.06	−1.84	2.39	−6.61 to 2.93	−.00	−.01	1.19	−2.39 to 2.37
Expression of Positive Emotions	.09	4.61	3.82	−3.01 to 12.23	−.01	−.14	1.85	−3.83 to 3.56

**t value = p < .001.

TABLE 5 Summary of Regression Analysis for Motivation Factors and Perpetration of Physical Aggression

Predictor variable	Minor physical aggression				Severe physical aggression			
	β	B	SE	CI	β	B	SE	CI
Expression of Negative Emotions	.36**	4.46	.88	2.71 to 6.21	.43**	1.70	.42	.86 to 2.54
Aggression as Response	−.09	−1.59	1.41	−4.41 to 1.23	−.24	−1.01	.64	−2.28 to .26
Communication	−.05	−.77	1.22	−3.19 to 1.65	−.00	.17	.59	−.10 to 1.34
Expression of Positive Emotions	−.05	−1.41	1.92	−5.24 to 2.41	−.01	−.41	.90	−2.20 to 1.38

**t value = $p < .001$.

DISCUSSION

The current study adds to the scant literature investigating the use, experience, and conceptualization of violence in African American college-age women. Similar to other studies identifying high rates of dating violence in college samples, the African American women in the current sample perpetrated and experienced high rates of IPV. Furthermore, as in previous studies (e.g., Straus, 2004), the current sample perpetrated and experienced similar frequencies of aggression; in fact, there were significant moderate to strong positive relationships between perpetration of aggression and victimization in the present study. The current results support the findings of previous studies (Hamberger & Potente, 1994; Swan & Snow, 2006) that women's perpetration almost always occurs in the context of their own victimization (only one person in the current sample who perpetrated reported no victimization). The finding that women reported perpetrating significantly more minor and severe psychological and minor physical aggression than they received from their partners may be due, in part, to the study's sampling strategy. Recall that to be included in the study, participants had to report one physical or verbal act of aggression (victim unspecified) in the past year. These women, selected based on their recent use of aggression, likely have engaged in more aggression than would be found in a general sample of college women.

However, the finding that women used more aggression against their partners than their partners used against them is also consistent with several other studies of college students (Allen, Swan, & Raghavan, 2008; Cercone et al., 2005; Graves et al., 2005; Straus, 2004). These include studies with female samples (similar to the present study), which found that women reported a greater frequency of physical aggression against partners than partners' aggression against them (Graves et al., 2005), as well as studies with male and female samples in which women reported committing more physical aggression against partners than men (Allen et al., 2008; Cercone et al., 2005; Graves et al., 2005; Straus, 2004). The results of the current study regarding African American women's greater aggression is also consistent with Archer's (2000) meta-analysis finding that women self-reported committing slightly more physical aggression against partners than men.

The findings of previous research (e.g., Barnett et al., 1997) suggest that women in the current sample should primarily be acting in "self-defense" or in retaliation for previous physical and emotional assaults against them; however, the findings of the current study did not support this assertion. That is, only 9.5% of the sample endorsed self-defense, identified on the MEQ as "to protect self," as the strongest motivation for their perpetration. Furthermore, even though some women identified self-defense as a motive, the Aggression as Response factor, which included "to protect self," was unrelated to women's perpetration of aggressive behavior. In contrast, the Expression of Negative Emotions factor was the only factor that was predictive of the perpetration of aggressive behavior. These findings suggest that it is the communication of negative emotions that are predominately driving African American women's severe psychological and minor and severe physically aggressive behavior in the current sample.

Moreover, while African American college women used their own aggressive behavior as a means of communicating negative emotions, the strongest motivations perceived for their partner's aggression against them were the inability to express themselves verbally, in retaliation for being hit first, and in retaliation for emotional hurt. Collectively these findings suggest that the African American women in the current sample were more likely to use violence not as defensive or even in retaliation for previous aggression against them, but primarily as a method of expressing negative emotions. Furthermore, the finding that women conceptualized their partners' violence against them as due to the partners' inability to express themselves verbally implies that African American college women may view violence in their relationships largely as a means of communicating, either through their own expression of negative emotions or their partners' use of violence to express themselves.

Nabors et al. (2006) asserted that holding beliefs supportive of violence against a partner is strongly associated with committing violent acts against partners. This idea, however, has not been tested with college-age women, and more specifically, African American women. In the current sample, the assertion was supported: increased justifications for aggression were associated with the perpetration of minor physical aggression, providing support for previous research that has suggested that acceptance of the use of violence is an important determinant for the use of aggressive behavior (e.g., Cauffman et al., 2000; Stets & Pirog-Good, 1987).

Still, the relationship between African American women's justifications for aggression and their own motivations for aggression may be more complex than anticipated. On the one hand, the more motivations participants had for their own aggression, the more justifications they had for aggression in general. However, when rating the acceptability of various reasons for aggression, the only item that was endorsed by a statistically significant proportion of the sample as a justifiable reason to use aggression against a partner was "in retaliation for being hit first." Thus it appears that African American women, at least in the current sample, are engaging in aggression for reasons that they themselves do not view as justifiable. These findings raise important questions about the relationship between general attitudes toward aggressive behavior and the actual act of engaging in aggressive behavior, in that the relationship may not be as linear as perceived. Social psychology research on the relationship between general, nonspecific attitudes and behavior has supported that the link between *general* attitudes and behavior is, at best, weak; however, it is equally clear that our attitudes toward *specific* behaviors do exert an important influence on those behaviors (Fiske, 2003). This complexity, particularly in the current sample, suggests that in therapeutic treatments with women who use violence toward their partners, more attention should be placed on exploring and addressing African American women's attitudes about aggression in addition to their actual behavior. A motivational interviewing/cognitive dissonance framework may be helpful as a method of pointing out inconsistencies between a woman's belief that violence against a partner is only justified if one is hit first and that her behavior is inconsistent with this belief (Miller & Rollnick, 2002). Motivational interviewing has been used with court-mandated male perpetrators of IPV (Eckhardt & Utschig, 2007; Neighbors, Walker, Roffman, Mbilinyi, & Edelson, 2008). Furthermore, focusing on women's attitudes toward aggression, even with women who have not engaged in the behavior, may serve to prevent future aggression.

On the one hand, it is positive that of the 24 possible justifications for violence, a statistically significant proportion of participants only perceived one justification, "in retaliation for being hit first," as acceptable. On the other hand, it is concerning that 72% of participants identified this as a justifiable reason for aggression. The belief that using violence is an appropriate response to violence against them may be putting these women at risk for retaliation from their partners. Indeed, when participants were asked what they believed their partners' motivation for using violence against them was, one of the primary perceived motivations for their partners' aggression against them was "in retaliation for being hit first." Participants' belief that violence is justifiable in response to being hit first is particularly disturbing when coupled with the high levels of women's aggression against their partners. Thus women in the current sample appear to be engaging in behavior that is harmful to their partners and may put the women themselves at risk for retaliation from their partners. Given the findings of previous research that has supported that men's use of aggression against women is more severe and injurious than women's aggression against their male partners (e.g., Cascardi et al., 1992), this approval of violence in retaliation may actually serve to put African American women at greater risk for victimization and injury. This claim is an obvious area for future research.

Although providing rich initial information about African American college-age women's use, experience, and conceptualization of IPV, the current study also has some limitations. First, the sample of women was self-selected based on recruitment materials specifically soliciting "aggressive" women (i.e., materials stated that the researchers were looking for women for a paid study on aggressive behavior). In addition, due to an interest in motivations for aggressive behavior specifically, only women who reported the use of some form of aggressive behavior in the past year were included in the study. Thus the current findings may not be generalizable to a broad population of African American college-age women. Future studies should investigate these variables in a more varied sample of African American women. Second, the reliability of some measures was low (specifically psychological perpetration and victimization, as well as the motives measure). In spite of these shortcomings, however, the current findings provide valuable information regarding African American college-age women and IPV.

The findings of the current study add significantly to our understanding of IPV in a continually underrepresented group, African American women. The women in this study used IPV primarily as a destructive method of communication. This suggests that treatments aimed at women who perpetrate IPV focusing on teaching communication skills may be warranted (see Tutty, Babins-Wagner, & Rothery, 2009, for research on an existing program for women). Furthermore, the acceptance of violence as retaliation in the current sample serves to put women at increased risk for victimization and injury, as well as allowing African American women to excuse their partners' violence if it is in retaliation for the women's previous aggression. Thus an area of emphasis in the prevention of dating violence is to convey the message of the nonacceptability of violence in relationships, regardless of the reason. Prevention messages should focus on more adaptive responses to conflict in relationships and teach young people that violence as a means of communication is never acceptable, and that violence as self-defense should be an absolute last resort, not a first response.

REFERENCES

Allen, C. T., Swan, S. C., & Raghavan, C. (2008). Gender symmetry, sexism, & intimate partner violence. *Journal of Interpersonal Violence*. Advance online publication. Retrieved December 23, 2008, from http://jiv.sagepub.com/pap.dtl

Archer, J. (2000). Sex differences in aggression between heterosexual partners: A meta-analytic review. *Psychology Bulletin, 126*, 651–680.

Bartlett, M. S. (1954). A note on the multiplying factors for various chi square approximations. *Journal of the Royal Statistical Society, Series B, 16*, 296–298.

Barnett, O. W., Lee, C. Y., & Thelen, R. E. (1997). Gender differences in attributions of self-defense and control in interpersonal aggression. *Violence Against Women, 3*, 462–481.

Caldwell, J. E., Swan, S. C., Allen, C. T., Sullivan, T. P., & Snow, D. L. (2009). Why I hit him: Women's reasons for intimate partner violence. *Journal of Aggression, Maltreatment & Trauma, 18*(7), 672–697.

Cascardi, M., Langhinrichsen, J., & Vivian, D. (1992). Marital aggression: Impact, injury, and health correlates for husbands and wives. *Archives of Internal Medicine, 152*, 1178–1184.

Cascardi, M., & Vivian, D. (1995). Context for specific episodes of marital violence: Gender and severity of violence differences. *Journal of Family Violence, 10*, 265–293.

Cauffman, E., Feldman, S. S., Jensen, L. A., & Arnett, J. J. (2000). The (un)acceptability of violence against peers and dates. *Journal of Adolescent Research, 15*, 652–673.

Cercone, J. L., Beach, S. R. H., & Arias, I. (2005). Gender symmetry in dating intimate partner violence: Does similar behavior imply similar constructs? *Violence and Victims, 20*, 207–218.

Clark, M. L., Beckett, J., Wells, M., & Dungee-Anderson, D. (1994). Courtship violence among African-American college students. *Journal of Black Psychology, 20*, 264–281.

Dekeserdy, W. S., Saunders, D. G., Schwartz, M. D., & Alvi, S. (1997). The meanings and motives for women's use of violence in Canadian college dating relationships: Results from a national survey. *Sociological Spectrum, 17*, 199–222.

DeKeseredy, W. S., & Schwartz, M. D. (1998). *Woman abuse on campus: Results from the Canadian National Survey*. Thousand Oaks, CA: Sage.

DeMaris, A. (1990). The dynamics of intergenerational transmission in courtship violence: A biracial exploration. *Journal of Marriage and the Family, 52*, 219–231.

Eckhardt, C. I., & Utschig, A. C. (2007). Assessing readiness to change among perpetrators of intimate partner violence: Analysis of two self-report measures. *Journal of Family Violence, 22*, 319–330.

Fiske, S. T. (2003). *Social beings: A core motives approach to social psychology* (1st ed.). New York: John Wiley & Sons.

Follingstad, D. R., Rutledge, L. L., Polek, D. S., & McNeill-Harkins, K. (1988). Factors associated with patters of dating violence toward college women. *Journal of Family Violence, 3*, 169–182.

Follingstad, D. R., Wright, S., Lloyd, S., & Sebastian, J. A. (1991). Sex differences in motivations and effects in dating violence. *Family Relations: Journal of Applied Family & Child Studies, 40*(1), 51–57.

Graham-Kevan, N., & Archer, J. (2005). Investigating three explanations of women's relationship aggression. *Psychology of Women Quarterly, 29*, 270–277.

Graves, K. N., Sechrist, S. M., White, J. W., & Paradise, M. J. (2005). Intimate partner violence perpetrated by college women within the context of a history of being victimized. *Psychology of Women Quarterly, 29*, 278–289.

Hamberger, L. K. (2005). Men's and women's use of intimate partner violence in clinical samples: Toward a gender-sensitive analysis. *Violence and Victims, 20*, 131–151.

Hamberger, L. K., Lohr, J. M., & Bonge, D. (1994). The intended function of domestic violence is different for arrested male and female perpetrators. *Family Violence and Sexual Assault Bulletin, 10*, 40–44.

Hamberger, L. K., & Potente, T. (1994). Counseling heterosexual women arrested for domestic violence: Implications for theory and practice. *Violence and Victims, 9*, 125–137.

Jackson, S. M. (1999). Issues in the dating violence research: A review of the literature. *Aggression and Violent Behavior, 4*, 233–247.

Kaiser, H. (1970). A second generation Little Jiffy. *Psychometrika, 35*, 401–415.

Kaiser, H. (1974). An index of factorial simplicity. *Psychometrika, 39*, 31–36.

Kernsmith, P. (2005). Exerting power or striking back: A gendered comparison of motivations for domestic violence perpetration. *Violence and Victims, 20*, 173–184.

Kurtz, D. (1993). Physical assaults by husbands: A major social problem. In R. J. Gelles & D. R. Loseke (Eds.), *Current controversies on family violence* (pp. 88–103). Newbury Park, CA: Sage.

Leisring, P. A. (2009). What will happen if I punch him? Expected consequences of female violence against male dating partners. *Journal of Aggression, Maltreatment & Trauma, 18*(7), 739–751.

Lewis, S. F., & Fremouw, W. (2001). Dating violence: A critical review of the literature. *Clinical Psychology Review, 21*, 105–127.

Miller, W., & Rollnick, S. (2002). *Motivational interviewing* (2nd ed.). New York: Guilford Press.

Nabors, E. L., Dietz, T. L., & Jasinski, J. L. (2006). Domestic violence beliefs and perceptions among college students. *Violence and Victims, 21*, 779–794.

Neighbors, C., Walker, D. D., Roffman, R. A., Mbilinyi, L. F., & Edelson, J. L. (2008). Self-determination theory and motivational interviewing: Complementary models to elicit voluntary engagement by partner-abusive men. *American Journal of Family Therapy, 36*, 126–136.

Osthoff, S. (2002). But, Gertrude, I beg to differ. A hit is not a hit is not a hit: When battered women are arrested for assaulting their partners. *Violence Against Women, 8*(12), 1521–1544.

Roscoe, B., & Benaske, N. (1985). Courtship violence experienced by abused wives: Similarities in patters of abuse. *Family Relations, 34*, 419–424.

Saunders, D. G. (1986). When battered women use violence: Husband-abuse or self-defense? *Violence and Victims, 1*, 47–60.

Stets, J. E., & Pirog-Good, M. A. (1987) Interpersonal control and courtship aggression. *Journal of Social and Personal Relationships, 7*, 371–394.

Straus, M. A. (2004). Prevalence of violence against dating partners by male and female university students worldwide. *Violence Against Women, 10*, 790–811.

Straus, M. A., Hamby, S. L., Boney-McCoy, S., & Sugarman, D. B. (1996). The revised Conflict Tactics Scales (CTS2): Development and preliminary psychometric data. *Journal of Family Issues, 17*, 283–316.

Stuart, G. L., Moore, T. M., Gordon, K. C., Hellmuth, J. C., Ramsey, S. E., & Kahler, C. W. (2006). Reasons for intimate partner violence perpetration among arrested women. *Violence Against Women, 12*, 609–621.

Sugarman, D. B., & Hotaling, G. T. (1989). Dating violence: Prevalence, context and risk markers. In M. A. Pirog-Good & J. E. Stets (Eds.), *Violence in dating relationships: Emerging social issues* (pp. 3–32). New York: Praeger.

Swan, S. C., & Snow, D. L. (2003). Behavioral and psychological differences among abused women who use violence in intimate relationships. *Violence Against Women, 9,* 75–109.

Swan, S. C., & Snow, D. L. (2006). The development of a theory of women's use of violence in intimate relationships. *Violence Against Women, 12,* 1026–1045.

Temple, J. R., Weston, R., & Marshall, L. L. (2005). Physical and mental health outcomes of women in nonviolent, unilaterally violent, and mutually violent relationships. *Violence and Victims, 20,* 335–359.

Tutty, L. M., Babins-Wagner, R., & Rothery, M. A. (2009). A comparison of women who were mandated and non-mandated to the "Responsible Choices for Women" group. *Journal of Aggression, Maltreatment & Trauma, 18*(7), 770–793.

West, C. (2002). Battered, black, and blue: An overview of violence in the lives of black women. In C. West (Ed.), *Violence in the lives of black women: Battered, black, and blue* (pp. 5–27). Binghamton, NY: Haworth Press.

West, C. (2004). Black women and intimate partner violence: New directions for research. *Journal of Interpersonal Violence, 19*(12), 1487–1493.

West, C. M., & Rose, S. (2000). Dating aggression among low income African American youth: An examination of gender differences and antagonistic beliefs. *Violence Against Women, 6,* 470–494.

An Exploratory Study of Women as Dominant Aggressors of Physical Violence in Their Intimate Relationships

LISA CONRADI

Rady Children's Hospital, San Diego, San Diego, California, USA

ROBERT GEFFNER

Alliant International University, San Diego, California, USA

L. KEVIN HAMBERGER

Medical College of Wisconsin, Racine, Wisconsin, USA

GARY LAWSON

Alliant International University, San Diego, California, USA

In the last 20 years, research has emerged that suggests that women may be violent in intimate relationships. This article describes a qualitative study focusing on women who were classified as dominant aggressors of violence in their intimate relationships. Ten subjects participated in a detailed clinical interview and completed five written measures to examine the factors that led to their later aggression, including sociocultural factors, history of trauma, gender role identification, and intergenerational transmission of violence. Seven major themes emerged, including a history of victimization and trauma, substance abuse, and a history of violence across relationships and situations. These results suggest that the violence committed by dominantly aggressive women may be explained by an integrated conceptual framework of domestic violence.

Multiple theories have often been used to explain the occurrence of intimate partner violence (IPV), including various sociocultural factors such as substance abuse (Stuart, Moore, Ramsey, & Kahler, 2003) and a history of violent behavior (Straus & Ramirez, 1999). Additional theories include those that focus on the intergenerational transmission of violence (Langhinrichsen-Rohling Neidig, & Thorn, 1995), trauma (Dutton, Saunders, Starzomski, & Bartholomew, 1994), and gender role identification (Thompson, 1991). However, many of these theories lack empirical support when examining women who have been arrested for IPV. The present study examined these factors as they relate to a particular subset of domestically violent women. Each of the following factors will be discussed in relation to female IPV.

SOCIOCULTURAL FACTORS

Various sociocultural factors may be related to women's use of IPV, including substance abuse and a history of violent behavior. Straus and Ramirez (1999) surveyed students and examined the extent to which those who physically assaulted a partner had a history of criminal activity, including other violent crime and property crime. They found that for both males and females, a history of early onset crime was related to assaulting a partner, but not later crime. Moffitt and Caspi (1999) conducted a longitudinal study examining partner violence among 1,037 men and women in New Zealand who were interviewed at various times from birth to age 21. They found that female perpetrators showed risk factors of harsh family discipline and histories of aggressive behavior. The strongest risk factor for female perpetrators of IPV was a record of physically aggressive delinquency before the age of 15.

Substance abuse may also play a role in women's use of IPV (Sullivan, Cavanaugh, Ufner, Swan, & Snow, 2009). Given that alcohol serves a disinhibitory effect, it is not surprising that several studies have found a link between alcohol abuse and IPV. Caetano, Schafer, and Cunradi (2001) found that 30% to 40% of the men and 27% to 34% of the women who perpetrated violence against their partners were drinking at the time of the event. The relationship between violence and substance abuse may apply to other drugs as well. Stuart et al. (2003) examined the relationship between women who had been court ordered to domestic violence treatment and substance use characteristics. They found that 25% of the women reported symptoms consistent with an alcohol abuse or dependence diagnosis and 25% of the women reported symptoms consistent with a drug-related diagnosis. According to this research, there appears to be a strong relationship between female perpetrators of IPV and current or recent substance abuse or dependence.

INTERGENERATIONAL TRANSMISSION OF VIOLENCE

Another explanation provided for the origins of IPV lies in social learning theory, or the intergenerational transmission of violence theory. This theory suggests that if an individual grows up witnessing violence or as the victim of violence, that individual is predisposed to becoming violent or the victim of violence in his or her own intimate relationships (Widom, 1989). It proposes that children learn about violence through witnessing it between their parents or experiencing it themselves. Some researchers have found that the association between witnessing parental violence and perpetrating partner violence is stronger for males (Marshall & Rose, 1988). Others have found the relationship to be stronger for females (Langhinrichsen-Rohling et al., 1995), and about the same for both males and females (Tontodonato & Crew, 1992).

GENDER ROLE IDENTIFICATION

In the current study, the term "gender role identification" was used to describe various traits and behaviors associated with a particular gender. According to Bem (1981), individuals who identify with a feminine gender role are more likely to endorse that they believe they have a more expressive orientation, or an affective concern for the welfare of others and the harmony of the group. On the other hand, individuals who identify with a masculine gender role are more likely to endorse an instrumental orientation, or a cognitive focus on getting the job done or the problem solved. Some researchers have proposed a "masculinity argument" of male violence (Huselid & Cooper, 1994) that anticipates an interaction between gender and gender role identification. This expectation suggests that physical violence is related to men's traditional role norms. Therefore men with a strong, traditional masculine orientation are more likely to be more aggressive in dating relationships. Thompson (1991) examined the effect of a masculine gender role orientation on women's and men's physical aggression while dating by giving the Bem Sex Role Inventory (BSRI; Bem, 1974) to 352 male and female undergraduate college students. They found that gender role orientation was independently related to IPV in dating relationships.

HISTORY OF TRAUMA

Recently, many researchers have suggested that individuals who have a significant trauma history experience difficulty modulating their anger, which may be manifested in their use of violence in intimate relationships. Therefore they are more likely to behave in an angry and violent manner with their partner. Trauma theory was initially explored using veterans with combat-related posttraumatic stress disorder (PTSD). Chemtob, Hamada, Roitblat, and Muraoka (1994) found an association between anger and combat-related PTSD in veterans.

Various explanations have been suggested to relate to women's anger responses, including the notion that, as children, they were taught it is unsafe or unacceptable for women to express angry feelings. As a result, their anger responses build up and are often expressed inappropriately. Scott and Day (1996) examined the relationship between abuse-related symptoms and style of anger expression for female survivors of childhood incest. They found that adult female survivors of childhood incest who suppress their anger report significantly more symptoms on a measure of inwardly directed anger than do survivors who appropriately express their angry feelings. It is suggested that victims of abuse, sexual trauma in this particular instance, learned that it was dangerous to express anger toward their perpetrator or those who were supposed to protect them. Given findings such as these, it is important to understand the trauma history of women who are dominant aggressors, that is, those who have expressed their anger outward, rather than inward.

TYPES OF FEMALE VIOLENCE IN INTIMATE RELATIONSHIPS

While there are many theories that may be used to explain women's use of violence in intimate relationships, very little research has been done to date focusing solely on the context, motivation, and typologies of violent female offenders. In their groundbreaking work, Swan and Snow (2002) differentiated three types of female offenders: (a) women as victims, (b) women as aggressors, and (c) bidirectional violence. Victims were classified as women who primarily used violence as a form of self-defense or retaliation against their more violent partner. Bidirectional violence occurs in relationships where both partners are violent with one another. In the third category, labeled "women as aggressors," a woman was classified as the dominant aggressor in the relationship if she committed more acts of severe violence and coercive control than her partner committed against her. Furthermore, the acts of violence by these women cannot fit the previously defined criteria of self-defense. In other words, she was the significant aggressor of relationship violence and did not act primarily in self-defense (Swan & Snow, 2002).

Studies have indicated that dominant aggression by women in intimate relationships is a relatively rare phenomenon. Swan and Snow (2002) found that only 13 of 104 participants, or 12% of the women in their studies, could be defined as the dominant aggressor, based on their own self-report of aggressive acts in the previous 6-month period. From these results, they distinguished two subtypes of female dominant aggressors. Type A aggressors were the women who committed more of all types of partner violence than her partner committed against her, including moderate violence and emotional abuse; this type accounted for 7% of their sample. Type B aggressors were the women who committed greater levels of severe violence and coercion, but the partner committed more moderate violence and emotional abuse; this type accounted for the remaining 5% of their sample. Female aggressors (both Type A and B) committed an average of 64 more abusive behaviors than their male partners in the previous 6-month period. However, the results in this study were not corroborated by the male victim's reports, so it is difficult to determine if women were actually more abusive than their male counterparts, if they were more likely to report their own use of abusive behaviors, or if they were more likely to perceive their own behavior as abusive.

Using the same sample, Swan and Snow (2003) expanded on their previous research by examining the relationship between the female offender's typology and various behavioral and psychological indicators, including anxiety, depression, and PTSD. They found that "abused aggressors" (their term for dominant aggressors who also display a significant victim history) were more likely to have experienced traumatic childhood abuse than other types of female offenders. Furthermore, abused aggressors reported the lowest level of control over their anger. They also reported that they were more likely to inflict injury on their partner and use violence as a form of power and control over their partners. These women displayed greater levels of overall anxiety, depression, and PTSD symptoms than members of the other categories. Finally, women in the abused aggressor type were usually the first to use violence with their partner overall whenever violence occurred in the relationship. While these results are limited due to the small sample size ($n = 13$), they indicate that women who serve as the dominant aggressors of IPV in their relationships present with a variety of unique psychological and behavioral issues that should be explored more deeply in research.

While many theorists have proposed possible explanations for the incidence of female violence, very few researchers have explored the experiences of women who are classified as dominant aggressors of physical violence in their intimate relationships. The present study examined the factors that led to the participant's later aggression, including sociocultural factors, history of trauma, gender role identification, and intergenerational transmission of violence.

METHOD

Participants

Ten heterosexual women who were court ordered to attend treatment for domestic violence offenders participated in this research. The study was limited to heterosexual women who had committed violence against their male partners, since findings from previous research (Bernhard, 2000) have suggested that the perpetration and experience of violence varies between heterosexual and lesbian women. In particular, lesbian women reported experiencing greater degrees of nonsexual violence. A total of 138 women were screened prior to their court-ordered treatment group; 12 women met the inclusion criteria and were invited to participate in the study. One participant later declined participation and another could not be reached to reschedule her interview, resulting in 10 interview participants. The average age of the participants was 32 years and their length of attendance at the treatment program ranged from 7 weeks to completion of the program (52 weeks). None of the women had ever been homeless. Table 1 provides a listing of the participants' assigned code numbers, ages, race, income, number of weeks in treatment, marital status, number of children, whether or not they were still with the partner with whom they committed the violent act, and a brief history of the arresting incident. The ethnicity and annual income were extremely varied. In seven cases, the participant was arrested for perpetrating violence against a current partner. In three cases, the participant was arrested for perpetrating violence against a former partner. According to self-reports, all but one of the participants had been violent with their partners within the past 15 months. For one participant, there was a 4-year lag between her last reported violent incident and the interview due to her serving time in prison for the offense.

In order to be selected to participate in the study, the participants needed to qualify as the dominant aggressor of physical violence in their heterosexual intimate relationship. In order to be considered a dominant aggressor, potential participants met the following criteria: (a) the police report identified the individual as the dominant aggressor or equivalent, (b) more extensive injuries were sustained by the other partner, (c) the presence of fear in the partner of the aggressor at the time of arrest (based on participant self-report), and (d) a history of similar behavior with this partner or other partners in the past. These criteria were assessed by a self-report measure created by the researcher termed the Partner Aggression Style Screening Questionnaire (PAASQ). The PAASQ is a two-page, paper-and-pencil screener developed by the researchers in an attempt to operationalize the definition of dominant aggressor. It was used to determine if a woman could be classified as the dominant aggressor of IPV in her relationship according to the definition of dominant aggressor defined previously. It contained questions assessing the following factors: initiation of violence; commission of various violent acts; fear; and pattern of violent acts, including the commission of violence on more than one occasion with more than one partner.

TABLE 1 Demographic Information of the Participants

ID no.	Age	Ethnicity/ race	Annual income	Weeks in treatment	Marital status	No. of children	With partner?	Description of violent episode
P1	40	Caucasian	Less than $9,999	7	Single/committed	1	Yes	Throwing things, slapping him
P2	22	Caucasian	$10,000–$19,999	9	Single	0	No	Kicked and bit him
P3	50	African American	$10,000–$19,999	14	Single/committed	2	Yes	Threw hot grease and oil on him; convicted of attempted murder
P4	25	Caucasian	$10,000–$19,999	42	Single/committed	0; pregnant	Yes	Throwing things at him in public
P5	32	Hispanic	$40,000–$49,999	19	Married	1	Yes	Threw ceramic mugs at him
P6	23	African American	$10,000–$19,999	52	Divorced	0	No	Violation of restraining order; numerous incidents of throwing things and hitting him with objects
P7	34	Hispanic	$30,000–$39,999	10	Married	3	Yes	Threw wine glass, shards cut his chest
P8	39	Caucasian	$20,000–$29,999	21	Single/committed	2	Yes	Broke elbow, throwing things at him
P9	33	Hispanic	$40,000–$49,999	49	Married	0	Yes	Slapped and scratched
P10	27	Mixed Race	$50,000–$74,999	51	Single	0	No	Broke a bottle on his head

Procedure

The researcher approached batterer intervention programs in the San Diego County area and invited group members to complete the PAASQ. Women who fit all of the criteria were classified as the dominant aggressor and asked to participate in the research study. All individuals were provided with candy as an incentive to complete the screening measure. Individuals were notified immediately if they met the criteria to participate in the study. If they agreed, they were scheduled for a 3-hour block of time to meet with the researcher for the interview and completion of measures.

At the appointed time, the first author met with the participant and had her complete the informed consent, written measures, and interview. Each participant completed the following measures: BSRI (Bem, 1974), Detailed Assessment of Posttraumatic Stress (DAPS; Briere, 2001), Drug Abuse Screening Test (DAST; Skinner, 1983), and the Michigan Alcoholism Screening Test (MAST; Selzer, 1971). After completing the written measures, the researcher conducted the semistructured interview. The interview questions concerned the participants' experiences of abuse as a child, adolescent, or in previous intimate relationships; history of violent behavior both within and outside of intimate relationships; description of the arresting incident; history of drug and alcohol abuse; criminal history; and their own understanding of why they have used violence and aggression. The interview questions were based on themes suggested by the literature on women's use of violence in intimate relationships and on female gender socialization, as well as information from clinical experience with women who are perpetrators of IPV. The interview lasted approximately 2 hours.

Measures

Bem sex role inventory

The BSRI (Bem, 1974) is a 60-item paper-and-pencil self-report measure designed for conducting empirical research on psychological androgyny. The BSRI contains 60 distinct personality trait descriptors. Twenty of the descriptors are stereotypically feminine (e.g., affectionate, gentle, understanding, sensitive to the needs of others), 20 are stereotypically masculine (e.g., ambitious, self-reliant, independent, assertive), and 20 are filler items. The participant was asked to indicate on a 7-point scale how well each of the 60 characteristics described her. The items were scored on independent dimensions of masculinity and femininity, as well as androgyny and undifferentiated classifications. Those who rated high on masculinity and femininity were described as "androgynous." Those scoring low on masculinity and femininity were "undifferentiated." Those high on masculinity and low on femininity were "masculine," and those high on femininity and low on masculinity were "feminine." In the current study, the BSRI was used to explore if the participants identified more strongly with a masculine, androgynous, undifferentiated, or feminine gender role.

The DAPS (Briere, 2001) is a measure designed to assess trauma exposure and posttraumatic stress in individuals who have a history of exposure to one or more events that can be considered traumatic. The inventory contains 104 statements that an individual can mark in one of five categories: "in the last day," "more than a day ago, but in the last month," "between 1 and 3 months ago," "more than 3 months ago, but in the last year," or "a year ago or longer." The DAPS has two validity scales and 11 clinical scales. It includes three PTSD symptom clusters (reexperiencing, avoidance, hyperarousal) and three associated features of PTSD (dissociation, substance abuse, suicidality) related to a particular trauma event. Two validity scales identify overreporting and underreporting of psychological symptoms. The results on the DAPS generate a tentative diagnosis of PTSD or acute stress disorder (ASD).

In the current study, the DAPS was used to provide information on the level of posttraumatic symptoms experienced by each participant. This information was used in conjunction with the semistructured interview to provide an overall picture of each participant and her responses to previous victimization.

MICHIGAN ALCOHOLISM SCREENING TEST

The MAST (Selzer, 1971) is a 24-item self-report measure designed to detect alcoholism in a population that frequently denies problems with alcohol. The respondent is asked to answer yes or no to each statement as it applies to them. The items on the MAST were selected on the basis of review of several other approaches to investigating alcohol abuse. A few items were developed to be sufficiently neutral so that people who are reluctant to see themselves as problem drinkers may reveal their alcoholic symptoms. Items regarding amounts of alcohol consumed were not included because that information is notoriously unreliable. Four points indicates possible alcoholism and five points or more is indicative of alcoholism (Selzer, 1971).

In the current study, the MAST was used to provide a measure of each participant's level of alcohol abuse in the past 12 months. This information was used in conjunction with the semistructured interview to provide an overall picture of the individual's use of alcohol and the role that use played in their perpetration of IPV.

DRUG ABUSE SCREENING TEST

The DAST (Skinner, 1983) is a 28-item instrument that yields a quantitative index of the range of problems associated with misuse of prescription drugs and illegal drug use. The questions on the DAST are based on items comprising the MAST. Thus the DAST also has some items that are neutral enough to accurately assess for substance use despite the fact that this population tends to be defensive and deny problems associated with substance use. Individuals scoring five or more points are very likely to be substance abusers or substance dependent.

In the current study, the DAST provided a measure of each participant's level of drug abuse problems in the past 12 months. This information was used in conjunction with the semistructured interview to provide an overall picture of the individual's use of substances and the role that use played in their perpetration of IPV.

Analysis of Data

The interview data were formally analyzed using Maykut and Morehouse's (1994) "constant comparative method" in order to identify some of the themes present in lives and relationships of women who are identified as dominant aggressors in IPV. Each interview was transcribed and the data were then scanned several times using a line-by-line analysis, paying attention to recurrent and important key words or phrases used by the participants. Each one of these ideas and concepts was coded as a "unit of meaning." Each unit of meaning was compared to all other units of meaning. Themes and concepts that overlapped with one another were combined. One prominent idea (word/phrase) was selected and written on an index card. This word/phrase became the first provisional category. If a second data card also fit the first category, the researcher reread the first data card and compared it to the second. If the second card "looked like" or "felt like" the meaning of the first card, it was included under the first provisional category. If the data card did not fit the first provisional category, it was placed under another provisional category. If a data card was found that did not fit under any of the provisional categories, a new category was created and named. After six to eight cards accumulated in a category, a rule of inclusion was written to serve as the basis for including (or excluding) subsequent data cards in the category. This rule of inclusion was written as a prepositional statement and was intended to convey the meaning contained in the data cards included under a category name. Additional data cards that satisfied the rules were included and those that did not were categorized elsewhere. Data analysis continued until all data cards were categorized into a substantive category and overlap was reduced. The researcher analyzed relationships and patterns across the provisional categories, identifying salient themes (see Table 2).

In order to provide independent validation of the themes mentioned, three persons not involved in the present research each reviewed the same two manuscripts and analyzed them for units of meaning. They provided the researcher with a list of the units of meaning they found, who then

TABLE 2 Major Themes Discussed by Participants.

Theme no.	Theme name	Subtheme no.	Subtheme name	P1	P2	P3	P4	P5	P6	P7	P8	P9	P10
1	History of victimization	1a	Physical abuse by parent/caregiver	X		X	X		X			X	X
		1b	Exposed to domestic violence in childhood	X		X	X	X	X	X		X	X
		1c	Victim of domestic violence in past relationship	X	X	X				X	X		
		1d	Met criteria for PTSD on DAPS	X	X						X		
2	Gender role identification	2a	Identified with masculine gender traits in interview	X	X	X	X	X	X	X	X		X
		2b	Identified with masculine gender role on BSRI	X		X			X	X	X		X
3	Problems related to substance abuse	3a	Substance abuse in family of origin	X		X		X	X	X	X	X	X
		3b	Participant history of substance abuse			X	X		X	X	X		X
		3c	Intoxicated at time of offense			X	X	X	X				X
		3d	Met criteria for alcoholism on MAST				X			X	X		X
		3e	Met criteria for drug abuse on DAST		X								X
4	Reported emotional abuse by partner			X	X	X				X	X	X	X
5	Viewed self as dominant in relationship				X	X	X	X	X	X		X	X
6	History of violent behavior across situations			X	X		X			X	X	X	X
7	Personal belief of inherent aggressiveness			X		X	X	X	X	X	X	X	X

compared that list to the units of meaning previously found by the researcher. If the units were not on the list of those found by the researcher, they were added. A total of 10 units of meaning were added to the first interview and 7 units were added to the second interview. A total of 11 units of meaning were added to the overall list of units of meaning. The overall list of units of meaning and two additional interviews were then given to three additional persons not involved in the research. These three people examined each unit of meaning and noted whether the unit of meaning was evident in the manuscript. The consistency or agreement between the researcher and outside readers was 92% for the first interview and 92% for the second interview. Conclusions regarding the research questions were drawn from the themes extrapolated during the data analysis combined with a qualitative review of the participants' answers on each of the measures.

RESULTS

Emergent Themes

HISTORY OF VICTIMIZATION

All 10 women described being victimized in their past. Victimization primarily occurred in three forms: (a) physical abuse as a child; (b) exposure to domestic violence between parents or caregivers; and (c) being the victim of domestic violence by a former partner. Six women described incidents of physical abuse by a parent or caregiver as a child. These responses ranged from a single incident of physical abuse to a long history of physical abuse by a caregiver.

Seven of the women discussed exposure to domestic violence between their parents or caregivers as a child. One woman discussed her exposure to her mother's violence and indicated that she believed that this is where she learned to be violent. Others indicated that they "jumped in" to protect their mother from the physical violence. Five of the women reported that they had previously been a victim of domestic violence. Three of the five women stated that they had previously been victimized by the same partner on which they perpetrated their violence. However, none of their partners had been violent within the prior 2-year period. These women indicated that they often used their partner's violence against him, believing that he would never do it again.

Since a history of victimization is somewhat related to PTSD, participants' scores on the DAPS were first used to determine if they were experiencing symptoms of PTSD. In addition, their profiles were examined to see if there were any general trends compared to the other participants in the study. The data obtained from the DAPS suggested that 4 of the 10 participants met the diagnostic criteria for PTSD. It is possible that two of the protocols may not be valid due to inflated negative bias scores, or an attempt to present oneself as especially symptomatic. However, even those who did not meet the criteria appeared to be experiencing some psychological distress related to traumatic experiences in their lives. While many women did not meet the criteria for PTSD, they had experienced significant levels of trauma, and often shared how that trauma affected their current level of functioning.

IDENTIFICATION WITH MASCULINE GENDER TRAITS

Nine of the 10 women indicated that they often got along better with boys than girls in childhood, adulthood, or both. On the BSRI, their overall scores for masculinity and femininity were computed and compared to the median in the population. Five of the participants more closely identified with a masculine gender role; three of the participants closely identified with an undifferentiated gender role; and only one participant closely identified with an androgynous or feminine gender role.

PROBLEMS RELATED TO SUBSTANCE ABUSE

All 10 of the women indicated that substance abuse had played a significant role in their lives that often led to their own violence or violence within their family of origin. Eight of the 10 women indicated that one or both of their parents were substance abusers (e.g., alcohol, illegal drugs, or prescription medication). Seven of the 10 women discussed the abuse of alcohol or drugs in their interview. Four of these 10 women indicated that they were using alcohol or drugs at the time of the offense. All four of these women believed that their use of substances played a role in their violence. However, while some understood that they were still responsible for their actions, one participant dismissed her violence due to her drunkenness, stating that it would not happen again.

For the MAST and DAST, a total number of positive responses were computed and those scores were compared to those in the general population to determine whether the participant had a problem with drugs or alcohol. On the MAST, five of the women had scores in the range that indicates alcoholism. Two of the participants had scores that suggested that the participant may currently have a problem with alcoholism. Three of the participants had scores indicating that they do not have problems with alcohol. On the DAST, only one participant scored higher than a 5 (indicative of drug abuse) on the DAST. No other participants had scores indicative of a drug problem on the DAST.

While many of the participants indicated that they did not believe their substance abuse was a problem, all of these particular participants had inflated scores on the MAST or DAST, which suggests that they had issues with substance abuse at the time of assessment. Alternatively, one participant admitted to daily use of marijuana in the interview, although she did not endorse that on the DAST. Furthermore, another participant reported an extensive personal and criminal history related to her use of drugs, which played a direct role in her violent incident. However, she had been clean and sober for 4 years at the time of the interview, so her previous history of drug use was not reported on the DAST, which focuses on drug use in the previous 12 months.

EMOTIONAL ABUSE BY PARTNER AS MOTIVATION FOR VIOLENCE

Seven of the 10 women indicated that they believed their physical aggression against their partner was somewhat justified because of the emotional abuse they received from him. While all of these women were classified as dominant aggressors of physical violence, many of them described feelings of victimization due to their partner's emotional abuse.

VIEW OF THEMSELVES AS DOMINANT IN THE RELATIONSHIP

Eight of the 10 women viewed themselves as the dominant partner in their relationship. They viewed their partners as weak and in need of protection. They reported that they often felt their job was to stand up for their partner and protect him from others who might take advantage of him. Many women indicated that they had always viewed their partner as weak and that their partner had been abused in previous relationships.

HISTORY OF VIOLENT BEHAVIOR

Seven of the 10 women indicated that they had a history of initiating violence across situations with a different variety of people, not only with their partners. Examples of such violence included fighting extensively with their siblings, fights in bars while intoxicated, or fights in public places with strangers.

PERSONAL BELIEF OF INNATE AGGRESSIVENESS

When asked about the reasons for their violence and aggression, 9 of the 10 women viewed their aggression and violence as one of the characteristics of their personality. Many indicated that they had been aggressive their whole lives across a variety of situations and were often seen as the aggressive and violent child within their families of origin.

DISCUSSION

The current research study provided information on a previously neglected group of women—those who have been classified as dominant aggressors of physical violence in their intimate relationships. The findings suggested that these women often believed their violence was justified based on their partner's actions. A set of seven themes emerged from the participants' responses. The themes suggested that many of these women have shared experiences and behaviors that may play a role in their aggressive and violent behavior. These themes supported some of the principles and tenets of various theoretical perspectives and previous research findings, including trauma theory, the intergenerational transmission of violence theory, gender role identification theory, and various sociocultural factors.

Trauma Theory

The findings supported principles of trauma theory when examining participants' history of victimization, such as being physically abused by a parent or caregiver as a child, reported emotional abuse by their partner, and previous domestic violence in the current or past relationships where they were classified as the victim. The participants shared that their experiences of trauma and abuse played a significant role in the way in which they coped with stressful events, including emotional abuse from their partner. Many stated that they never learned to express their feelings in an assertive way because they felt emotionally detached from others and had difficulty forming close relationships. These findings are consistent with findings from male offenders of IPV. Recently, researchers have begun to address the individual issues among male perpetrators of IPV and found that their history of trauma, shaming, and insecure attachment form a triad that constitutes a powerful trauma source (Dutton, 1999). Evidence from the current study suggests that traumatic events may have a similar influence on women who use violence in their intimate relationships, given the significant amount of trauma experienced by many of the participants in the current study.

Further, the women interviewed for the current study closely resembled Swan and Snow's (2003) subtype of abused aggressors. In their study, they found that abused aggressors experienced a high degree of traumatic childhood abuse, reported the lowest level of control over their anger, and used violence as a form of power and control over their partners. These women displayed greater levels of overall anxiety, depression, and PTSD symptoms than those who were classified as victims or in mixed-violence relationships. Clearly, a history of trauma, when combined with other factors, plays a powerful role in the potential use of physical aggression among these women.

Intergenerational Transmission of Violence

The intergenerational transmission of violence theory was evident in the number of women who were exposed to domestic violence in their family of origin. Many of the women reported that they often watched or were exposed to the effects of abuse their mother endured at the hands of their father or stepfather and they made a conscious decision never to be victimized in a similar way. One participant reportedly saw her mother as the initiator of violence. In that situation, it is possible that she identified with the aggressor and decided not to become a victim, just as her mother decided not to become a victim.

There exists very little research on women who are violent in their intimate relationships in general and even less on the relationship between female exposure to domestic violence as children and later becoming dominant aggressors. Most of the research has focused on women repeating the pattern set by their mothers and becoming the victim of violence by their partner. The results from the current study support the findings of Foshee, Bauman, and Linder (1999), who examined the relationship between exposure to family violence and adolescent dating violence. They found that, for females in particular, having an aggressive response style to conflict was positively related to witnessing parental violence and receiving physical violence from their mother.

Gender Role Identification

Perhaps one of the most striking findings of the current study is that 9 of the 10 women stated that they had traditionally gotten along better with males than females in childhood or adulthood and were identified with masculine gender traits. While five of the women were found to identify with masculine gender traits on the BSRI, only one of the women identified with feminine gender traits. These findings strongly contradict the societal norm suggesting that women are more likely to identify with feminine gender traits while males are more likely to identify with masculine gender traits. In addition, three of the women were classified as low on both masculine and feminine traits, while one classified as androgynous, which is relatively rare in the general population. It is possible that the women who qualified as either undifferentiated or androgynous are experiencing difficulty identifying themselves with any particular gender role. That is, they fit criteria for both masculine and feminine traits equally. Since 9 of the 10 women in the current study did not closely identify with feminine gender traits, the women in the current study have defied the societal norm suggesting that women should be feminine.

The results of the current study support those by Thompson (1991), who found that gender role identification was independently related to who inflicts and sustains physical aggression while dating for both men and women. He suggested that sex and gender role were categorically different and may be mutually exclusive for many individuals. For the women in the current study, that appears to be the case. Furthermore, the current results offer support to the study by Campbell, Mackenzie, and Robinson (1987), who examined incarcerated female offenders. They found that women who identified with a masculine gender role in terms of aggressiveness, assertiveness, and dominance were more likely to be serving time for violent offenses. While no prior research has examined identification with masculine gender traits of female perpetrators of IPV, the current study suggests that there may very well exist a relationship between those women who are the predominant aggressors of IPV and their gender identification.

Sociocultural Factors

Various shared sociocultural factors were also present in this sample of women, including a history of violent behavior, substance abuse either within themselves or their family of origin, personal belief about their own inherent aggressiveness, and view of themselves as dominant in the relationship. Only 4 of the 10 women indicated that they had an early criminal history, including running away, stealing a car, drug use, and destruction of property. While there does not appear to be a major trend among these women of committing criminal acts, there does appear to be a history of aggression and committing violent acts, such as getting into fights in bars or parking lots or fighting with other children at school when they were younger. It is possible that these women adopted a coping strategy for dealing with conflict early in their childhood that included engaging in physical fights either to protect themselves or others. It is suggested that they continued these coping strategies into adulthood and used physical violence as a method of communicating with partners or others when they did not feel heard and did not feel that their needs were being met. In addition, these women reported that they felt more dominant in the relationship than their partner, providing further support that their personal individual factors played a role in their justification of physical violence against their "weaker" partner.

In addition, many of the women who participated in the current study exhibited problems with substance abuse either in themselves or their family of origin. They reported only using violence against partners who had a history of violence, suggesting that past abuse from a partner may also mediate the effect of alcohol on IPV. Women who were previously victims were not more likely to be intoxicated at the time of the offense. However, it appeared that many of the women who were intoxicated at the time of the offense believed alcohol or drugs lowered their inhibitions, resulting in violence against their partner. These women used substances as an excuse to be physically aggressive with their partners during conflict rather than being passive.

Integrative Conceptual Framework

The results of the current study suggest that a single model or way of looking at IPV is not sufficient. Researchers, clinicians, and theorists need to adopt an integrative conceptual framework when examining IPV, one that includes trauma theory, the intergenerational transmission of violence, gender roles, and sociocultural factors. According to the women interviewed, they felt that they exerted the power and control in the relationship and viewed their partner as weaker than them. Most of the women interviewed had a significant history of trauma and victimization from either a past partner or in their childhood. They had felt powerless on many occasions, whether it was through the murder of their mother by their stepfather or through long-term sexual abuse. These women made a conscious decision not to be victims again and defeat the oppression that they experienced as children or in past relationships.

Treatment Recommendations

The findings of the current study suggest that women who are classified as dominant aggressors of IPV have unique needs that should be addressed during treatment. Effective treatment for these women may focus on providing a balance of power and control within their intimate relationships and teaching the women to become aware of how they abuse their power when they become violent. Therefore it is very important that treatment programs assess an individual's history of trauma for both male and female offenders and address symptoms of trauma in the treatment. These women clearly experience a disconnect between their thoughts, feelings, and actions and resort to physical aggression when emotionally overwhelmed. A treatment program that teaches women to identify their emotions and appropriate ways of sharing them with their partners is strongly recommended (Goldenson, Spidel, Greaves, & Dutton, 2009).

CONCLUSION

It is proposed that a conceptual framework of domestic violence combining our understanding of trauma theory, the intergenerational transmission of violence, gender role identification, and sociocultural factors will provide a more accurate understanding of women who are dominant aggressors of physical violence in their intimate relationships. Thus a bioecological or biopsychosocial framework is likely more helpful in dealing with these complex issues and situations. According to the bioecological model of human development, an individual's behavior results from interactions with various systems that interrelate and affect one another. These subsystems include the individual system, family system, sociostructural system, and the sociocultural system (Bronfenbrenner, 1979).

Similarly, a biopsychosocial model includes components of biology, cognitions, and sociocultural factors (Rosenbaum, Geffner, & Benjamin, 1997). Application of either the bioecological or biopsychosocial models to female offenders of IPV allows for an understanding of both the individual and how that particular individual interacts with her environment (Carlson, 1984; Rosenbaum et al., 1997). Given the complex histories and motivations of women in the present study, the importance of an interactive, multidimensional model of human understanding is essential. The current research has provided preliminary, qualitative data on this topic, but more research is warranted. Determining the characteristics, motivations, and perceptions of women who are dominant aggressors of IPV is an essential component for effective treatment and prevention efforts for this population.

This article has indicated that, for the most part, women who are classified as dominant aggressors share a variety of traits, motivations for violence, and familial factors that play a role in their violence. Many of these women possess personality characteristics that make them particularly prone to violence across a variety of situations. It is important to note that most of these women did not view themselves as physically violent, although they had been physically violent with various individuals across a variety of situations. All of the women felt justified in their use of violence and aggression, whether it was because of their partner's emotional abuse or a desire to get their partner's attention. They all viewed their violence and aggression as distinct incidents rather than part of a general trend, although their history clearly indicated otherwise. It is interesting to note that much of the above self-descriptions are similar to what is stated by male IPV offenders (MacLaurin, 2007).

In a qualitative study such as this one, a statistical relationship cannot be drawn between women who can be classified as dominant aggressors in their intimate relationships and factors associated with their use of violence. In addition, the current study does not allow the researcher to compare these participants with other women who have used violence in their intimate relationships, particularly those who are in relationships that are consistently bidirectionally violent and women who use violence in self-defense. However, inferences can be made based on the shared experiences of the participants. The findings indicate that a multifaceted mix of personal characteristics, historical factors, perceptions of others' behavior, and an understanding of oneself combine to create women who are particularly prone to resorting to violence in their intimate relationships.

REFERENCES

Bem, S. L. (1974). The measurement of psychological androgyny. *Journal of Consulting and Clinical Psychology, 42*(2), 155–162.

Bem, S. L. (1981). *Bem Sex Role Inventory manual.* Redwood City, CA: Consulting Psychologists Press.

Bernhard, L. A. (2000). Physical and sexual violence experienced by lesbian and heterosexual women. *Violence Against Women, 6*(1), 68–79.

Briere, J. (2001). *Detailed Assessment of Posttraumatic Stress (DAPS).* Odessa, FL: Psychological Assessment Resources.

Bronfenbrenner, U. (1979). *The ecology of human development: Experiments by nature and design.* Cambridge, MA: Harvard University Press.

Caetano, R., Schafer, J., & Cunradi, C. B. (2001). Alcohol-related intimate partner violence among white, black, and Hispanic couples in the United States. *Alcohol Research and Health, 25*(1), 58–65.

Campbell, C. S., Mackenzie, D. L, & Robinson, J. W. (1987). Female offenders: Criminal behavior and gender-role identity. *Psychological Reports, 60,* 867–873.

Carlson, B. (1984). Causes and maintenance of domestic violence: An ecological analysis. *Social Service Review, 58,* 569–587.

Chemtob, C. M., Hamada, R. S., Roitblat, H. L., & Muraoka, M. Y. (1994). Anger, impulsivity and anger control in combat related posttraumatic stress disorder. *Journal of Consulting and Clinical Psychology, 62*(4), 827–832.

Dutton, D. G. (1999). Traumatic origins of intimate rage. *Aggression and Violent Behavior, 4*(4), 431–445.

Dutton, D. G., Saunders, K., Starzomski, A., & Bartholomew, K. (1994). Intimacy-anger and insecure attachment as precursors of abuse in intimate relationships. *Journal of Applied Social Psychology, 24*(15), 1367–1386.

Foshee, V. A., Bauman, K. E., & Linder, G. F. (1999). Family violence and the perpetration of adolescent dating violence: Examining social learning and social control processes. *Journal of Marriage and the Family, 61*(2), 331–342.

Goldenson, J., Spidel, A., Greaves, C., & Dutton, D. (2009). Female perpetrators of intimate partner violence: Within-group heterogeneity, related psychopathology, and a review of current treatment with recommendations for the future. *Journal of Aggression, Maltreatment, & Trauma, 18*(7), 752–769.

Huselid, R. F., & Cooper, M. L. (1994). Gender roles as mediators of sex differences in expressions of pathology. *Journal of Abnormal Psychology, 103*(4), 595–603.

Langhinrichsen-Rohling, J., Neidig, P., & Thorn, G. (1995). Violent marriages: Gender differences in levels of current violence and past abuse. *Journal of Family Violence, 19*(2), 159–176.

MacLaurin, J. L. (1997). *Understanding repeat offenders and barriers to change: Treatment implications for domestic violence intervention programs.* Unpublished doctoral dissertation. California School of Professional Psychology, Alliant International University, San Diego, CA.

Marshall, L. L., & Rose, P. (1988). Family of origin violence and courtship aggression. *Journal of Counseling and Development, 66,* 414–418.

Maykut, P., & Morehouse, R. (1994). *Beginning qualitative research: A philosophic and practice guide.* London: Routledge.

Moffitt, T. E., & Caspi, A. (1999). Findings about partner violence from the Dunedin Multidisciplinary Health and Development Study. In *National Institute of Justice: Research in brief* (pp. 1–12). Washington, DC: National Institute of Justice. Accessed February 10, 2009, from www.ncjrs.gov/pdffiles1/170018.pdf.

Rosenbaum, A., Geffner, R., & Benjamin, S. (1997). A biopsychosocial model for understanding relationship aggression. *Journal of Aggression, Maltreatment, & Trauma, 1*, 57–79.

Scott, R. I., & Day, H. D. (1996). Association of abuse-related symptoms and style of anger expression for female survivors of childhood incest. *Journal of Interpersonal Violence, 11*(2), 208–220.

Selzer, M. L. (1971). The Michigan Alcohol Screening Test: The quest for a new diagnostic instrument. *American Journal of Psychiatry, 127*(12), 89–94.

Skinner, H. A. (1983). The drug abuse screening test. *Addictive Behaviors, 7*(4), 363–371.

Straus, M. A., & Ramirez, I. L. (1999, November). *Criminal history and assault of dating partners: The role of gender, age of onset, and type of crime.* Paper presented at the American Society of Criminology Annual Meeting, Toronto, Ontario, Canada.

Stuart, G. L., Moore, T. M., Ramsey, S. E., & Kahler, C. W. (2003). Relationship aggression and substance use among women court-referred to domestic violence intervention programs. *Addictive Behaviors, 28*(9), 1603–1610.

Sullivan, T. P., Cavanaugh, C. E., Ufner, M. J., Swan, S. C., & Snow, D. L. (2009). Relationships among women's use of aggression, their victimization, and substance use problems: A test of the moderating effects of race/ethnicity. *Journal of Aggression, Maltreatment, & Trauma, 18*(6), 646–666.

Swan, S. C., & Snow, D. L. (2002). A typology of women's use of violence in intimate relationships. *Violence Against Women, 8*(3), 286–319.

Swan, S. C., & Snow, D. L. (2003). Behavioral and psychological differences among abused women who use violence in intimate relationships. *Violence Against Women, 9*(1), 75–109.

Thompson, E. H. (1991). The maleness of violence in dating relationships: An appraisal of stereotypes. *Sex Roles, 24*(5/6), 261–278.

Tontodonato, P., & Crew, B. K. (1992). Dating violence, social learning theory, and gender: A multivariate analysis. *Violence and Victims, 7*, 3–14.

Widom, C. S. (1989). Does violence beget violence? A critical examination of the literature. *Psychological Bulletin, 106*(1), 3–28.

What Will Happen if I Punch Him? Expected Consequences of Female Violence Against Male Dating Partners

PENNY A. LEISRING

Quinnipiac University, Hamden, Connecticut, USA

Women's use of physical violence within college dating relationships is common, yet we know far less about aggressive women than we do about aggressive men. The current study examined expected consequences of using physical aggression against dating partners among aggressive and nonaggressive college women. More than half of the women in the current study had used physical aggression against a romantic partner during an argument. Aggressive women were more likely than nonaggressive women to expect that using aggression would result in winning an argument/getting their way and were more likely to expect retaliation by a partner. Among the aggressive women, perpetrator guilt was negatively correlated with the frequency of using physical aggression. Clinical implications of this study are discussed.

Intimate partner violence (IPV) within romantic relationships is a major social problem and public health issue (Douglas & Straus, 2006; Luthra & Gidycz, 2006). Partner violence is common and has negative physical and psychological consequences for victims (Cascardi, Langhinrichsen, & Vivian, 1992). Most research on IPV has focused on married couples. However, if we are to develop early intervention programs to stop partner violence, then we need to also attend to partner violence within younger dating samples, since aggressive patterns start early on. Rates of dating violence in college relationships range from 25% to 40% when students are asked whether they have engaged in specific aggressive acts toward partners (Foo & Margolin, 1995). Studies examining rates of dating violence find that women engage in aggression nearly as often as men in dating relationships and they seem to initiate acts of aggression at higher rates (for a review, see Lewis & Fremouw, 2001). A study examining rates of violence among social science students across 16 countries found that college dating violence is even more common than marital violence (Straus, 2004). About 29% of the college students engaged in physical dating aggression in the past year and about 9.4% of college students engaged in severe physical dating violence (Straus, 2004). Female-perpetrated IPV rates were higher than male-perpetrated violence rates at 21 of the 31 universities in this international study.

There has been much controversy about women's use of violence in romantic relationships. Numerous studies point out that women engage in equal or higher rates of IPV compared to men (see the meta-analysis by Archer, 2000). However, it is recognized that identical acts committed by women and men have very different effects on victims. A woman may be quite frightened as a result of being slapped by a male partner, while the same behavior perpetrated by a woman may not instill fear in a man. The motivation, context, and results of violence by women can be quite different than those for men. Most, but not all, aggressive women are in bidirectionally aggressive relationships (Leisring, Dowd, & Rosenbaum, 2005; Ross & Babcock, 2009; Straus & Gelles, 1990; Swan & Snow, 2002, 2006), and self-defense is often viewed as one of several motivations for women's use of aggression, along with anger, stress, jealousy, and a desire to retaliate against one's partner (Caldwell, Swan, Allen, Sullivan, & Snow, 2009; Cascardi & Vivian, 1995; Follingstad, Wright, Lloyd, & Sebastian, 1991; Foshee, Bauman, Linder, Rice, & Wilcher, 2007; Hettrich & O'Leary, 2007; Stuart et al., 2006).

Additional research examining women's use of aggression is sorely needed if we are to prevent and treat this form of partner violence. While female victims of male violence are more apt to be physically injured or to suffer psychological consequences as a result of IPV (Cascardi et al., 1992), negative consequences for male victims of IPV do exist. According to a meta-analysis, 32% of those physically injured by heterosexual partner violence are male (Archer, 2000). Male victims of IPV can also suffer from psychological sequelae like depression and stress (Hines & Douglas, 2009; Hines & Malley-Morrison, 2001). Women's use of violence may also have negative consequences for the women themselves. Longitudinal studies have found that women's use of aggression increases the likelihood that women will be victimized in the future by their male partners (Feld & Straus, 1989; Murphy & O'Leary, 1989). Women's psychological aggression has been found to predict men's future use of violence, even for couples in which the man had not previously been physically violent (Murphy & O'Leary,

1989). Straus (1993) indicated that women's use of aggression may give men the idea that aggression is acceptable within their relationship. This does not imply that women are to be blamed for their own victimization. Men are to be held responsible when they use aggression against partners. Likewise, women are being held responsible when they choose to use partner aggression. As states have implemented mandatory arrest laws for partner violence, there has been an increase in the number of women being arrested on domestic violence charges (Henning, Martinsson, & Holdford, 2009; Hirschel & Buzawa, 2002). Some of these arrested women are being court-mandated to intervention programs, and information about partner aggressive women is needed to inform such programs.

Social learning is one of the main theories used to explain IPV, especially violence committed by males. According to this theory, modeling and cognitive factors play a central role in the development and maintenance of aggressive behavior. Outcome expectations (e.g., payoffs) can affect the development and maintenance of behavior (Breslin, Riggs, O'Leary, & Arias, 1990). Breslin et al. (1990) examined actual and expected consequences for male and female college students. Aggression was followed by both positive and negative consequences. When asked to consider what might happen if they "behaved aggressively" toward a partner, aggressive individuals expected fewer negative consequences than their nonaggressive counterparts. Unfortunately, Breslin et al. (1990) combined men and women's responses, preventing the examination of gender-specific results; it is also unclear how respondents interpreted the words "behaved aggressively." In addition, the Breslin et al. (1990) study examined 53 expected consequences separately, which increased the likelihood of false-positive (i.e., Type I) errors.

Riggs and Caulfield (1997) extended the work of Breslin et al. (1990) by developing a specific measure, the Survey of Consequences to Aggression in Relationships (SCAR), to assess 15 expected consequences for three specific aggressive acts (slapping, shoving, and punching). They used a sample of college men and found that partner aggressive men were more likely to expect that using dating violence would result in winning an argument and they were less likely to expect that dating violence would result in their relationship ending. Riggs and Caulfield (1997) did not include women in their sample.

Foshee, Bauman, and Linder (1999) also examined outcome expectations for dating violence, but did so in a sample of 13- and 14-year-olds who had "been on a date" at least once. Foshee et al. (1999) created a six-item measure to assess outcome expectations for hitting a dating partner. Three positive outcomes and three negative outcomes were assessed. They provided examples of two of the items in their article: "My friends would think I was cool" (positive outcome) and "My partner would break up with me" (negative outcome). The other four outcomes assessed in the measure were not described. Results were conducted separately for each gender. For both genders, aggressive students were more likely to expect positive outcomes and less likely to expect negative outcomes than were the nonaggressive students.

The present study sought to add to the existing literature by examining expected consequences for dating violence perpetrated by college women. The purpose was to determine whether college women who use aggression against men differ in their outcome expectations from nonaggressive women. Based on previous findings with a younger sample (Foshee et al., 1999) and with college men (Riggs & Caulfield, 1997), it was hypothesized that aggressive women would expect more positive consequences for aggression (e.g., winning an argument) than would nonaggressive women.

METHOD

Participants

Participants in this study were 232 college women recruited for a study on "close relationships." Participants were recruited from 100- and 200-level psychology courses at a small, private New England university. One hundred thirteen participants were removed from the sample since, at the time of the study, they were not currently in a romantic relationship. One bisexual woman was also removed from the study, leaving a sample of 118 heterosexual women. The mean age of women in the sample was 18.8 years (SD = .8). Ninety-three percent of the sample were Caucasian, 3% were Hispanic, 2% were Asian, and 2% were of mixed race. The mean length of the longest romantic relationship reported by participants was 26 months (SD = 14 months). The mean length of the current romantic relationship reported by participants was 18 months (SD = 15 months).

Measures

REVISED CONFLICT TACTICS SCALE (CTS2)

This 78-item measure of IPV contains subscales for physical aggression, psychological aggression, sexual aggression, injuries, and negotiation (Straus, Hamby, Boney-McCoy, & Sugarman, 1996). The 12 physical aggression items from the CTS2 were of primary interest in the current study. The "mild" physical aggression items from the CTS2 are (a) threw something at your partner that could hurt, (b) twisted your partner's arm, (c) pushed or shoved your partner, (d) grabbed your partner, and (e) slapped your partner. The "severe" physical aggression items are (a) used a knife or gun on your partner, (b) punched or hit your partner with something that could hurt, (c) choked your partner, (d) slammed your partner against a wall, (e) beat up your partner, (f) burned or scalded your partner, and (g) kicked your partner.

Participants indicated how many times they had engaged in each behavior during an argument in their romantic relationships using a scale ranging from 0 times to more than 20 times. Participants also indicated how many times a partner had engaged in each behavior against them during an argument in their romantic relationships using the same scale. Dichotomous scoring of the CTS2 was used to indicate whether respondents endorsed any of the items on the physical aggression scale. Continuous scoring was used to estimate the frequency with which respondents used physical aggression in their relationships. Within the current sample, Cronbach's alpha for the continuous physical aggression scale was .85.

SURVEY OF CONSEQUENCES TO AGGRESSION IN RELATIONSHIPS (SCAR)

A slightly modified version of this survey originally created by Riggs and Caulfield (1997) was used. The SCAR contains items that assess five general areas of outcomes following partner aggressive behavior. These five areas include relationship interrupted, perpetrator wins, perpetrator guilty, partner upset, and partner retaliates. Participants were asked, "Which of the following do you think would happen if you were to shove your partner during an argument?" This was followed by a list of 15 possible consequences (see individual items in Tables 1 and 2). Respondents indicated which of the consequences they would expect to occur by placing a check next to the consequence. After the checklist, the directions and consequence list were repeated for two other aggressive acts: "Which of the following do you think would happen if you were to slap [punch] your partner?" Multiple consequences could be checked for each aggressive act. The responses

TABLE 1 Factor Structure of the Survey of Consequences to Aggression in Relationships

Item	Relationship interrupted	Perp. wins	Perp. guilty	Partner upset	Partner retaliates
Partner stops talking to you	**.80**	.01	.15	−.20	−.03
Partner breaks up	**.74**	−.17	.07	−.01	.10
Partner avoids you	**.69**	.09	.29	−.26	.15
You make up	**.60**	.07	.33	−.28	−.06
You get your way	−.06	**.89**	−.00	−.02	−.03
You win argument	−.07	**.85**	−.09	−.05	−.06
You feel guilty	.14	.05	**.81**	−.06	.09
You apologize	−.02	−.21	**.73**	.13	−.21
Partner is physically hurt	.24	.25	**.43**	−.34	.22
Partner cries	.09	.00	−.06	**−.74**	−.05
Partner becomes depressed	.13	.00	.26	**−.72**	−.10
Partner calls police/campus security	−.09	.24	−.33	**−.58**	.23
Partner hits you	−.22	.14	−.13	−.05	**.66**
Partner yells at you	.30	−.06	.31	−.01	**.66**
Argument stops	−.20	.31	.22	−.25	**−.58**

Note: Bold figures indicate the factor summary score on which the item was included.

TABLE 2 Percentage of Women Expecting Various Consequences for Their Use of Aggression

Consequence	Entire sample N = 118	Aggressive N = 60	Nonaggressive N = 58
You apologize	98.3	98.3	98.3
You feel guilty	95.8	95	96.6
Partner yells at you	71.2	81.7	60.3
Partner stops talking to you	71.2	70	72.4
You make up	61.9	60	63.8
Partner avoids you	58.5	55	62.1
Partner is physically hurt	42.4	45	39.7
The argument would stop	36.4	28.3	44.8
Partner breaks up	34.7	33.3	36.2
Partner becomes depressed	24.6	25	24.1
Partner cries	12.7	16.7	8.6
You get your way	7.6	15	0
Partner hits you	5.9	10	1.7
You win argument	3.4	5	1.7
Partner calls police/campus security	2.5	3.3	1.7

Note: Numbers are percentages of women that expected each consequence for any of the aggressive acts (shove, slap, punch) on the SCAR.

were summed across the three aggressive behaviors so that each of the 15 consequences received a score ranging from 0 (expected consequence for none of the aggressive behaviors) to 3 (expected consequence for all of the aggressive behaviors). Note that the "partner would call the police" item from the original SCAR was changed in the current study to "partner would call the police or campus security." This was the only modification made to the original survey.

Procedure

Participants completed questionnaires on as voluntary basis during their regularly scheduled psychology class period. Questionnaires were completed anonymously and participation was uncompensated. Participants received a consent form to keep that described the study, its risks and benefits, the participants' rights as human subjects, and a phone number for the university counseling center in case they wanted to discuss any emotional discomfort with a trained counselor.

RESULTS

Prevalence of Dating Aggression

Fifty-one percent of the women reported having used physical aggression against a dating partner at least once during their romantic relationships. Of these aggressive women, 70% had used physical aggression more than twice against a partner and 32% had engaged in severe aggression as defined by the CTS2. Of the aggressive women, 77% reported that they had been physically aggressed against by a dating partner during their romantic relationships.

Factor Analysis of the SCAR

A principal-components factor analysis with oblique rotation was conducted on the responses to the SCAR. Oblique rotation was used because it was anticipated that consequence scores would be correlated (Tabachnick & Fidell, 2001) and to be consistent with the rotation used by Riggs and Caulfield (1997). Five expected consequence factors were extracted from the 15 items. All five factors had eigenvalues greater than 1 and a five-factor solution was consistent with a scree test. Thus a five-factor model was used. The factors accounted for 60% of the variance in the items (see Table 1). The five factors were labeled (a) Relationship Interrupted, (b) Perpetrator Wins, (c) Perpetrator Guilty, (d) Partner Upset, and (e) Partner Retaliates. Summary scores were derived for each of the five factors. Each item was included only in the summary score for the factor on which it loaded most heavily (see Table 1). Summary scores for Relationship Interrupted and Partner Retaliates were correlated, $r = .20, p < .05$.

Expected Consequences and Dating Violence

A multivariate analysis of variance (MANOVA) was conducted comparing aggressive women ($n = 60$) to nonaggressive women ($n = 58$) on the five SCAR summary scores. Results indicated a significant group difference, $F(5, 112) = 4.49, p < .01$. Follow-up univariate analysis of variance indicated that aggressive women had higher Perpetrator Wins, $F(1, 116) = 5.75$, $p < .05$, and Partner Retaliates scores, $F(1, 116) = 8.71, p < .01$, compared to nonaggressive women. Correlations were conducted within the aggressive women group ($n = 60$) to determine if the SCAR factor scores correlated with the frequency of aggression perpetrated by women. Results revealed that the frequency with which the aggressive women used violence was negatively correlated with Perpetrator Guilt, $r = -.34, p < .01$.

Prevalence of Expected Consequences

Frequencies were conducted to illustrate the percentage of women who expected the 15 SCAR consequences for any of the three hypothetical acts of aggression (shove, slap, punch). Frequencies were conducted for the overall sample and then again separately for aggressive and nonaggressive women. The frequencies for each expected consequence can be seen in Table 2. Women's most commonly expected consequences for their use of aggression were the following items: you apologize, you feel guilty, partner yells at you, partner stops talking to you, you make up, partner avoids you, and partner is physically hurt.

DISCUSSION

Expectations for positive consequences do seem to play a role in the use of violence for college women. Aggressive women were more likely to report believing that aggression would result in the women getting their way/winning an argument than nonaggressive women. This is consistent with findings that some women engage in instrumental aggression (Babcock, Miller, & Siard, 2003; Johnson, 2006; Swan & Snow, 2002). Similar findings were found for aggressive college males in the Riggs and Caulfield (1997) study and for younger aggressive males and females in the Foshee et al. (1999) study. Thus evidence is accumulating that suggests that women and men may use partner aggression at times to achieve outcomes that they perceive as positive.

Aggressive women in the current sample were also more likely to expect that using violence would result in retaliation from their partner (e.g., getting hit or yelled at) than were nonaggressive women. This may reflect the actual results of previous aggressive behavior engaged in by the women. Previous research has indicated that women who use aggression are at risk for being aggressed against by their partners (Dasgupta, 1999; Feld & Straus, 1989; Murphy & O'Leary, 1989; O'Leary & Slep, 2006). While aggressive women did view retaliation as a more likely consequence than nonaggressive women, overall only 6% of women in the current study expected that their partners would hit them if they used violence. Women may be underestimating the likelihood that their partners would physically retaliate against them.

Expecting one's partner to contact the police or campus security was extremely rare in the current study (under 3% of women reported expecting this to happen). This result is in line with reports that most IPV goes unreported to authorities (Dutton, 1987) and with the fact that men are less likely than women to be injured or fearful as a result of partner violence (Cascardi et al., 1992). Nevertheless, perhaps women need to recognize that while partner aggression perpetrated by a woman is not the same as aggression by a man, both are considered criminal acts.

Forty-two percent of women thought that their partners might be physically hurt if they shoved, slapped, or punched them. This rate is actually higher than one might expect given that women are on average less strong than men. It has been suggested that women may have high approval ratings of women's use of violence since they do not expect men to be hurt by the violence (Greenblatt, 1983, as cited in Straus, 2006). The current study suggests that some women do think that they have the capability to "physically hurt" their partners despite the fact that men are typically injured less often and less severely than are female victims of IPV.

It is interesting to note that an extremely high number of women in the current study, even the aggressive women, believed that negative consequences would occur if they used violence against a partner (e.g., feeling guilty, partner yelling, partner ceasing to talk to the woman). Despite these expected negative consequences, more than half of the sample had engaged in aggression against dating partners. It is possible, however, that the beliefs about negative consequences developed as a result of actual consequences to the aggressive women's use of violence. Since the data in this study are cross-sectional, we do not know whether the beliefs preceded or followed the use of violence for the aggressive women. Positive outcome expectations for women's use of violence, though more likely to be held by aggressive women, were still uncommon for both aggressive and nonaggressive women. Not a single nonaggressive woman expected that aggression would result in her getting her way, and only 15% of the aggressive women expected this consequence. Thus, while positive outcome expectations discriminate between groups, it should be noted that many aggressive women did not hold these beliefs.

The CTS2 was used to measure aggression in the current study. This is an improvement over the use of the first version of the CTS in the Riggs and Caulfield (1997) study. The CTS2 is more comprehensive in its approach and has 12 items to measure physical aggression, compared to 7 items on the previous version. Critics of the CTS2 and the CTS, however, point out that by simply counting whether acts occur or not does not provide meaningful context for the aggression (Dekeserdy, 2006). The use of the CTS2 in the present study, however, is justified in that the author was primarily interested in dividing the sample into two groups based on whether any acts of aggression had been perpetrated by the respondent. Furthermore, some limited context of women's aggression was yielded with the CTS2 by investigating the percentage of aggressive women who had also been victimized by partners (77%) and by examining what percentage of women had used violence against a partner three or more times (70%).

The five labels given to the SCAR factors from the factor analysis were identical to those used in the Riggs and Caulfield (1997) study with male college students, but the structure of the factors differed slightly in the current study. Factor structure was examined since women were not included in the original sample when the SCAR was developed. Four of the 15 items loaded on different factors in this study compared with the Riggs and Caulfield (1997) study. It should be pointed out that both studies only examined expected consequences of aggression that were contained on the

SCAR. It is quite possible, and likely, that other unmeasured consequences for women's aggression exist. For example, it is possible that using aggression against one's partner could negatively impact one's sense of dignity and integrity.

A limitation of the current study was the lack of diversity among the participants. Future research should use samples with more respondents from underrepresented groups. Another issue to note in the current sample is that the women were involved in somewhat lengthy romantic relationships. The mean length of the women's current relationship was 18 months. It is possible that expected consequences for IPV could differ depending on how new or established the romantic relationships are. It is possible, for example, that women might be more likely to expect that violence would lead to a breakup in a less established relationship.

The rate at which women in the current study reported using violence (51%) is somewhat higher than we would expect given the findings of other studies (e.g., Straus, 2004), but this study differed from others in some critical ways. First, the current study asked women to report about whether they had engaged in the physical aggression items within their romantic relationships and they were not asked only about aggression within the past 12 months. Also, analyses were conducted only on women who reported that they were currently in a dating relationship. It is possible that by doing this, the rate of aggression was inflated since those who have never dated (and thus could not have aggressed against a dating partner) were removed from the sample.

The rates of partner aggression within dating samples across studies are alarming. Prevention and intervention efforts that target both men's and women's use of aggression should be more widespread. Results from interventions targeting male batterers are extremely discouraging (see Babcock, Green, & Robie, 2004). We do not yet know whether we will be any more successful at helping women to cease their own use of violence in relationships. It has been suggested previously that aggressive women should be taught to consider the consequences of their actions (Leisring, Dowd, & Rosenbaum, 2003). While some of the short-term consequences of using aggression may be perceived as positive (e.g., getting one's way and winning an argument), emphasis should be placed on the numerous possible negative costs of being violent (e.g., physical retaliation by one's partner, relationship strain or loss, guilt, stress, violation of one's dignity and integrity, and negative physical and psychological effects for one's partner). Also, since beliefs about getting one's way/winning an argument differ for aggressive and non-aggressive women, perhaps we need to teach college students nonviolent methods for getting their way/arguing. Communication and assertiveness skills are likely warranted.

Guilt was negatively correlated with the frequency with which the aggressive women used violence in the current study. In addition, almost all of the women indicated that they would feel guilty for using at least one of the violent acts on the SCAR. However, approval ratings for women's use of violence from other studies are quite high (see Douglas & Straus, 2006). It is unclear at this time how to reconcile these findings. Prevention and intervention efforts should emphasize that using violence against one's partner is morally unacceptable for both men and women. Feelings of guilt after engaging in aggression are appropriate unless the aggression was used to protect oneself or someone else from imminent harm.

The percentage of college women expecting specific consequences for their use of partner aggression has not previously been reported and this information adds to the existing empirical literature regarding women's use of violence. Findings from the current study suggest that expected consequences of aggression are important to attend to in our theoretical models of dating violence. Understanding the factors that contribute to partner aggression perpetrated by women will likely help us to decrease this type of aggression.

REFERENCES

Archer, J. (2000). Sex differences in aggression between heterosexual partners: A metaanalytic review. *Psychological Bulletin, 126*(5), 651–680.

Babcock, J. C., Green, C. E., & Robie, C. (2004). Does batterers' treatment work? A meta-analytic review of domestic violence treatment. *Clinical Psychology Review, 23*(8), 1023–1053.

Babcock, J. C., Miller, S. A., & Siard, C. (2003). Toward a typology of abusive women: Differences between partner-only and generally violent women in the use of violence. *Psychology of Women Quarterly, 27*, 153–161.

Breslin, F. C., Riggs, D. S., O'Leary, K. D., & Arias, I. (1990). Family precursors, expected and actual consequences of dating aggression. *Journal of Interpersonal Violence, 5*, 247–258.

Caldwell, J. E., Swan, S. C., Allen, C. T., Sullivan, T. P., & Snow, D. L. (2009). Why I hit him: Women's reasons for intimate partner violence. *Journal of Aggression, Maltreatment & Trauma, 18*(7), 672–697.

Cascardi, M., Langhinrichsen, J., & Vivian, D. (1992). Marital aggression: Impact, injury, and health correlates for husbands and wives. *Archives of Internal Medicine, 152*, 1178–1184.

Cascardi, M., & Vivian, D. (1995). Context for specific episodes of marital violence: Gender and severity of violence differences. *Journal of Family Violence, 10*(3), 265–293.

Dasgupta, S. D. (1999). Just like men? A critical view of violence by women. In M. F. Shepard & E. L. Pence (Eds.), *Coordinating community responses to domestic violence: Lessons from Duluth and beyond* (pp. 195–222). Thousand Oaks, CA: Sage.

Dekeserdy, W. S. (2006). Future directions. *Violence Against Women, 12*(11), 1978–1085.

Douglas, E. M., & Straus, M. A. (2006). Assault and injury of dating partners by university students in 19 countries and its relation to corporal punishment experiences as a child. *European Journal of Criminology, 3*(3), 293–318.

Dutton, D. (1987). The criminal justice response to wife assault. *Law and Human Behavior, 11*(3), 189–206.

Feld, S. L., & Straus, M. A. (1989). Escalation and desistance of wife assault in marriage. *Criminology, 27*, 141–161.

Follingstad, D. R., Wright, S., Lloyd, S., & Sebastian, J. A. (1991). Sex differences in motivations and effects in dating violence. *Family Relations, 40*, 51–57.

Foo, L., & Margolin, G. (1995). A multivariate investigation of dating aggression. *Journal of Family Violence, 10*, 351–377.

Foshee, V. A., Bauman, K. E., & Linder, G. F. (1999). Family violence and the perpetration of adolescent dating violence: Examining social learning and social control processes. *Journal of Marriage and the Family, 61*, 331–342.

Foshee, V. A., Bauman, K. E., Linder, G. F., Rice, J., & Wilcher, R. (2007). Typologies of adolescent dating violence. *Journal of Interpersonal Violence, 22*(5), 498–519.

Henning, K., Martinsson, R., & Holdford, R. (2009). Gender differences in risk factors for intimate partner violence recidivism. *Journal of Aggression, Maltreatment & Trauma, 18*(6), 623–645.

Hettrich, E., & O'Leary, K. D. (2007). Females' reasons for their physical aggression in dating relationships. *Journal of Interpersonal Violence, 22*(9), 1131–1143.

Hines, D. A., & Douglas, E. M. (2009). Women's use of intimate partner violence against men: Prevalence, implications, and consequences. *Journal of Aggression, Maltreatment & Trauma, 18*(6), 572–586.

Hines, D. A., & Malley-Morrison, K. (2001). Psychological effects of partner abuse against men: A neglected research area. *Psychology of Men and Masculinity, 2*(2), 75–85.

Hirschel, D., & Buzawa, E. (2002). Understanding the context of dual arrest with directions for future research. *Violence Against Women, 8*(12), 1449–1473.

Johnson, M. P. (2006). Conflict and control: Gender symmetry and asymmetry in domestic violence. *Violence Against Women, 12*(11), 1003–1018.

Leisring, P. A., Dowd, L., & Rosenbaum, A. (2003). Treatment of partner aggressive women. *Journal of Aggression, Maltreatment & Trauma, 7*, 257–277.

Leisring, P. A., Dowd, L., & Rosenbaum, A. (2005). Abuse histories and symptoms of posttraumatic stress in partner aggressive women. *Family Violence and Sexual Assault Bulletin, 21*(1), 5–12.

Lewis, S. F., & Fremouw, W. (2001). Dating violence: A critical review of the literature. *Clinical Psychology Review, 21*(1), 105–127.

Luthra, R., & Gidycz, C. A. (2006). Dating violence among college men and women: Evaluation of a theoretical model. *Journal of Interpersonal Violence, 21*(6), 717–731.

Murphy, C. M., & O'Leary, K. D. (1989). Psychological aggression predicts physical aggression in early marriage. *Journal of Consulting and Clinical Psychology, 57*, 579–582.

O'Leary, S. G., & Slep, A. M. S. (2006). Precipitants of partner aggression. *Journal of Family Psychology, 20*(2), 344–347.

Riggs, D. S., & Caulfield, M. B. (1997). Expected consequences of male violence against their female dating partners. *Journal of Interpersonal Violence, 12*(2), 229–240.

Ross, J. M., & Babcock, J. C. (2009). Gender differences in partner violence in context: Deconstructing Johnson's (2001) control-based typology of violent couples. *Journal of Aggression, Maltreatment & Trauma, 18*(6), 604–622.

Straus, M. A. (1993). Physical assaults by wives: A major social problem. In R. J. Gelles & D. R. Loseke (Eds.), *Current controversies on family violence* (pp. 67–87). Newbury Park, CA: Sage.

Straus, M. A. (2004). Prevalence of violence against dating partners by male and female university students worldwide. *Violence Against Women, 10*(7), 790–811.

Straus, M. A. (2006). Future research on gender symmetry in physical assaults on partners. *Violence Against Women, 12*(11), 1086–1097.

Straus, M. A., & Gelles, R. J. (1990). How violent are American families? In M. A. Straus & R. J. Gelles (Eds.), *Physical violence in American families: Risk factors and adaptations to violence in 8,145 families* (pp. 95–112). New Brunswick, NJ: Transaction Publishers.

Straus, M. A., Hamby, S. L., Boney-McCoy, S., & Sugarman, D. B. (1996). The revised conflict tactics scale (CTS2): Development and preliminary psychometric data. *Journal of Family Issues, 17*, 283–316.

Stuart, G. L., Moore, T. M., Gordon, K. C., Hellmuth, J. C., Ramsey, S. E., & Kahler, C. W. (2006). Reasons for intimate partner violence perpetration among arrested women. *Violence Against Women, 12*(7), 609–621.

Swan, S. C., & Snow, D. L. (2002). A typology of women's use of aggression in intimate relationships. *Violence Against Women, 8*(3), 286–319.

Swan, S. C., & Snow, D. L. (2006). The development of a theory of women's use of violence in intimate relationships. *Violence Against Women, 12*(11), 1026–1045.

Tabachnick, B. G. & Fidell, L. S. (2001). *Using multivariate statistics* (4th ed.). Boston: Allyn & Bacon.

TREATMENT IMPLICATIONS AND APPROACHES FOR FEMALE OFFENDERS OF INTIMATE PARTNER VIOLENCE

Female Perpetrators of Intimate Partner Violence: Within-Group Heterogeneity, Related Psychopathology, and a Review of Current Treatment with Recommendations for the Future

JULIE GOLDENSON

Forensic Psychiatric Services Commission, Toronto, Ontario, Canada

ALICIA SPIDEL

University of British Columbia, Vancouver, British Columbia, Canada

CAROLINE GREAVES

Simon Fraser University, Vancouver, British Columbia, Canada

DONALD DUTTON

University of British Columbia, Vancouver, British Columbia, Canada

Female perpetrators of intimate partner violence (IPV) are now beginning to receive some scholarly attention both in Canada and the United States, particularly with zero tolerance policies and the increasing number of female arrestees. This article reviews research on the relative prevalence of IPV (comparing males and females) and the context and motivation for perpetration and female perpetrators' general psychopathology (e.g., their attachment issues, trauma experiences, and personality organization). We not only examine intergroup comparisons between women and men, but also highlight some of the intragroup heterogeneity within female perpetrators of the IPV population. The aim of this review is also to describe some of current treatment approaches and provide recommendations for the future.

Despite widely held beliefs about females traditionally being victims of intimate partner violence (IPV), an increasing number of studies have reported that females perpetrate IPV at rates similar to males (for a review, see Dutton, Nicholls, & Spidel, 2005). For the most part, these findings are fairly consistent regardless of the nature of the romantic relationship (dating, cohabiting, or married). There is also some research suggesting that across genders there is a similar breakdown in terms of the types of perpetrators (those people who are the dominant aggressors, mutually/bidirectionally violent, or predominantly victims; Dutton et al., 2005). These studies, paired with mandatory arrest policies across Canada and the United States, have led to some urgency with regard to further investigations of possible similarities and differences between female and male perpetrators of IPV, with the aim of tailoring appropriate treatment. The review that follows highlights some of the findings on the prevalence of female-perpetrated IPV, the context and motivation for women's use of violence, the characteristics and psychopathology of these women, current treatment, and recommendations to help inform the development of future treatment strategies.

PREVALENCE RATES, CONTEXT, AND MOTIVATION

Admittedly, the prevalence of domestic violence can be difficult to gauge, as it is often a private event (i.e., occurring within the home). Nonetheless, studies of prevalence have typically demonstrated that irrespective of the population examined (e.g., university undergraduates, the general population, or people in court-ordered treatment), there have been relatively high rates of IPV perpetration not only among males, but also among females. A study completed more than two decades ago by Bernard and Bernard (1983) served to highlight the extent to which females perpetrated IPV. These researchers examined 168 male and 293 female undergraduate students and found similar rates of perpetration and victimization across genders. Overall, 30% of the students reported having either perpetrated against or having been victimized by their respective partners. Specifically regarding perpetration, 15% of the men reported that they had abused a partner, compared to 21% of the women.

More recently, Nicholls, Desmarais, Spidel, and Koch (2004) compared the prevalence and nature of victimization and abuse in a sample of undergraduate males and females from a Canadian university. Results evidenced no gender differences in the perpetration of abuse. Notable in this study was that both genders reported similar rates of victimization with regard to psychological abuse (women = 78.8%; men = 69.2%); physical abuse (women = 26.9%; men = 23.1%); and sexual coercion (women = 42.3%; men = 46.2%). Nicholls et al. (2004) found that the most severe abuse (i.e., psychological, physical, sexual coercion, any injury, and severe injury) was experienced more often by women than men.

Although the studies cited thus far were conducted with undergraduate samples, research utilizing community samples of people in married or cohabiting relationships have also yielded findings suggestive of similar rates of abuse perpetrated by males and females. In fact, Archer's (2000, 2002) meta-analytic study of gender and violence concluded that females in all types of relationships, including married or cohabiting relationships, were somewhat more violent than males. In addition, Kwong, Bartholomew, and Dutton (1999) found that men and women in marital relationships reported similar rates of violence.

While these research findings certainly suggest the possibility of gender symmetry in the commission of IPV, it is important to note that criminal databases estimate that 10 times the number of women are victims of domestic violence as compared to men (Babcock, Miller, & Siard, 2003). These divergent findings may be due to the fact that fewer female-perpetrated assaults come to police attention in comparison with male-perpetrated assaults. Another consideration when examining research findings has to do with a widely used measure of violence—the Conflict Tactics Scale (CTS; see Straus, 1996)—about which there has been lively debate. While the CTS has been revised (CTS2; Straus, 1996) in an attempt to include items measuring sexual violence and consequences of violent behavior (i.e., injury/physical outcome items), some researchers argue that the CTS2 still does not fully remedy many of the initial problems, including establishing the context and motivation for the violent acts (DeKeseredy & Schwartz, 1998).

Despite controversies over prevalence and measurement limitations, it is clear that women are responsible for committing IPV, and several studies have reported that not only are women often the partner who initiate these incidents, but they also do so for reasons other than self-defense. Bland and Orn (1986), for example, reported that as many as 73.4% of women who used violence against their husbands stated that they had used violence first. Stets and Straus (1992) reported that 52.7% of the women in their sample initiated IPV. Similar proportions were also found among college students in dating relationships (Fiebert & Gonzalez, 1997).

In some of the cases in which women initiated violence, it seems they did so toward partners who were never abusive. Using data from a U.S.

national survey, Stets and Straus (1990) reported that females were three times more likely than males to perpetrate severe violence against a nonviolent partner. More specifically, these researchers found that 9.6% of the women in married relationships and 13.4% of the women in cohabiting couples reported being the sole perpetrators of IPV in their relationships. In contrast, these researchers found that only 2.4% and 1.2% of men in married and cohabitating relationships, respectively, reported being exclusively responsible for IPV. Lewis, Travea, and Fremouw (2002) examined female perpetration of violence in dating relationships utilizing a sample of 300 undergraduate women, reporting that 7% of the women were the sole perpetrators of abuse and that 16% of the women engaged in bidirectional violence (i.e., they both perpetrated and were the victims of violence). More recently, Goldenson, Geffner, Foster, and Clipson (2007) completed a study comparing 33 women who were in court-mandated domestic violence group treatment with a clinical control group of 32 women who had not perpetrated domestic violence but were receiving psychological treatment. They found that 24% of the women in court-mandated treatment were the dominant aggressors (this was operationalized as women who primarily initiated violence for reasons other than self-defense); 55% of the women were involved in bidirectional aggression (i.e., both the women and their respective partners were equally responsible for violence in the relation-ship); and 21% reported being largely the victims of violence. Research on the prevalence of IPV in lesbian relationships (Bernhard, 2000) also seems to raise doubt about earlier propositions regarding women largely being the victims of violence or using violence exclusively for self-defense.

While there remains a paucity of literature on this subject, women's motives for perpetrating IPV, including but certainly not limited to self-protection, are increasingly the subject of empirical attention. Follingstad, Wright, Lloyd, and Sebastian (1991) found that a greater number of women than men reported using aggression to feel powerful (3.4% vs. 0%), to establish a sense of perceived control over their partner (22.0% vs. 8.3%), or to punish their partner for "wrong behavior" (16.9% vs. 12.5%). Further-more, they found no significant difference in the percentage of men (17.7%) and women (18.6%) who endorsed using aggression for the purpose of self-defense. In their contribution to furthering the understanding of motivation, Fiebert and Gonzalez (1997) reported that a proportion of women in their study used violence or abusive tactics to gain attention from their partners.

As will be reviewed in more detail below, Babcock et al. (2003) and Ross and Babcock (2009) were one of the few research teams that specifi-cally investigated subtypes of female perpetrators of domestic violence and their respective motivations for IPV. These researchers found that generally violent (GV) women or those women who behaved violently both within and outside the context of their romantic relationships were more likely to report motivations for violence, including but not limited to a desire to "push their partner's buttons," "give partner what he/she deserved," or due to "feeling frustrated/losing control." In contrast, partner only (PO) women (i.e., women who used violence solely in the context of their romantic relationships) reported motivations that were more likely to be related to self-defense. Overall, the GV group reported using violence in a more instrumental manner as a means to control their partners. These women were also more likely to resort to using violence in response to verbal abuse or due to jealousy.

To summarize the aforementioned literature, not only are women included as perpetrators of domestic violence, but they at times may initiate such violence and may do so for a variety of motives, not limited to self-defense. Furthermore, while some women are indeed the sole victims of relational violence, there is a population of women who are the dominant aggressors (Conradi, Geffner, Hamberger, & Lawson, 2009) or who are engaged in mutually violent relationships. While not nearly as sizable as the research on male perpetrators of IPV, there is burgeoning research that is beginning to explore the specific characteristics of the female perpetrator population. Some preliminary findings on within-group differences in this population, as well as some global findings on the types of psychopathology found within the broader group of IPV perpetrators, are outlined below.

WITHIN-GROUP HETEROGENEITY

Research has been carried out that has led to the creation of typologies for male perpetrators of IPV. Holtzworth-Munroe and Stuart (1994), for example, proposed three types of male batterers: family-only, dysphoric borderline, and generally violent/antisocial. In their investigation of similar female typologies, Babcock et al. (2003) examined the context of and motivation for women's perpetration of IPV using a sample of 52 women referred to domestic violence group treatment (as noted above, the sample was divided a priori into PO aggressors and GV aggressors). Based on self-reports, GV women were more psychologically abusive, physically abusive, used more severe forms of abuse, and caused their partners more injury over the course of the past year as compared to PO women.

Swan and Snow (2002) grouped women into a typology based on dimensions of violence and levels of coercive control. They studied 108 women who had used some form of physical violence within the last 6 months. The sample was recruited from mandated domestic violence treatment programs, health clinics, family court, and women's shelters. These women were given a variety of measures that relied not only on the women's reports of their own abusive behavior, but also on their partners' reports regarding the women's use of IPV in their respective relationships.

The authors found 34% of the women met the classification as victims (i.e., when these women did use violence, it was reported to have occurred solely in the context of self-defense). The authors additionally identified 12% of the women as dominant aggressors. These individuals used more violence than their male counterparts. The women in this category committed an average of 113 abusive behaviors over the course of 6 months. Finally, 50% of the relationships were, using Swan and Snow's (2002) terminology, "mixed" (i.e., while one partner was more physically violent, the other partner was more coercive). Coercion, as defined in this study, referred to nonphysical means of exerting control; for example, using intimidation, isolation, and control over finances. Thirty-two percent of these relationships were mixed-male coercive; that is, the women used greater or equal violence as compared to their partners who were, in turn, more coercive. The remaining 18% of the relationships were mixed-female coercive, which occurred when the males' use of violence was greater or equal to their female partner's; however, the females used more coercion. While the percentages cited above show that overall there were more women identified as victims as opposed to aggressors, this could be due in part to the fact that some women were recruited from shelters. It is notable that contrary to the author's expectations, when women were the aggressors they were as physically abusive as the male perpetrators of IPV.

In 2001, Abel examined relationship characteristics of 67 women attending domestic violence treatment programs and 51 women receiving services for victims of domestic violence. Those in the former group were more often in dating relationships, whereas the women in victim intervention programs were significantly more likely to be married. Both groups reported similarly high rates of lifetime victimization, and the batterers reported more victim-related exposure (e.g., being threatened, coercive sex, etc). Despite the differing level of exposure, the female victims in Abel's (2001) study reported significantly more trauma symptomology than the female perpetrators.

To summarize the findings on heterogeneity in this population, research thus far appears to suggest that, similar to male offenders, there may be different subtypes of female offenders. For example, women who are victimized by their partners can be distinguished from women who have been identified primarily/solely as abusers. Further, women who are violent only in their intimate relationships appear to be different from women who also commit aggression in other contexts. This is consistent with conclusions drawn from the male batterer literature.

PSYCHOPATHOLOGY AMONG WOMEN WHO COMMIT IPV

Dutton (1998) reported that combinations of fearful attachment, borderline traits, and chronic trauma symptoms came together to generate what he termed an "abusive personality" in males. Recently, these factors have begun to be studied among female perpetrators of IPV.

A slowly growing body of literature is now developing around female offenders' attachment styles. Researchers have used this theory as a framework to help understand and explain the cognitive, affective, and behavioral elements of relationship distress in adult romantic relationships (Carnelley, Pietromonaco, & Jaffe, 1994; Dutton, Saunders, Starzomski, & Bartholomew, 1994). Findings suggest that individuals with an insecure attachment style typically tend to perceive their partners to be less reliable and available. While people with an insecure style may crave nurturing, they often feel less comfortable/more ambivalent about depending on their partners for support (Fraley, Waller, & Brennan, 2000). Research findings also suggest that people with attachment insecurity (particularly people with a more anxious as compared to avoidant style) experience anxiety in their romantic relationships, have a greater fear of being abandoned, have poorer emotional regulation, and in general they experience more jealousy, greater distress, and poorer communication (Kobak & Hazan, 1991).

There have been a number of studies conducted with male-only samples that have found that a substantial proportion of male domestic violence offenders suffer from insecure attachment (Dutton et al., 1994; Holtzworth-Munroe, Stuart, & Hutchinson, 1997). While studies focusing exclusively on female perpetrators of domestic violence have been fewer in number, many have also found a predominance of attachment insecurity in this population (Carney & Buttell, 2005; Goldenson et al., 2007; Orcutt, Garcia, & Pickett, 2005). Of note, Orcutt et al. (2005) found that bidirectionally violent women (those who were both perpetrators and victims of domestic-violence) reported the highest levels of attachment anxiety. Further, females who reported high attachment anxiety subscale scores and low attachment avoidance subscale scores were more likely to report perpetrating violence than females with high scores on both subscales. This may suggest that attachment anxiety (i.e., distress over fears of abandonment, poorer emotional regulation, jealousy) may be more critical to perpetration of IPV than an avoidant attachment style. Although these findings are informative and theoretically consistent with the research on the attachment style of male perpetrators of IPV, further research is most definitely required to support this assertion.

Insecure attachment has been linked with vulnerability to a variety of psychopathologies, including borderline personality (Fonagy et al., 1996) and antisocial personality disorder (Allen, Hauser, & Borman-Spurral, 1996). It may not be surprising then that some research exists showing that Cluster B personality traits (often characterized by a persisting pattern of impulsivity, manipulation, mood lability, and unstable/volatile interpersonal relationships) have been found in both male and female perpetrators of IPV. As with most variables, there has been more research conducted with males (Beasley & Stoltenberg, 1992; Dutton et al., 1994) than their female counterparts.

A widely used measure to examine both male and female perpetrator's personality is the Millon Clinical Multiaxial Inventory (MCMI; Millon, Davis, & Millon, 1997). A number of studies conducted with male domestic violence offenders have consistently found that these men, as a group, were more elevated on particular subscales (e.g., Borderline, Antisocial, Narcissistic, Passive-Aggressive, Aggressive/Sadistic) compared to nonoffending control groups (Beasley & Stoltenberg, 1992; Dutton & Starzomski, 1994).

Emergent research on female-perpetrated IPV also seems to suggest a common pattern of personality-related psychopathology concerning the women involved (Goldenson et al., 2007; Orcutt et al., 2005; Simmons, Lehmann, Cobb, & Fowler, 2005; Stuart, Moore, Gordon, Ramsey, & Kahler, 2006). In a recent study by Goldenson et al. (2007), for example, female perpetrators of domestic violence were found to have clinically significant elevations (i.e., suggestive of the potential for a personality disorder diagnosis) on subscales that tapped into borderline, antisocial, and narcissistic traits. Most of the research on female offenders that has employed the MCMI III has found women to have elevations on multiple subscales. It is possible that any combination of the above noted and other personality features (e.g., dependent and histrionic) may be related to female-perpetrated IPV.

Another issue that has received scholarly attention in the IPV literature has been the experience of trauma. As noted above, there is a growing body of research that shows the majority of female perpetrators of IPV have themselves been victims of violence (e.g., in their family of origin, in their romantic relationships; Abel, 2001; Babcock et al., 2003; Goldenson et al., 2007; Stuart et al., 2006). Stuart et al. (2006), for example, found that 44% of their sample of female perpetrators of IPV referred to court-mandated treatment experienced symptoms of posttraumatic stress disorder (PTSD).

The psychological symptoms of trauma can include, but are not limited to, anger, intrusive experiences, and difficulty regulating emotion (American Psychiatric Association, 2000). Furthermore, the experience of IPV carries the possibility of developing traumatic brain injuries (Valera & Berenbaum, 2003). This is an area that has received virtually no scholarly attention in relation to female perpetrators of IPV; however, it is an area of clear and substantial import, as traumatic brain injuries can cause a host of neurocognitive symptoms (e.g., reduced impulse control, emotional dysregulation, lowered frustration tolerance, and problems with planning, memory, and attention; Valera & Berenbaum, 2003). Not surprisingly, given these symptoms, brain injuries have been linked to the perpetration of violence in general, and domestic violence in particular, although the extant studies have been carried out using male-only samples (e.g., Turkstra, Jones, & Toller, 2003). The possibility of brain injury in female perpetrators of IPV has largely been overlooked; however, certainly behavioral outcomes associated with traumatic brain injuries would have implications for assessment and treatment.

CURRENT PERSPECTIVES ON TREATMENT

Previously the literature was scant concerning females' role as perpetrators of IPV, and although the past few years have yielded valuable information in terms of similarities and differences within and across genders, more research is needed to refine our understanding. This need is especially prominent considering it has been and apparently remains the case that convicted female perpetrators are mandated to interventions designed for males (Carney, Buttell, & Dutton, 2007; Dowd, 2001). Remarkably, few studies to date have examined the generalizability and efficacy of programs designed for male batterers in treating females. That there is also limited outcome research on treatment with male perpetrators leaves the treatment data with females in a particularly inadequate state. Accordingly, to complete a review of what information does exist, this section will touch on some of the literature examining treatment modalities and effectiveness with male samples. A number of psychological variables for consideration in the development of treatment for females will be highlighted throughout. The few studies that have examined the effectiveness of treatment for females will be reported, which will serve to illuminate the paucity of the treatment outcome literature base in general, and with regard to females in particular.

As mentioned, the efficacy of IPV treatment has received surprisingly little scientific consideration. This neglect has likely contributed to the fact that there is no top contender as the "treatment of choice," as no known research has been able to show consistent effectiveness of one treatment strategy over another (Dutton & Sonkin, 2003). In fact, as Carney et al. (2007) very recently noted, experimental evaluations conducted on the efficacy of male batterer intervention programs show them to have little to no positive effect. Whether such interventions are appropriate for females, and are even effective for males, needs to be the focus of a great deal more empirical attention.

To date, a feminist psychoeducational approach continues to underlie the most prominent type of clinical intervention, the Duluth model (see Dutton & Sonkin, 2003). This model tends to focus on reeducation (as opposed to therapy) and it integrates cognitive-behavioral techniques (e.g., challenging rationales for violence, communication skills training) toward the development of more adaptive attitudes, improving communication proficiency, and ultimately eliminating violent behavior. The main emphasis of this approach stresses the role of patriarchal male privilege of dominance and control, and accordingly it is sometimes difficult to give merit to its application to female perpetrators. Considering what current literature points to regarding the contributions of attachment-related issues, personality, and general psychopathology and trauma, it is not completely unexpected that the Duluth approach has not been highly effective at curbing recidivism (see Healey, Smith, & O'Sullivan, 1998, as cited in Babcock, Canady, Graham, & Schart, 2006).

Much is still left to be teased apart regarding women's roles in violent conflict (i.e., context of and motivation for violence). It appears that one of the most effective treatment strategies in general may come from differentially targeting treatment based on the likely etiology of the behavior; that is, differentiating between IPV that seems largely to arise due to situational variables and relationship dynamics within dyads as compared to IPV that seems more temperamentally driven (i.e., arising more due to someone's characterological makeup; see Babcock et al., 2006).

Although no known research to date has compared the efficacy of couples' therapy in female-perpetrated situationally related violence, there is some limited but promising evidence that certain modalities of couples' therapy may be effective for treating male-perpetrated situationally related violence. For instance, partners who were attending multicouple versus individual couples' therapy had lower rates of recidivism and improved relationship satisfaction (Stith, Rosen, McCollum, & Thomsen, 2004).

While situationally aggressive perpetrators of IPV, both males and females alike, may benefit from approaches/techniques that address couple-specific issues (e.g., communication strategies and problem solving), treatment may need to be differentially targeted when treating individuals who perpetrate IPV stemming from a manifestation of their characterological makeup. As this review has illustrated, a substantial proportion of IPV perpetrators suffer from psychopathology of some form. Indeed, research suggests it is often the case that both attitudes and behavior are symptoms of deeper personality issues (Dutton & Sonkin, 2003). Even at this early stage in the investigation into female perpetrators of IPV, there is evidence to suggest that, at least to some degree, female-perpetrated IPV may stem from a similar set of factors as does that of males. Specifically we refer to attachment, personality pathology, and even childhood witnessing and experiencing abuse (see Carney et al., 2007).

Theoretical work by Dutton (1995), Sonkin and Dutton's (2003) review of the literature, and studies such as Carney and Buttell's (2005) have helped to establish attachment-related problems as a central issue in the psychological makeup of IPV perpetrators. Issues surrounding interpersonal dependency and abandonment fears appear to be particularly salient, and accordingly could be a logical treatment target. Sonkin and Dutton (2003) created a treatment model for male domestic violence offenders based on attachment theory that addresses many of these issues, and this approach may also be applicable when treating female offenders. One of their many premises is that the therapeutic alliance is vitally important to create a feeling of safety among these offenders. Their framework involves (a) helping offenders better understand the impact that their upbringing has had on their patterns of behavior in romantic relationships, and (b) teaching self-regulation during periods of attachment-related anxiety instead of the offenders' typical responses of distancing, clinging, or approach-avoidance.

Research with males has led to the suggestion that perpetrators of IPV displaying borderline features may benefit from Dialectal Behavioral Therapy (DBT; Linehan, 1993) as an element of treatment (Babcock et al., 2006). DBT is expanding into use with clinical populations that are generally difficult to treat. More specifically, DBT is being used to treat people who have multiple diagnoses (Linehan, 2000) and who may be facing problems with emotional dysregulation, substance use, and PTSD (see Waltz, 2003), all of which have been discussed in relation to perpetrators of IPV. If borderline features are as salient an issue with female perpetrators of IPV as with males (as our review would suggest), it is reasonable to assume that shame, guilt, and fears of abandonment may similarly act as precursors in female-perpetrated violence. Emotional dysregulation also features prominently in this disorder, and can emerge as maladaptive responses, especially when women encounter perceived or actual rejection or abandonment. DBT serves to target emotional dysregulation through skill development to handle difficult emotions more effectively. The DBT model assumes that the client possesses oversensitivity to emotion-provoking events and that their emotional responses will be intense, long-lasting, and difficult for the individual to regulate. Thus DBT was designed to help the client develop and generalize adaptive behaviors/skills and to address obstacles to obtaining these skills by way of a clinician team-oriented approach (see Waltz, 2003, for an overview).

Waltz (2003) drew attention to the fact that DBT (as it pertains to IPV) may not be necessary for those who are situationally or less frequently or severely aggressive, nor for those displaying minimal psychopathology. In these cases, she pointed out that more traditional forms of intervention may be more suitable, especially when the realities of limited monetary and specialized personnel resources are taken into consideration. Further, clinical trials have yet to be conducted to assess any effects of DBT on IPV. However, Koons et al. (2001) found that decreases in the expression of anger in female veterans with borderline personality disorder could be attributed to DBT, lending some promise to this mode of therapy as a treatment option. With the emergence of research examining female-perpetrated IPV in its own right, clinicians and treatment teams can now start to look to the literature for the base for developing or refining effective interventions (e.g., DBT).

Although many similarities between female and male perpetrators are becoming apparent, it is also apparent that female clients present their own unique features with clinical implications. For instance, Stuart et al. (2006) found that female court-referred perpetrators of IPV were also frequent victims of physical, psychological, and sexual abuse. As previously mentioned, these women also display elevated levels of PTSD symptoms. Arguably, then, any effective treatment strategy should include a mode to address this trauma. This may also be an important consideration in light of previous findings with male offenders that PTSD may be associated with an increased likelihood of engaging in subsequent violent acts (Pollock, 1999). Indeed, Dutton and Sonkin (2003) clearly stated that an acknowledgment of attachment, shaming, and trauma precursors to battering should become an integral part of treatment. Unfortunately, this generally does not appear to be the reality.

Clearly, empirically based and widely used manualized treatment protocols have yet to be developed for female perpetrators of IPV. That said, strides are being made toward refining our understanding of the characteristics and needs of this complex population. Burgeoning research appears to offer the potential to inform treatment strategies, especially with regard to revising treatment protocols for male batterers that have been applied to females without sufficient empirical grounding. Leisring, Dowd, and Rosenbaum (2003), for example, made six specific suggestions to modify the typical treatment components used with men for use with women. They recommend that there is a need to (a) increase emphasis on treatment group members' safety; (b) attend to women's hierarchy of needs; (c) focus on PTSD symptoms; (d) focus on conditions leading to mood stability; (e) assist women in the development of parenting skills; and (e) decrease the emphasis on power and control issues.

Clinicians' reports of experiences with female perpetrators of IPV suggest that these women's treatment needs may exceed the needs of their male counterparts and may specifically include referrals for depression, PTSD, substance use, and parenting skills (Leisring et al., 2003). While it is possible that these women have greater treatment requirements, this population's treatment prognosis may be enhanced by a number of factors. Leisring et al. (2003) referred to some potential strengths evident among this population, including their tendency to be less resistant than males in initial sessions; their greater willingness to accept responsibility for their actions; their tendency to be more supportive and helpful toward their fellow treatment group members; and finally, female perpetrators' concern for their children has been cited as a powerful motivator for change.

It is largely unknown what proportion of women receiving treatment subsequently go on to reoffend after treatment completion. While, in large part, treatment programs for female perpetrators of IPV have yet to be subjected to evaluation, there is some reason to believe that people who complete treatment reduce their use of physical force (e.g., Carney & Buttell, 2004). Further research into characteristics of female perpetrators as a whole, as well as their intragroup differences, could serve to help distinguish those women who complete versus drop out of treatment prematurely. Such an understanding of this population would serve to highlight possible areas of adjustment that could be made to the interventions to help reduce attrition and, as alluded to above, further develop and refine effective treatment strategies overall.

In sum, personality psychopathology and situational versus characterological dynamics appear to remain as substantive considerations in the current treatment modalities with male perpetrators of IPV. Recently emerging empirical studies with male IPV groups indicate that attachment and borderline personality pathology are two factors that cannot be overlooked in the development of effective treatment interventions. Indeed, these issues are now being found with female IPV groups, along with a number of additional variables (e.g., PTSD, depression, and abuse history). Although strides have been made in terms of recognizing the importance of accompanying psychological issues, there definitely appears to be a dearth of knowledge in the domain of treatment outcome overall, and this should hopefully serve to fuel further research efforts. Certainly DBT, as one of the strongest current contenders, warrants continued empirical attention.

CONCLUSIONS AND RECOMMENDATIONS

The literature review above elucidates some areas that have direct implications for treatment of female perpetrators of IPV. The research suggests that female perpetrators are likely to present a variety of issues, some of which have implications for intimate relationships (e.g., attachment) and others which are more pervasive, relating to the women's own psychopathology (e.g., trauma symptoms, personality psychopathology). Attachment-related issues, certain types of personality psychopathology (e.g., borderline features) and trauma symptomology often share a constellation of symptoms, including anger, impulsivity, and difficulty regulating emotion. Individuals with attachment-related anxiety or borderline personality disorder also tend to experience excessive distress surrounding perceived abandonment. To date, there have been some approaches to treatment that address these issues (e.g., Sonkin & Dutton, 2003).

Self-regulation appears to be an important concept in treating not only attachment-related issues, but also personality psychopathology. Because many offenders have elevations on Cluster B traits, learning to self-soothe, modulate emotion, and reduce impulsive behavior would be appropriate and important. It is also critical to recognize the difficulties in treating personality psychopathology, and would likely require rigorous ongoing therapy. As mentioned previously, one modality that has proven to be particularly effective for treating personality disorders, especially borderline personality disorder, is DBT (Linehan, 1993). Such a model is quite involved, requiring the constant monitoring and coordinated input of a treatment and consultation team. Clients with borderline personality disorder are well known in the clinical community as being among those most difficult and time consuming to treat, and DBT was developed to match and address their therapeutic needs accordingly. With the issue of limited resources in mind, Waltz (2003) made the suggestion of further adapting DBT techniques for application in a group format, but only after screening for those individuals with relevant psychopathological issues. One immediate question arising from this may be whether subtherapeutic levels (or DBT interventions versus DBT groups) will have sufficient potency to address these long-standing personality issues. Again, further treatment evaluations will be needed to assess this.

While there has been some work exploring trauma symptoms in perpetrators and victims of IPV, a relatively understudied topic among female domestic violence offenders is traumatic brain injuries. Clearly people with impaired memory functioning, difficulty planning, attention problems, and issues with emotional regulation, etc., may have different and perhaps more medically oriented/rehabilitative treatment needs than non-brain-injured clients.

Overall, the heterogeneous nature of female perpetrators of IPV appears to have growing empirical support. More specifically, research suggests that there are within-group differences regarding severity and frequency of violence and the context and motivation for this population's use of violence. While some cursory work has been done, what has yet to be explored in great detail is whether there are within-group variations in terms of other psychopathology (e.g., in personality organization, trauma, attachment, and other psychological issues). Such research would be important to inform the treatment needs of these women. While it may not be cost effective or efficient to have separate groups or to provide individually tailored therapy, it also may not be effective or even worthwhile to treat women who are predominantly victims and women who are predominantly aggressors employing the same protocol. With increased numbers of IPV arrestees, it may be more useful to tailor different groups to meet the needs of the differing types of perpetrators.

Based on what is currently known, more rigorous pretreatment psychological testing with emphasis on personality assessment, trauma symptomology, and neurocognitive impairment may be necessary in order to serve the respective needs of each perpetrator. A more formally developed assessment strategy to determine females' context and motivation for offending and their respective offender type (dominant aggressors/bidirectionally violent or predominantly victim) would also be beneficial, particularly with respect to treatment group assignment.

To conclude, empirically supported treatment of female perpetrators of IPV has yet to be developed. What research has been done suggests that one size may not fit all for this highly heterogeneous group and that these women may benefit from an intervention tailored to their specific situational and characterological needs. Clearly the review of the literature speaks to the need for further research on female perpetrators of IPV and, more specifically, a need for research regarding within-group differences. Greater strides in knowledge would also be made from a more thorough and empirical evaluation of treatment outcomes. Employing the above suggestions appears essential to the provision of effective treatment to this seemingly growing population of female arrestees.

REFERENCES

Abel, E. M. (2001). Comparing the social service utilization, exposure to violence and trauma symptomology of domestic violence female "victims" and female "batterers." *Journal of Family Violence, 16*, 401–420.

Allen, J. P., Hauser, S. T., & Borman-Spurral, E. (1996). Attachment theory as a framework for understanding sequelae of severe adolescent psychopathology: An 11-year follow-up study. *Journal of Consulting and Clinical Psychology, 64*, 254–263.

American Psychiatric Association. (2000). *Diagnostic and statistical manual of mental disorders* (Text Revision; 4th ed.). Washington, DC: Author.

Archer, J. (2000). Sex differences in aggression between heterosexual partners: A meta-analytic review. Psychological Bulletin, 126(5), 651–680.

Archer, J. (2002). Sex differences in physically aggressive acts between heterosexual partners: A meta-analytic review. Aggression and Violent Behavior, 7(4), 313–351.

Babcock, J. C., Canady, B. E., Graham, K., & Schart, L. (2006). The evolution of battering interventions: From the dark ages into the scientific age. In J. Hamel, & T. Nicholls (Eds.), *Family therapy for domestic violence: A practitioner's guide to gender-inclusive research and treatment* (pp. 215–244). New York: Springer.

Babcock, J., Miller, S., & Siard, C. (2003). Toward a typology of abusive women: Differences between partner-only and generally violent women in the use of violence. *Psychology of Women Quarterly, 27*, 151–161.

Beasley, R., & Stoltenberg, C. (1992). Personality characteristics of male spouse abusers. *Professional Psychology: Research and Practice, 23*, 310–317.

Bernard, M. L., & Bernard, J. L. (1983). Violent intimacy: The family as a model for love relationships. *Family Relations, 32*, 283–286.

Bernhard, L. A. (2000). Physical and sexual violence experienced by lesbian and heterosexual women. *Violence Against Women, 6*, 68–79.

Bland, R., & Orn, H. (1986). Family violence and psychiatric disorder. *Canadian Journal of Psychiatry, 31*, 129–137.

Carnelley, K. B., Pietromonaco, P. R., & Jaffe, K. (1994). Depression, working models of others, and relationship functioning. *Journal of Personality and Social Psychology, 66*, 127–140.

Carney, M., & Buttell, F. (2004). A multidimensional evaluation of a treatment program for female batterers: A pilot study. *Research on Social Work Practice, 14*, 249–258.

Carney, M. M., & Buttell, F. P. (2005). Exploring the relevance of attachment theory as a dependent variable in the treatment of women mandated into treatment for domestic violence offenses. *Journal of Offender Rehabilitation, 41*(4), 33–61.

Carney, M., Buttell, F., & Dutton, D. (2007). Women who perpetrate intimate partner violence: A review of the literature with recommendations for treatment. *Aggression and Violent Behavior, 12*(1), 108–115.

Conradi, L. M., Geffner, R., Hamberger, L. K., & Lawson, G. (2009). An exploratory study of women as dominant aggressors of physical violence in their intimate relationships. *Journal of Aggression, Maltreatment & Trauma, 18*(7), 718–738.

DeKeseredy, W. S., & Schwartz, M. D. (1998). *Woman abuse on campus: Results from the Canadian National Survey.* Thousand Oaks, CA: Sage.

Dowd, L. (2001). Female perpetrators of partner aggression: Relevant issues and treatment. *Journal of Aggression, Maltreatment & Trauma, 5*(2), 73–104.

Dutton, D. (1995). *The batterer: A psychological profile.* New York: Basic Books.

Dutton, D. (1998). *Violence and control in intimate relationships: The abusive personality.* New York: Guilford Press.

Dutton, D., Saunders, K., Starzomski, A., & Bartholomew, K. (1994). Intimacy, anger and insecure attachment as precursors of abuse in intimate relationships. *Journal of Applied Social Psychology, 24*(15), 1367–1386.

Dutton, D. G., & Starzomski, A. (1994). Psychological differences between court mandated and self referred wife assaulters. *Criminal Justice and Behavior, 21*(2), 203–222.

Dutton, D., & Sonkin, D. J. (2003). Introduction: Perspectives on the treatment of intimate violence. *Journal of Aggression, Maltreatment & Trauma, 7,* 1–6.

Dutton, D. G., Nicholls, T. L., & Spidel, A. (2005). Female perpetrators of intimate abuse. *Journal of Offender Rehabilitation, 41*(4), 1–31.

Fiebert, M. S., & Gonzalez, D. M. (1997). College women who initiate assaults on their male partners and the reasons offered for such behavior. *Psychological Reports, 80*(2), 583–590.

Follingstad, D. R., Wright, S., Lloyd, S., & Sebastian, J. A. (1991). Sex differences in motivations and effects in dating violence. *Family Relations, 40*(1), 51–57.

Fonagy, P., Leigh, T., Steele, M., Steele, H., Kennedy, R., Mattoon, G., et al. (1996). The relationship between attachment status, psychiatric classification and response to psychotherapy. *Journal of Consulting and Clinical Psychology, 64,* 22–31.

Fraley, R. C., Waller, N. G., & Brennan, C. L. (2000). An item response theory analysis of self report measures of adult attachment. *Journal of Personality and Social Psychology, 78,* 350–365.

Goldenson, J., Geffner, R., Foster, S., & Clipson, C. (2007). Female domestic violence offenders: Their attachment security, trauma symptoms, and personality organization. *Violence and Victims, 22*(5), 530–543.

Holtzworth-Munroe, A., & Stuart, G. L. (1994). Typologies of male batterers: Three subtypes and the differences among them. *Psychological Bulletin, 116*(3), 476–497.

Holtzworth-Munroe, A., Stuart, G., & Hutchinson, G. (1997). Violent versus nonviolent husbands: Differences in attachment patterns, dependency and jealousy. *Journal of Family Psychology, 11,* 314–331.

Kobak, R., & Hazan, C. (1991). Attachment in marriage: Effects of security and accuracy of working models. *Journal of Personality and Social Psychology, 60*, 861–869.

Koons, C. R., Robins, C. J., Tweed, J. L., Lynch, T. R., Gonzalez, A. M., Morse, J. Q., Bishop G. K. A. Y., Butterfield, M. I., & Bastian, L. A. (2001). Efficacy of dialectical behavior therapy in women veterans with borderline personality disorder. *Behaviour Therapy, 32*, 371–390.

Kwong, M. J., Bartholomew, K., & Dutton, D. G. (1999). Gender differences in patterns of relationship violence in Alberta. *Canadian Journal of Behavioural Science, 31*(3), 150–160.

Leisring, P. A., Dowd, L., & Rosenbaum, A. (2003). Treatment of partner aggressive women. *Journal of Aggression, Maltreatment & Trauma, 7*, 257–276.

Lewis, S. F., Travea, L., & Fremouw, W. J. (2002). Characteristics of female perpetrators and victims of dating violence. *Violence and Victims, 17*(5), 593–606.

Linehan, M. M. (1993). *Cognitive behavioral therapy of borderline personality disorder.* New York: Guilford Press.

Linehan, M. M. (2000). Commentary on innovations in Dialectical Behavior Therapy. *Cognitive and Behavioral Practice, 7*, 478–481.

Millon, T., Davis, R., & Millon, C. (1997). *Millon Clinical Multiaxial Inventory III* (2nd ed.). Minneapolis, MN: NCS Pearson.

Nicholls, T. L., Desmarais, S., Spidel, A., & Koch, W. (2004, March). "Common couple violence" and "intimate terrorism": A study of Johnson's typologies. Poster presented at the American Psychology–Law Society, Division 41 of APA, Scottsdale, Arizona.

Orcutt, H., Garcia, M., & Pickett, S. (2005). Female-perpetrated intimate partner violence and romantic attachment style in a college student sample. *Violence and Victims, 20*(3), 287–302.

Pollock, P. H. (1999). When the killer suffers: Post-traumatic stress reactions following homicide. *Legal and Criminological Psychology, 4*, 185–202.

Ross, J. M., & Babcock, J. C. (2009). Gender differences in partner violence in context: Deconstructing Johnson's (2001) control-based typology of violent couples. *Journal of Aggression, Maltreatment & Trauma, 18*(6), 604–622.

Simmons, C., Lehmann, P., Cobb, N., & Fowler, C. (2005). Personality profiles of women and men arrested for domestic violence: an analysis of similarities and differences. In F. Buttell & M. Carney (Eds.), *Women who perpetrate relationship violence* (pp. 63–83). New York: Haworth Press.

Sonkin, D. J., & Dutton, D. (2003). Treating assaultive men from an attachment perspective. *Journal of Aggression, Maltreatment & Trauma, 7*, 105–133.

Stets, J., & Straus, M. A. (1992). Gender differences in reporting marital violence and its medical and psychological consequences. In M. A. Straus & R. J. Gelles (Eds.), *Physical violence in American families: Risk factors and adaptations in 8,145 American families* (pp. 151–166). New Brunswick, NJ: Transaction Books.

Stith, S. M., Rosen, K. H., McCollum, E. E., & Thomsen, C. J. (2004). Treating intimate partner violence within intact couple relationships: Outcomes of multi-couple versus individual couple therapy. *Journal of Marital and Family Therapy, 30*, 305–318.

Straus, M. A. (1996). The revised Conflict Tactics Scales (CTS2). *Journal of Family Issues, 17*(3), 283–317.

Stuart, G., Moore, T., Gordon, K., Ramsey, S., & Kahler, C. (2006). Psychopathology in women arrested for domestic violence. *Journal of Interpersonal Violence, 21*, 376–389.

Swan, S. C., & Snow, D. L. (2002). A typology of women's use of violence in intimate relationships. *Violence Against Women, 8*(3), 286–319.

Turkstra, L., Jones, D., & Toller, L. (2003). Brain injury and violence. *Brain Injury, 17*(1), 39–47.

Valera, E., & Berenbaum, H. (2003). Brain injury in battered women. *Journal of Consulting and Clinical Psychology, 71*(4), 797–804.

Waltz, J. (2003). Dialectical Behavior Therapy in the treatment of abusive behavior. *Journal of Aggression, Maltreatment & Trauma, 7*, 75–103.

A Comparison of Women Who Were Mandated and Nonmandated to the "Responsible Choices for Women" Group

LESLIE M. TUTTY

University of Calgary, Calgary, Alberta, Canada

ROBBIE BABINS-WAGNER

Calgary Counselling Centre, Calgary, Alberta, Canada

MICHAEL A. ROTHERY

University of Calgary, Calgary, Alberta, Canada

Since 1995, the Calgary Counselling Centre has offered a group treatment program for women who behave abusively to intimate partners or children. This article describes the group format, the demographic characteristics of the 293 women who began the Responsible Choices for Women program based on whether they were mandated to treatment or not, and a comparison of those who completed treatment versus those who dropped out. Data from a total of 154 women found significant improvements on almost all outcome measures. Women's status as mandated or nonmandated did not affect treatment outcomes, despite the fact that the nonmandated women reported more scores in the clinical range at pretest. The clinical implications of these results are described.

The major focus in intimate partner violence (IPV) has appropriately been on male perpetrators, the most common offenders. A focus on women who have been charged with domestic assault and mandated to treatment could be seen as unnecessary and even misguided by some. However, with new dual-arrest policies common across North America, women are increasingly being charged with partner abuse and mandated to treatment. Other women seek treatment themselves for being aggressive with intimate partners or children.

We currently know little about the characteristics of aggressive women and how they might respond to treatment (Abel, 2001). To enhance this understanding, this article reviews the literature on the extent and nature of violence perpetrated by women in intimate relationships. It reports an evaluation of "Responsible Choices for Women," a group developed for women who have abused intimate partners, both male and female, or children.

IPV BY MEN AND WOMEN

Even the most vocal critics who argue that the abuse of men is not a significant social issue (e.g., DeKeseredy, 1993) do not deny that some men are abused by women partners. The existence of such abuse is not at issue; the debate is with respect to how commonly it occurs and the degree of harm that results. Numerous studies worldwide, many of which used a sociological measure (the Conflict Tactics Scales [CTS]; Straus, 1979), repeatedly conclude that similar proportions of women use violence against male partners as men do against women (i.e., Lupri & Grandin, 2004). The concept of equally perpetrated violence is known as "gender symmetry" (Belnap & Melton, 2005). The debate about whether men are equally abused as women is perhaps the most contentious in the field of IPV (Osthoff, 2002; Sarantakos, 2004; Saunders, 2002; Straus, 2009; Tutty, 1999).

In the latest Canadian national study on IPV, the 2004 General Social Survey on Victimization (Statistics Canada, 2005), men reported being victimized by women in the past 5 years to a similar degree as women have been victimized by men (an estimated 7% of Canadian women and 6% of men). However, this survey, which also uses CTS-like questions, added important queries about the context and consequences of the violent acts (Johnson, 2006). Looking at the responses to these items, it becomes clear that abuse against women by male partners is more often repetitive and life threatening, with 44% of women reporting being injured, more than twice as many as the men reporting injuries (19%).

Hamberger and Guse (2002), Osthoff (2002), and others have questioned the validity of the interpretation of the community CTS survey studies that women are "equally" as violent as men. They suggest looking beyond studies in which one literally "counts hits" to understanding the complexities of abuse in intimate relationships. These criticisms do not deny that women use violent tactics, but suggest that the results of at least some female violence need to be perceived differently and is less likely to have the same serious consequences as that used by men. For example, even where partners are "mutually" violent, women are often defending themselves from attack and are significantly more likely to be injured than men (Stets & Straus, 1990).

Kimmel (2002) added other reasons why the national incidence studies using the CTS overestimate the extent of male victimization. First, the CTS questions are couched in a framework of dealing with marital conflict; thus the violence is presented as in response to an argument, an "expressive" reaction. In contrast to expressive or reactive violence, such as heated responses to marital arguments, violence can be "instrumental" (Cornell et al., 1996). Instrumental violence is intentional, goal oriented, and used to control, and while it may occur during marital spats, it also is used outside of this context. This distinction has been used primarily in looking at criminal offenders for crimes other than domestic assaults, but may prove invaluable to IPV research.

Kimmel (2002) likened the two types of violence to Johnson's (1995) distinction between common couple violence (expressive or reactive violence that occurs relatively commonly and involves less severe acts of violence, such as pushing and shoving) and Johnson's terms "patriarchal terrorism," which includes not only control through physical violence, but "economic subordination, threats, isolation, and other control tactics" (p. 284). Instrumental violence need not occur often. A beating that occurred several years ago need only be threatened again to control the behavior of one's partner. According to Kimmel, a second reason that the CTS studies overestimate male abuse is that the first version of the CTS (used in most studies) does not include questions about sexual assault, an important component of woman abuse.

With a clear understanding of the difficulties presented when interpreting the CTS studies, Belnap and Melton (2005) conducted a thorough review of the gendered nature of IPV, concluding that perhaps 5% of cases represented woman-to-man violence. Dasgupta (2002) and Hamberger (1997) provided a compelling rationale for concluding that many women who behave aggressively to their male partners are themselves abused. Across studies, about eight times more cases of woman abuse come to the attention of authorities than the opposite. For example, Canadian police statistics note that 84% of reported spousal abuse cases involve women victims, while 16% of cases involve men (Ogrodnik, 2007). Similar patterns of differences in the abusive behaviors of men and women were found in Melton and Belknap's (2003) study of a large sample of domestic violence cases in the United States.

This distinction between violence against male partners and violence against female partners is not made to obscure or ignore the suffering of male victims of abuse, but to address the claims of those who would argue that women have been unfairly provided with services and societal support, ignoring men's requests for help. While the nature of the abusive behaviors of men compared to women seems conceptually different, no abuse should be tolerated.

THE CRIMINAL JUSTICE RESPONSE TO WOMEN CHARGED WITH DOMESTIC ASSAULTS

With new criminal justice approaches to domestic violence aimed at taking these offenses more seriously, a new population of women charged with domestic violence offenses has created the need to offer counseling for those mandated to treatment. Nevertheless, researchers and community professionals have become increasingly concerned about the numbers of dual arrests (or cross-charging) that have recently been documented (Frye, Haviland, & Rajah, 2007). A dual arrest (or cross-charge) is when both individuals involved in a domestic violence incident are arrested.

Some researchers have conceptualized dual arrests as a negative side effect of the proarrest laws that were meant to protect women (Finn, Sims Blackwell, Stalans, Studdard, & Dugan, 2004; Osthoff, 2002). In Canada, dual arrests have increased slightly in some jurisdictions since the advent of proarrest policies. Winnipeg saw dual arrests increase 2% (from 6% to 8%) in the 4-year period from 1992/1993 to 1996/1997; similarly, Alberta saw an increase of 2% (from 4% to 6%) from 1999 to 2000, although there was a 1% decrease (from 6% to 5%) from 2000 to 2001 (Ad Hoc Federal-Provincial-Territorial Working Group, 2003).

Dual arrests occur for a number of reasons. While some authors purport that dual arrests reflect the reality that women are equally as violent as men (Mills, 2003), most emphasize the need to understand the contextual factors that influence dual arrests. Hirschel and Buzawa (2002) called for an examination of the possible responses available to police, the political and social climate within which they exist, and the policies and leadership under which they operate.

In the city of Calgary, Alberta, Canada, the site of the current evaluation, a specialized community and court process, called HomeFront, was initiated in 2001 (Tutty, McNichol, & Christensen, 2008). One of the major actions of the specialized first-appearance court was to offer low-risk accused who were willing to take responsibility for their actions the opportunity to be mandated to treatment. In an analysis of 3 years of justice data from 2001 to 2004 (Tutty et al., 2008), 2,243 individuals were charged with domestic violence–related offenses, 9.7% (217) of which were dual charges in which both members of the couple were charged by the police. Of the 315 women charged, 205 (65%) were solely charged, while 110 (43%) were charged as well as their male partners. One of the programs to which the women accused were mandated was the Responsible Choices for Women group.

MANDATED COUNSELING FOR WOMEN CHARGED WITH DOMESTIC ASSAULTS

In comparison to the vast research on male abusers, we know relatively little about the characteristics of aggressive women and how they respond to treatment (Abel, 2001). Dasgupta (1999) interviewed 32 women who had been referred to the Duluth, Minnesota program because of aggression toward partners. All had also been abused by either current partners or in past close relationships. The women's aggression was often psychological rather than physical and rarely resulted in the men being afraid. Instead, the women tried to limit their partner's contacts with relatives or friends, but seldom achieved total control. Although some women withheld sexual access as a control mechanism, the impact of this could not compare to the marital rape often experienced by abused women (Bergen, 2004).

Babcock, Miller, and Siard (2003) compared generally violent women to partner abuse–only women, finding that generally violent women reported more trauma symptoms, used more instrumental violence, and were more likely to have witnessed their mother's being physically aggressive. Abel (2001) compared female participants in groups for perpetrators of IPV and victims of IPV. Significantly more of the women in the perpetrator groups were non-White and were less likely to have sought help from services such as shelters (only one-third of the women had utilized such resources). The perpetrator group clients reported significantly lower levels of trauma symptomatology (with the exception of the depression and overall trauma subscales) than the abused women; however, the trauma scores of the women in the perpetrator groups were significantly higher than the nonabused women. Both studies suggest the importance of a trauma assessment in working with women mandated to treatment for abusive partners.

Several recent studies have documented high rates of substance abuse among women who are court referred to domestic violence treatment (Stuart, Moore, Ramsey, & Kahler, 2003, 2004). As Gondolf (2002) has suggested with respect to men's treatment, these authors also highlight the importance of substance screening and offering adjunct substance abuse treatment.

Still, we are only in the beginning stages of understanding the differences between male- and female-perpetrated violence. If we are to offer effective interventions, we must understand more about the dynamics of female-perpetrated abuse. While there is an increase in research on the characteristics of abusive women, there is virtually none on their treatment. Aggressive women may either seek counseling or be mandated to attend programs to change their behaviors. With dual-arrest policies common across North America, women are increasingly being charged with partner abuse and mandated to treatment (Finn et al., 2004; Hirschel & Buzawa, 2002). Few treatment programs are described in the literature.

U.S. clinicians Hamberger and Potente (1996) developed a treatment program for women arrested for abusing their partners. While the content areas appeared similar to those in many men's treatment programs, the authors found that, "Most of women who resort to violence against their partners do so as a direct outgrowth of violence and oppression perpetrated against them in a context that has permitted or encouraged violence to be used as a problem-solving strategy. Of the 67 women treated to date, only three clearly exhibited primary perpetrator characteristics and battered their male partners" (p. 70). As such, in addition to presenting information on dealing with anger and aggression, the groups included sessions on safety planning, children's issues, and assertiveness training commonly utilized in support groups for victims of woman abuse.

Buttell (2002) evaluated treatment with 91 women court ordered into treatment for partner violence. At pretest, they were assessed as employing a level of moral reasoning (a contentious outcome variable) two standard deviations below norms for adults in general. At posttest, however, there were no significant improvements in moral reasoning, raising questions about the impact of the group.

A previous evaluation of the Responsible Choices for Women program offered by the Calgary Counselling Centre (Tutty, Babins-Wagner, & Rothery, 2006) showed that, at pretest, these mostly nonmandated women reported levels of physical and nonphysical abuse of partners that was serious. The greater use of nonphysical abuse by women asking for treatment for aggressive behavior is identical to that reported by other practitioners who have conducted research with such women (Dasgupta, 1999; Hamberger & Potente, 1996) and their partners (Tutty, 1999). The Responsible Choices for Women group members reported clinically significant problems in many areas of their lives, including stress, depression, low self-esteem, and serious marital and family relations. After treatment, they significantly improved in several areas: less nonphysical abuse, higher self-esteem, more contentment, less clinical stress, and higher assertion.

In summary, our knowledge about both specialized treatment models and the efficacy of programs for women mandated to treatment for abusing intimate partners is in its infancy. Simply revamping men's group models will likely be ineffective, and addressing trauma and possible substance abuse is recommended (Abel, 2001; Tutty et al., 2006).

THE RESPONSIBLE CHOICES FOR WOMEN PROGRAM

The Calgary Counselling Centre in Alberta, Canada has provided family violence programs and services since 1981, including the Responsible

Choices for Men program developed for males who use physical or psychological violence and control tactics in intimate relationships (McGregor, Tutty, Babins-Wagner, & Gill, 2002). The agency also offers groups for women who have been abused by intimate partners and recently developed groups for male victims of IPV.

In the early 1990s, increasing numbers of women in same-sex relationships who were abusing partners began requesting services and the Centre saw an increase in referrals of women who were abusive to male partners. Initially the Centre offered groups for women in same-sex relationships, but these are no longer available because the demand decreased. We now offer groups for women who are abusive in intimate relationships in which both lesbians and heterosexual women are included. The Responsible Choices for Women program, a narrative-informed approach modeled after the men's program, began in 1995. This program is unique compared to most family violence treatment groups described in the literature. The interventions are based on an approach by Australian family therapist Alan Jenkins (1991), and differ substantially from some of the models widespread in North America, especially anger management, a cognitive behavioral approach.

The primary goal of Responsible Choices for Women is to assist women who are abusive in intimate relationships to become violence free. The major objectives include decreasing all forms of abusive behavior, accepting responsibility for one's behavior, increasing self-esteem, increasing assertive behavior, improving family relations, decreasing stress, increasing empathy toward those who have been impacted by abusive behavior, and assisting parents to cease physically abusing their children.

Prior to entering the Responsible Choices for Women group, clients must be engaged with a primary therapist in the agency. This therapist assesses the client's readiness for change and the degree of violence, and determines treatment goals. During the assessment process, it is important to distinguish between women who are acting in self-defense and require a victim's group (the You're Not Alone Group) and those who are perpetrating abuse against their male or female intimate partners or children (Responsible Choices for Women). The women need not necessarily be involved in a relationship at the time of the group. However, should they have a partner, the therapist will meet with him or her during the assessment phase.

The Responsible Choices for Women groups are 30-hour groups conducted over 14 weeks, in weekly 2-hour sessions, except for the first and last groups, which are 3 hours each. The groups typically comprise 6 to 12 women, both self- and court referred, and employ both an unstructured psychotherapeutic and a structured psychoeducational component. Covering the key themes is considered crucial; however, the facilitators have the flexibility to focus on an alternate issue should one emerge, allowing group members input into the agenda.

The model adopts methods and techniques of social learning and cognitive behavioral theory, including cognitive restructuring, stress and relaxation techniques, communication skill building, and sex role socialization strategies. Additional techniques include modeling appropriate behavior, monitoring or conflict situations through "responsible choices logs," timeouts, role playing, and the use of audio and audio-visual material. In addition, contact with the women's partners occurs at three points throughout the woman's participation in the group. These partner checks are conducted both to monitor the women's progress in the group and to assess the partner's safety.

A female–male team facilitates the groups, with at least one leader a senior therapist experienced in working with domestic violence and group work. A mixed-gender team provides modeling for conflict negotiation between men and women and resolving problems in nonabusive ways. In addition, a mixed-gender team prevents a "female only" mindset and assists in helping confront stereotypes about both male and female roles.

Some Responsible Choices for Women groups work with a reflecting team comprised of three to six individuals who observe sessions from behind a one-way mirror. The reflecting team members join the therapy group in the last 20 minutes of each session and talk among themselves about the group process and their observations of individual members or themes. The reflections allow for a multiplicity of ideas to be presented not only to the members of the groups, but to the facilitators as well. The reflections may act as therapeutic interventions and provide group supervision in a supportive environment. Finally, the opportunity to be a member of the reflecting team provides training to new staff and facilitators.

Given the paucity of treatment programs for abusive women and the lack of evaluation of those that are available, the current study was initiated to address several questions: What are the demographic, referral and clinical characteristics of the clients attending the Responsible Choices for Women program? What variables distinguish women who complete the program from those who drop out? Finally, do women change as a result of participating in the group?

METHOD

Research Design and Measures

The study employed a two-group pretest, posttest design. As with most research conducted in the community, it was not feasible to include a comparison group. While this limits the generalizability of the research results and means that any improvements identified in the group members cannot be attributed to the program alone, given the unique nature of the intervention and the relatively large sample size, a more exploratory research design was considered a logical first step.

The following 11 standardized measures were chosen to reflect the previously identified objectives of the Responsible Choices for Women program. Three of the scales were administered only at pretest and were not considered outcome measures but added important descriptive information on this population of women: The Personality Assessment Screener, the Trauma Symptom Checklist-40, and the University of Rhode Island Change Assessment – Domestic Violence (URICA-DV). The remaining eight measures were administered at both pretest and posttest as representing variables that might improve as a result of attending the group intervention.

THE TRAUMA SYMPTOM CHECKLIST-40 (TSCL-40; ELLIOT & BRIERE, 1992)

This 40-item inventory was specifically developed for research designed to measure the long-term sequelae of sexual abuse, including posttraumatic stress symptoms such as anxiety, depression, dissociation, sexual abuse trauma, sexual problems, and sleep disturbance. The internal consistency for the total score is an alpha of .90, with alphas greater than .62 for all of the subscales. Norms on a group of 2,833 professional women have been collected. Each of the subscales differentiated between women who have and who have not been sexually abused (Elliot & Briere, 1992; Gold, Milan, Mayall, & Johnson, 1994).

PERSONALITY ASSESSMENT SCREENER (PAS; MOREY, 2007)

The PAS is a 22-item screening tool that provides an index of how likely important clinical elevations would be found on the Personality Assessment Inventory, a much longer, more comprehensive measure. Clinical interpretations are recommended when the PAS total P score exceeds 47.

UNIVERSITY OF RHODE ISLAND CHANGE ASSESSMENT–DOMESTIC VIOLENCE (URICA-DV; LEVESQUE, GELLES, & VELICER, 2000)

The URICA-DV is a 20-item questionnaire that assesses stages of change according to the Transtheoretical Model (Prochaska, 1995). Items employ a 5-point Likert response format ranging from 1 (strongly disagree) to 5 (strongly agree). The URICA-DV is specific to partner violence, assessing readiness to change violent behavior toward intimate partners. Separate subscales are provided for Precontemplation (i.e., "The violence in my relationship isn't a big deal"), Contemplation ("I'm beginning to see that the violence in my relationship is a problem"), Action ("I'm finally going to do something to end my violent behavior"), and Maintenance ("Although I haven't been violent in awhile, I know it's possible for me to be violent again").

Levesque et al. (2000) reported internal consistency estimates (coefficient alphas) ranging from 0.68 to 0.81. Eckhardt, Babcock, and Homack (2004) and Eckhardt (2007) reported similar estimates for these subscales. Principal component analyses of the URICA-DV have been conflicting. Levesque et al. (2000) found a four-factor solution including all four subscales, while Eckhardt et al. (2004) and Eckhardt (2007) suggested a three-factor solution with clearly defined Precontemplation, Action, and Maintenance subscales.

ABUSE OF PARTNER SCALES: PHYSICAL AND NONPHYSICAL (HUDSON, 1992)

These two 25-item measures assess the "degree or magnitude of perceived physical or nonphysical abuse that clients have imposed on a spouse or partner." The physical abuse scale (PAPS) contains items with respect to physical and forced sexual assault. The nonphysical abuse of partner scale (NPAPS) consists of items that reflect psychological abuse or coercive behavior. Items are rated on a 7-point scale ranging from "never" (0) to "all the time" (6). Final scores range from 0 to 100, with high scores indicating higher levels of abuse.

PARTNER ABUSE SCALES: PHYSICAL (PASPH) AND NONPHYSICAL (PASNP; HUDSON, 1992)

These (additional) two 25-item scales measure the perceived physical or nonphysical abuse that clients have experienced from their spouse or partner using the same items from the PAPS and NPAPS, but from a victim's perspective. The cutoff scores and the psychometric properties are similar. The internal consistency of both scales is greater than .90. With a clinical cutoff score of 2, the PASPH has 87.6% sensitivity and 96% specificity; a cutoff score of 15 with the PASNP has 98.9% sensitivity and 88% specificity (Attala, Hudson, & McSweeney, 1994).

GENERALIZED CONTENTMENT SCALE (HUDSON, 1992)

This 25-item scale measures the "degree, severity, or magnitude of non-psychotic depression" (p. 15). Items are rated on a 7-point scale ranging from "never" (0) to "all the time" (6), with scores ranging from 0 to 100. The scale has three cutoff scores: scores greater than 30 suggest a clinically significant problem, scores greater than 50 suggest some suicidal ideation, and scores greater than 70 suggest a strong possibility that suicide is being considered and the respondent is experiencing severe distress. The scale norms were developed with 2,140 individuals. The coefficient alpha is .92; 2-hour test-retest reliability is .94.

INDEX OF CLINICAL STRESS (HUDSON, 1992)

This 25-item scale measures the respondent's perceived level of personal stress. The items "were developed not as responses to specifically identified stressors events, but as general indicators of affective states associated with the experience of stress" (Hudson, 1992, p. 281). Each item is rated on a 7-point scale ranging from "never" (0) to "all the time" (6), with scores ranging from 0 to 100. The ICS has a Cronbach's alpha of .96 and has also demonstrated good construct and factorial validity.

ROSENBERG SELF-ESTEEM INDEX (ROSENBERG, 1965)

This 10-item measure uses a 4-point scale ranging from "strongly agree" (1) to "strongly disagree" (4). The psychometric properties suggest that the scale is a reliable and valid measure for adolescents and young adults. The possible scores range from 10 to 40, with higher scores indicating higher self-esteem. Scores less than 25 are suggested as clinically problematic.

MARLOWE-CROWNE SOCIAL DESIRABILITY TEST SHORT FORM (REYNOLDS, 1982)

Social desirability, which has also been termed "impression management," refers to endorsing items that make one appear more competent or able than is the case. Reynolds (1982) developed a 13-item short version (Form C) of the scale with acceptable internal reliability and that significantly correlates (r = .93) with the original measure. Scores range from 0 to 13, with higher scores representing greater social desirability. Andrews and Moyer (2003) collected norms on Form C with 1,096 individuals from forensic populations. There were no gender or education differences and the mean score was 7.61.

Procedures

All research participants attended at least the first session of the Responsible Choices for Women group between 1995 and 2008. The women were administered the instrument package in sessions 1 and 14 of the group. Each participant was provided informed consent, confidentiality, and the choice to participate or not, as approved by the University of Calgary Conjoint Faculties Research Ethics Board.

Data Analysis

Data were analyzed using either Pearson chi-square tests or mixed factorial analysis of variance, depending on the comparison. Because of the high number of statistical comparisons, with at least 10 scales involved in each analysis, a procedure to control the overall error rate was utilized (Ott, 1984). Utilizing this procedure to approximate an alpha of .10 (since all of the hypotheses were one-tailed), a p value of .009 is necessary to establish statistical significance in all analyses.

RESULTS

Descriptions of the Research Participants

While 294 women have participated in the Responsible Choices for Women groups since its inception in 1995, demographic data are available for only 261 women. (In many variables, the total is not 261, due to missing information.) The average age of the women was 31.5 years (SD = 8.3; range 18 to 60 years). The average length of relationship was 5.8 years (SD = 6.3; range 0 to 44 years). Less than half of the women continued in relationships with intimate partners while in group (113 of 260; 43.4%), being either married (56 of 260; 21.5%) or in common-law relationships (57 of 260; 21.9%). Another 14.6% (14 of 260) were separated, 7.3% (19 of 260) were divorced, and 32.3% (84 of 260) were single. Nine relationships (4%) were lesbian.

The average income of the women was $16,937 per year ($SD$ = $18,127; range $0 to $140,000). The majority of the women (65.3%) had from one to six children: most had one (23.4%) or two (25.9%). As one way to gauge the life stage of the family, we collected information on the age of the oldest child, which ranged from 0 to 38 years, with an average of 9.4 years (SD = 6.2). The first language of almost all of the research participants was English (96.6%).

The ages of the partners ranged from 17 to 62 years, with an average of 34.2 years (SD = 9.2). The income of 105 partners was listed as an average of $34,700 ($SD$ = $27,485; range $0 to $160,000). Most of the women reported that they had separated previously from their partners because of conflict (60.6%). Most had only separated once.

A majority of the women had previously been in counseling (79.8%; 205 of 257). A little less than one-third (29.1%; 74 of 254) self-reported a psychiatric history. Of the 62 women who specified the diagnosis, almost half sought counseling for depression (48.4%), 11.3% for suicidal ideation, and 8.2% for either substance or sexual addiction. A further 8.1% of the women had been sexually abused. When asked about substance abuse, 10.7% of the women indicated concerns (28 of 261). Almost one-third (30.7%; 80 of 261) reported medical problems, although these were unspecified. A large proportion of the women (62.2%; 158 of 254) reported histories of violence in their families as children.

The most frequent referral source to the Responsible Choices for Women program was the criminal justice system (court and probation), which accounted for one-third of the referrals (37.5%; 101 of 269). Child welfare authorities referred 18 women. The second largest referral group was self/family/friends (31.2%; 84 of 269), followed by counselors (21.2%; 57 of 269) and others (10%; 27 women). In total, then, 58% of the women (156) were self- or counselor-referred, compared to 42% (114 women) who were mandated either by the courts, probation, or child welfare.

Not surprisingly given the number of the women who were court mandated to treatment, a large number (40.5%; 104 of 257) reported previous police involvement. Further, almost half had some type of legal order (such as a restraining order, no contact order, or emergency protection order) in place (47.9%; 123 of 257).

The Nature of the Abuse

At assessment for entry into the Responsible Choices for Women group, each woman was asked additional questions about the physical abuse of their part-ner (18 items) and the psychological abuse of their partner (18 items). Although these scales are not normed or validated, because so little is known about women who behave abusively, the scores are reported to provide additional information about the nature of the abuse. The scores of each item were compared based on whether the women were mandated versus nonmandated.

Notably, the information about physically and psychologically abusive behaviors provides no relationship context, such as the actions of the partner and whether some may have been in self-defense. With this caveat in mind, with respect to physically abusive behaviors (see Table 1), the most commonly endorsed items were pushing/shoving (63%), slapping with an open hand (46.4%), grabbing (39.5%), and punching with a closed fist (38.6%). The nonmandated women in the Responsible Choices for Women program were statistically more likely to self-report four physically abusive behaviors: poking, pushing/shoving, grabbing, and pulling hair.

Regarding psychologically abusive behaviors, the most commonly men-tioned were name calling (63%), making degrading/critical comments (58%), unfair accusations or interrogation (40.3%), and glaring at partner (40.2%; see Table 2). Once again, the women not mandated to attend treatment were more likely to self-disclose using psychologically abusive behaviors than the women who were mandated to the program. The nonmandated women reported using the following five behaviors significantly more often than the mandated women: name calling (63%), making degrading/critical comments (58%), unfair accusations or interrogation (52%), threatening to use violence (34%), and withholding sex from your partner (35%).

Pretest Scores on the Standardized Outcome Measures

The URICA-DV scores at pretest are of interest in assessing the extent to which the women were prepared and motivated for treatment. A Pearson's

TABLE 1 Women's Self-Reported Physical Abuse Behaviors to Partner

Item	Mandated (n = 87)	Nonmandated (n = 123)	Chi-square (p value)	Eta
Poking*†	9%	34.1%	15.7 (.001)	.273
Pushing/shoving*	51.7%	70.7%	7.9 (.005)	.19
Grabbing*	27.6%	49.6%	10.2 (.001)	.22
Pulling hair*	10.3%	25.3%	7.3 (.007)	.19
Restraining with hands	19.5%	24.4%	0.68 (.41)	.057
Restraining with object	1.1%	2.4%	0.45 (.50)	.046
Choking	7%	17.9%	5.18 (.023)	.158
Choking to unconsciousness	0%	0%	—	—
Yanking/twisting arms	8%	12.2%	.935 (.33)	.067
Pinning to ground/wall/bed	12.6%	21.1%	2.53 (.11)	.11
Pushing to ground	13.8%	14.6%	0.03 (.86)	.012
Attacking with knife/gun/other weapon	12.6%	6.5%	2.33 (.15)	.105
Scratching/gouging	20.7%	24.4%	0.39 (.53)	.043
Kicking	22.1%	38.2%	6.09 (.014)	.171
Slapping with open hand	37.2%	53.7%	5.49 (.019)	.16
Punching with a closed fist	31%	44.7%	4.00 (.045)	.138
Biting	16.1%	16.3%	0.00 (.94)	.002
Other physical violence	11.5%	26%	6.72 (.010)	.179

†Because of the number of comparisons, and since all of the hypotheses were one-tailed, a p value of .009 establishes statistical significance at an alpha level of .10.
*Indicates a statistically significant difference as explained above.

TABLE 2 Women's Self-Reported Psychological Abuse Against Partner

	Mandated (n = 87)	Nonmandated (n = 123)	Chi-square (p value)	Eta
Name calling*	52.9%	71%	7.2 (.007)	.185
Unfair accusations/interrogation*	25.3%	52.4%	15.5 (.000)	.271
Degrading/critical comments*	39.1%	71.8%	22.5 (.000)	.326
Trailing/following partner	25.3%	29.8%	0.53 (.47)	.050
Threatening you will use violence*	14.9%	33.9%	9.5 (.002)	.212
Control partner's access to money	5.2%	15.3%	1.72 (.19)	.09
Withholding sex from partner*	16.1%	34.7%	8.95 (.003)	.206
Screening telephone calls	9.2%	8.9%	.007 (.95)	.006
Direct threats of violence/death	5.7%	13.7%	3.47 (.062)	.128
Glaring at partner	33.3%	45.2%	2.97 (.085)	.119
Blocking partner's path	28.7%	35.5%	1.06 (.30)	.071
Spying/watching partner	8.0%	11.3%	0.60 (.438)	.053
Harassment at partner's job, public places	8.0%	6.5%	0.19 (.66)	.031
Threats to commit suicide if partner leaves	10.3%	21.8%	4.72 (.03)	.15
Threats to leave/divorce partner	33.3%	29.8%	0.29 (.59)	.037
Threats to take children away	8.0%	13.7%	1.63 (.20)	.088
Limiting friendship	18.4%	24.2%	1.01 (.32)	.069
Other verbal/emotional abuse*	12.1%	33.1%	10.9 (.001)	.229

*Indicates a statistically significant difference with a p value ≤ .009.

chi-square analysis indicated significant differences between the stages of changes with respect to the women mandated versus those not mandated to the Responsible Choice for Women group, χ^2 (4; N = 179) = 20.8; p < .001; η = .34, indicating a moderate effect. As can be seen in Table 3, the women who were not mandated by the legal system or child welfare were largely beyond contemplation or precontemplation and had moved into the preparation or action phases. Notably, about one-fifth (19.8%) were in the action–high relapse category, which means that although they were actively seeking change, they were at risk of relapse.

However, almost 25% were in the action–low relapse stage at pretest. This difference likely reflects the impact of the pregroup individual sessions with the primary counselor at the agency. The nonmandated women had more individual sessions before beginning group, although the difference was not statistically significant (7.7 individual counseling sessions compared to 5.3 sessions for the mandated women, t[200] = 2.3; p = .03).

In contrast, the women mandated to the program were more evenly spread across the stages of change. A larger proportion of them were in precontemplation and contemplation (48.4%) than the nonmandated women (27.9%). Notably, only 3.2% were in the action–high relapse category and another almost one-third were in action–low relapse, perhaps supporting the impact of the criminal justice system in motivating at least some women.

The pretest scores on the standardized measures of 275 women (see Table 4) are in the clinical range for all of the measures that provided clinical cutoff scores, including clinical stress, generalized contentment, self-esteem, partner abuse physical, partner abuse psychological, being abused by partner physical, and being abused by partner nonphysical.

As mentioned previously, at pretest we utilized two scales as further descriptors of the women (the TSCL-40 and the PAS). The TSCL-40 has no clinical cutoff; however, when we compared the current scores to large samples in Elliot and Briere's (1992) research, the average score of the women in the Responsible Choices groups was much higher than a community sample of professional women (20.91) and a group of women with histories of child sexual abuse (26.02), suggesting the relevance of trauma symptoms. Also notable is that the average score on the PAS was 48.2, slightly above the suggested P value of concern, 47. This indicates that half of the women were in the clinical range and additional assessment was suggested using a more comprehensive measure such as the Personality Assessment Inventory.

Finally and notably, the scores on the Marlowe-Crown Social Desirability Scale (Form C) were lower than the average score of 7.61 as reported by Andrews and Moyer (2003) in forensic populations. This suggests that the women were not presenting themselves as significantly better than they are.

TABLE 3 URICA-DV Stages at Pretest ($N = 179$)

	Precontemplation	Contemplation	Preparation	Action–high relapse	Action–low relapse	Total
Mandated	24 (25.8%)	21 (22.6%)	15 (16.1%)	3 (3.2%)	30 (32.3%)	93
Not mandated	11 (12.8%)	13 (15.1%)	25 (29.1%)	17 (19.8%)	20 (23.3%)	86
Total	35 (19.6%)	34 (19%)	40 (22.3%)	20 (11.2%)	50 (27.9%)	179

TABLE 4 Responsible Choices for Women: Standardized Scale Scores at Pretest

Scale[†]	Pretest	Range	Standard deviation
Physical abuse against partner ($N = 245$)	5.6	0–74	9.0
Nonphysical abuse against partner ($N = 249$)	17.4	0–90	15.4
Partner physical abuse ($N = 188$)	5.8	0–76.7	11
Partner nonphysical abuse ($N = 191$)	23.6	0–90	21.1
Generalized contentment scale ($N = 273$)	38.1	0–81	17.5
Index of Clinical Stress ($N = 275$)	40.6	0–98.7	20.2
Rosenberg Self-Esteem ($N = 214$)	21.7	10–37	6.2
Trauma Symptom Checklist-40 ($N = 93$)	31.3	1–101	21.6
Marlowe-Crown Social Desirability ($N = 213$)	5.7	0–13	3.3
Personality Assessment Screener total ($N = 59$)	48.2	1.7–99	30.9

[†]The *ns* for each test differ because the assessment protocol has changes over time.

Comparison of Group Completers and Noncompleters

Of the 290 women for whom there is information with respect to whether they completed the Responsible Choices for Women group, almost two-thirds (185; 63.8%) finished the program. Independent *t* tests were used to identify whether any special variables characterized women who completed the group versus those that dropped out.

Not all of the women who completed the groups completed the measures at both pretest and posttest. The 177 women who both completed the group and the measures at pretest scored no differently than the 86 non-completers on any of the standardized measures at that time point. Similarly, none of the demographic characteristics, such as whether the women were mandated, their stage of change at pretest, age, length of relationship, previous counseling, or psychiatric history, differentiated those who completed group versus those who did not.

The Effects of Group Treatment

The analysis of the treatment effects used a mixed factorial design with mandated status as the between-subjects factor and pretest–posttest scores as the within subjects factor. Interestingly, the only variable that differentiated the mandated and nonmandated women was on the nonphysical abuse of partner measure (Hudson, 1992), with the mandated women reporting use of fewer abusive behaviors at pretest.

As can be seen in Table 5, the 154 women who completed both pre- and posttests reported statistically significant improvements on five variables: generalized contentment (depression), clinical stress, nonphysical abuse of partner, partner nonphysical abuse of the woman, and partner physical abuse of the woman. Self-esteem worsened significantly after the

TABLE 5 Responsible Choices for Women: Pre/Post Comparison of Mandated and Nonmandated Women

Scale	Nonmandated		Mandated		F test mandated (p value)	η²	F test outcome (p value)	η²
	Pre	Post	Pre	Post				
Physical abuse against partner	6.5 (n = 77)	10.6	5.9 (n = 51)	6.2	4.5 (.04)	.04	6.2 (.014)	.05
Nonphysical abuse against partner*	19.5 (n = 79)	3.3	13.3 (n = 52)	3.5	7.7 (.006)	.056	129 (.001)	.50
Partner physical abuse	5.8 (n = 49)	2.8	5.0 (n = 50)	2.6	0.2 (.68)	.002	10.9 (.001)	.10
Partner nonphysical abuse	22.9 (n = 50)	15.7	27 (n = 51)	17.5	.03 (.57)	.003	17.5 (.001)	.15
Generalized Contentment Scale	42.9 (n = 86)	33.9	29.7 (n = 67)	23.0	1.3 (.26)	.009	62.9 (.001)	.30
Index of Clinical Stress	46.0 (n = 88)	32.6	32.2 (n = 66)	22.9	2.5 (.12)	.02	72.5 (.001)	.32
Rosenberg Self-Esteem	24.1 (n = 56)	21.3	18.7 (n = 64)	17.1	1.8 (.18)	.015	28.4 (.001)	.20
Marlowe-Crowne Social Desirability	4.0 (n = 55)	5.3	7.4 (n = 61)	7.6	3.7 (.06)	.03	6.4 (.013)	.05

*Indicates a statistically significant difference at a p value ≤ .009.

group program and remained in the clinical range. Scores on social desirability increased slightly (such that the women were presenting themselves in a more favorable light), but not significantly so, and still at about the average score of the norm group of Andrew and Mayer's (2003) forensic sample.

Jacobson, Follette, and Revenstorf (1984) recommended an additional method to examine statistically significant improvements: identifying movement from the clinical into the normal range, especially in conjunction with statistical significance. From this perspective, the generalized contentment scales, clinical stress, partner physical abuse, and nonphysical abuse against partner scores moved from the clinical into the nonclinical range. Notably, although the scores on partner physical abuse decreased and nonphysical abuse by their partners did not decrease, these are not within the women's control and should be viewed descriptively only.

The physical abuse against partner scores of both the mandated and the nonmandated women increased, although not significantly. This likely reflects more honesty about their use of physically abusive behaviors after the group than before and is not uncommon with offender treatment. A similar pattern has been noted with men attending the Responsible Choices for Men program at the Calgary Counselling Centre (Babins-Wagner, Tutty, & Rothery, 2005).

Recently we added space on the outcomes package for the women to provide some written comments about the program. To conclude the results section, here are several of the comments collected to date (all positive) in response to the question, "What difference has coming to this program made for you?"

- Recognizing my problems and my part in violent relationships and learning ways to end the violence and make better choices in my behavior.
- It's helped me deal with issues I didn't realize I had.
- I feel calmer and have successfully avoided violence and verbal abuse for 4 months. It has increased my self-esteem because I have participated and completed the program.
- Huge. While I had a very keen awareness of myself already, how I got here, there were key skills I managed to acquire and new ideas to contemplate. I feel I have successfully changed that way I see myself now—a worthwhile person with loads of value with a few issues to work out vs. broken, unlovable, unworthy.

DISCUSSION

These study results must be interpreted cautiously because of limitations such as the lack of a control group, a design feature that is seldom feasible in community research. However, the number of group participants is relatively large and, given the paucity of research with respect to both the characteristics of women who behave abusively and their response to treatment, the study provides important suggestions for treatment providers and researchers alike.

Interestingly, there were relatively few differences in demographic characteristics and scores on the standardized measures at pretest of the women who were mandated to treatment by the courts or child welfare compared to those that were not. While the women who were mandated to treatment by the courts or child welfare self-reported using a few more physically and nonphysically abusive tactics and showed a different pattern of readiness for change, this factor did not differentiate treatment outcomes. The women attending the Responsible Choices for Women groups reported levels of physical and nonphysical abuse of their partners that were serious. The greater use of nonphysical abuse by the nonmandated women who were asking for treatment for aggressive behavior had been reported by other practitioners who have worked with or conducted research with women in similar circumstances (Dasgupta, 1999; Hamberger & Potente, 1996) and their partners (Tutty, 1999).

At the start of the program, the Responsible Choices for Women group members reported clinically significant problems in a number of areas of their lives, including stress, depression as documented by the Generalized Contentment Scale, low self-esteem, mental health distress symptoms as measured by the PAS, and trauma, in addition to self-reporting clinically significant levels of partner perpetration and victimization by their partners. Four of these variables significantly improved after the group, moving out of the clinical range on average: the women self-reported less depression, clinical stress, partner physical abuse, and nonphysical abuse against partner scores. Interestingly, their self-esteem scores remained in the clinical range, with the actual scores worsening significantly on average.

The Responsible Choices for Women groups are relatively short, and we must be cautious not to overestimate expectations for change in that brief length of time. Despite the relative brevity of the groups, the extent of change is encouraging. However, given the clinical nature of so many of the variables assessed in these women, the groups should probably not constitute the sole intervention. Additional interventions are strongly indicated, whether in second-stage groups or marital, family, or continued individual counseling (Tutty, 2006). At the Calgary Counselling Centre, after the Responsible Choices group the women meet once again with their primary therapist to determine the need for additional counseling.

Nevertheless, many questions remain about abusive women and the programs developed to assist them. First, it is not necessarily easy to distinguish women who behave aggressively in self-defense from those who act as the "major" perpetrator in a couple. Some of the women in the Responsible

Choices group clearly fit the former group rather than the latter. Second, most programs for women, including the current one, utilize models initially developed for men who abuse their intimate partners. One might question whether utilizing such models is the best fit for female aggressors. Groups designed specifically for women may take women's prescribed roles and behaviors into consideration and how women's abuse of intimate partners likely differs from men's. Several years ago, the Responsible Choices for Women groups were revised to include these perspectives.

Finally, the overall impact of dual arrests and subsequent mandating of women to treatment needs to be monitored closely and evaluated. It will be critical to assess the extent to which women may be secondarily victimized by legal intervention when they were primarily defending themselves from harm.

REFERENCES

Abel, E. M. (2001). Comparing the social service utilization, exposure to violence, and trauma symptomatology of domestic violence female "victims" and female batterers." *Journal of Family Violence, 16*(4), 401–420.

Ad Hoc Federal-Provincial-Territorial Working Group. (2003). *Spousal abuse policies and legislation: Final report*. Ottawa, ON: Author.

Andrews, P., & Moyer, R. G. (2003). Marlowe-Crowne Social Desirability Scale and Short Form C: Forensic norms. *Journal of Clinical Psychology, 59*(4), 483–492.

Attala, J. M., Hudson, W. W., & McSweeney, M. (1994). A partial validation of two short-form partner abuse scales. *Women and Health, 21*(2/3), 125–139.

Babcock, J. C., Miller, S. A., & Siard, C. (2003). Toward a typology of abusive women: Differences between partner-only and generally violent women in the use of violence. *Psychology of Women Quarterly, 27*, 153–161.

Babins-Wagner, R., Tutty, L., & Rothery, M. (2005, July). *A comparison of mandated to non-mandated men for the Responsible Choices for Men groups*. Presented at the 9th International Family Violence Research Conference, Portsmouth, NH.

Belnap, J., & Melton, H. (2005). Are heterosexual men also victims of intimate partner abuse? *VAWnet Applied Research Forum*. Retrieved March 20, 2009, from http://new.vawnet.org/Assoc_Files_VAWnet/AR_MaleVictims.pdf.

Bergen, R. K. (2004). Studying wife rape: Reflections on the past, present, and future. *Violence Against Women, 10*(12), 1407–1416.

Buttell, F. P. (2002). Levels of moral reasoning among female domestic violence offenders: Evaluating the impact of treatment. *Research on Social Work Practice, 12*(3), 349–363.

Cornell, D. G., Warren, J., Hawk, G., Stafford, E., Oram, G., & Pine, D. (1996). Psychopathy of instrumental and reactive violent offenders. *Journal of Consulting and Clinical Psychology, 64*, 783–790.

Dasgupta, S. D. (1999). Just like men? A critical view of violence by women. In M. Shepard & E. Pence (Eds.), *Coordinating community responses to domestic violence: Lessons from Duluth and beyond* (pp. 195–222). Thousand Oaks, CA: Sage.

Dasgupta, S. D. (2002). A framework for understanding women's use of non-lethal violence in intimate heterosexual relationships. *Violence Against Women, 8*(11), 1364–1389.

DeKeseredy, W. S. (1993). *Four variations of family violence: A review of sociological research*. Ottawa, ON: National Clearinghouse on Family Violence.

Eckhardt, C. I. (2007). Assessing readiness to change among perpetrators of intimate partner violence: Analysis of two self-report measures. *Journal of Family Violence, 22*(5), 319–330.

Eckhardt, C. I., Babcock, J., & Homack, S. (2004). Partner assaultive men and the stages and processes of change. *Journal of Family Violence, 19*(2), 81–93.

Elliot, D., & Briere, J. (1992). Sexual abuse trauma among professional women: Validating the Trauma Symptom Checklist-40 (TSC-40). *Child Abuse & Neglect, 16*, 391–398.

Finn, M. A., Sims Blackwell, B., Stalans, L. J., Studdard, S., & Dugan, L. (2004). Dual arrest decisions in domestic violence cases: The influence of departmental policies. *Crime & Delinquency, 50*(4), 565–589.

Frye, V., Haviland, M., & Rajah, V. (2007). Dual arrest and other unintended consequences of mandatory arrest in New York City: A brief report. *Journal of Family Violence, 22*, 397–405.

Gold, S., Milan, L., Mayall, A., Johnson, A. (1994). A cross-validation study of the Trauma Symptom Checklist: The role of mediating variables. *Journal of Interpersonal Violence, 9*(1), 12–26.

Gondolf, E. (2002). *Batterer intervention systems: Issues, outcomes, and recommendations*. Thousand Oaks, CA: Sage.

Hamberger, L. K. (1997). Female offenders in domestic violence: A look at their actions in their context. *Journal of Aggression, Maltreatment & Trauma, 1*(1), 117–129.

Hamberger, L. K., & Guse, C. E. (2002). Men's and women's use of intimate partner violence in clinical samples. *Violence Against Women, 8*, 1301–1331.

Hamberger, L. K., & Potente, T. (1996). Counseling heterosexual women arrested for domestic violence: Implications for theory and practice. In L. K. Hamberger & C. Renzetti (Eds.), *Domestic partner abuse* (pp. 53–75). New York: Springer.

Hirschel, D., & Buzawa, E. (2002). Understanding the context of dual arrest with directions for future research. *Violence Against Women, 8*(12), 1449–1473.

Hudson, W. (1992). *The WALMYR assessment scales scoring manual*. Tempe, AZ: WALMYR.

Jacobson, N., Follette, W., & Revenstorf, D. (1984). Psychotherapy outcome research: Methods for reporting variability and evaluating clinical significance. *Behavior Therapy, 17*, 308–311.

Jenkins, A. (1991). Intervention with violence and abuse in families: The inadvertent perpetuation of irresponsible behaviour. *Australian and New Zealand Journal of Family Therapy, 12*(4), 186–195.

Johnson, H. (2006). *Measuring violence against women: Statistical trends 2006*. Ottawa, ON: Minister of Industry. Retrieved December 9, 2008, from http://www.statcan.ca/Daily/English/061002/d061002a.htm.

Johnson, M. P. (1995). Patriarchal terrorism and common couple violence: Two forms of violence against women. *Journal of Marriage and the Family, 57*, 283–294.

Kimmel, M. S. (2002). "Gender symmetry" in domestic violence: A substantive and methodological research review. *Violence Against Women, 8*(11), 1332–1363.

Levesque, D. A., Gelles, R. J., & Velicer, W. F. (2000). Development and validation of a stages of change measure for men in batterer treatment. *Cognitive Therapy and Research, 24*(2), 175–199.

Lupri, E., & Grandin, E. (2004). *Intimate partner abuse against men: Overview paper.* Ottawa, ON: National Clearinghouse on Family Violence. Retrieved February 11, 2009, from http://www.phac-aspc.gc.ca/ncfv-cnivf/familyviolence/maleabus_e.html.

McGregor, M., Tutty, L., Babins-Wagner, R., & Gill, M. (2002). The long term impact of group treatment for partner abuse. *Canadian Journal of Community Mental Health, 21*, 67–84.

Melton, H. C., & Belknap, J. (2003). He hits, she hits: Assessing gender differences and similarities in officially reported intimate partner violence. *Criminal Justice and Behavior, 30*(3), 328–348.

Mills, L. G. (2003). *Insult to injury: Rethinking our responses to intimate abuse.* Princeton, NJ: Princeton University Press.

Morey, L. C. (2007). *The Personality Assessment Inventory professional manual.* Lutz, FL: Psychological Assessment Resources.

Ogrodnik, L. (2007). Spousal violence and repeat police contact. In L. Ogrodnik (Ed.), *Family violence in Canada: A statistical profile 2006* (pp. 11–28). Ottawa: Centre for Justice Statistics.

Osthoff, S. (2002). But, Gertrude, I beg to differ, a hit is not a hit is not a hit: When battered women are arrested for assaulting their partners. *Violence Against Women, 8*(12), 1521–1544.

Ott, L. (1984). *An introduction to statistical methods and data analysis* (2nd ed.). Boston: Duxbury.

Prochaska, J. (1995). An eclectic and integrative approach: Transtheoretical therapy. In A. Gurman & S. Messer (Eds.), *Essential psychotherapies: Theory and practice* (pp. 403–440). New York: Guilford Press.

Reynolds, W. (1982). Development of a reliable and valid short form of the Marlowe-Crowne Social Desirability Scale. *Journal of Clinical Psychology, 38*, 118–125.

Rosenberg, M. (1965). *Society and the adolescent self-image.* Princeton, NJ: Princeton University Press.

Sarantakos, S. (2004). Deconstructing self-defense in wife-to-husband violence. *Journal of Men's Studies, 12*(3), 277–296.

Saunders, D. (2002). Are physical assaults by wives and girlfriends a major social problem? A review of the literature. *Violence Against Women, 8*(12), 1424–1448.

Statistics Canada. (2005). *Family violence in Canada: A statistical profile.* Ottawa, CA: Minister of Industry.

Stets, J., & Straus, M. (1990). Gender differences in reporting marital violence and its medical and psychological consequences. In M. Straus & R. Gelles (Eds.), *Physical violence in American families* (pp. 151–165). New Brunswick, NJ: Transaction Press.

Straus, M. A. (1979). Measuring intrafamilial conflict: The Conflict Tactics Scales (CTS). *Journal of Marriage and the Family, 41*, 75–88.

Straus, M. A. (2009). Why the overwhelming evidence on partner physical violence by women has not been perceived and is often denied. *Journal of Aggression, Maltreatment & Trauma, 18*(6), 552–571.

Stuart, G. L., Moore, T. M., Ramsey, S. E., & Kahler, C. W. (2003). Relationship aggression and substance use among women court-referred to domestic violence intervention programs. *Addictive Behaviors, 28*(9), 1603–1610.

Stuart, G. L., Moore, T. M., Ramsey, S. E., & Kahler, C. W. (2004). Hazardous drinking and relationship violence perpetration and victimization in women arrested for domestic violence. *Journal of Studies on Alcohol, 65*(1), 46–53.

Tutty, L. (1999). *Husband abuse: An overview of research and perspectives.* Ottawa, ON: National Clearinghouse on Family Violence. Retrieved April 24, 2008, from http://www.hc-sc.gc.ca/hppb/familyviolence/maleabuse.html.

Tutty, L. (2006). Identifying, assessing and treating male perpetrators and abused women. In R. Alaggia & C. Vine (Eds.), *Cruel but not unusual: Violence in Canadian families* (pp. 371–396). Waterloo, ON: Wilfrid Laurier.

Tutty, L., Babins-Wagner, R., & Rothery, M. (2006). Group treatment for aggressive women: An initial evaluation. *Journal of Family Violence, 21*(5), 341–349.

Tutty, L. M., McNichol, K., & Christensen, J. (2008). Calgary's HomeFront specialized domestic violence court. In J. Ursel, L. Tutty, & J. LeMaistre (Eds.), *What's law got to do with it? The law, specialized courts and domestic violence in Canada* (pp. 152–171). Toronto, ON: Cormorant Press.

Index

Page numbers in *Italics* represent tables.
Page numbers in **Bold** represent figures.